MANUAL OF

Neonatal Surgical Intensive Care

Second Edition

Anne R. Hansen, MD, MPH
Medical Director
Neonatal Intensive Care Unit
Children's Hospital
Harvard Medical School
Boston, Massachusetts

Mark Puder
Associate
Children's Hospital
Harvard Medical School
Boston, Massachusetts

2009
People's Medical Publishing House
Shelton, Connecticut

People's Medical Publishing House
2 Enterprise Drive, Suite 509
Shelton, CT 06484
Tel: 203-402-0646
Fax:203-402-0854
E-mail: info@pmph-usa.com

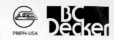

09 10 11 12 / PMPH / 9 8 7 6 5 4 3 2 1

ISBN 978-1-60795-002-8
Printed in China by People's Medical Publishing House of China
Production Manager: Paula Mucci, Copyeditor/Typesetter: Diacritech,
Cover Designer: Mary McKeon

Sales and Distribution

United States
BC Decker Inc
P.O. Box 785
Lewiston, NY 14092-0785
Tel: 905-522-7017; 800-568-7281
Fax: 905-522-7839; 888-311-4987
E-mail: info@bcdecker.com
www.bcdecker.com

Canada
McGraw-Hill Ryerson Education
Customer Care
300 Water St.
Whitby, Ontario L1N 9B6
Tel: 1-800-565-5758
Fax: 1-800-463-5885

Foreign Rights
John Scott & Company
International Publishers' Agency
P.O. Box 878
Kimberton, PA 19442
Tel: 610-827-1640
Fax: 610-827-1671
E-mail: jsco@voicenet.com

Japan
United Publishers Services Limited
1-32-5 Higashi-Shinagawa
Shinagawa-Ku, Tokyo 140-0002
Tel: 03 5479 7251
Fax: 03 5479 7307

UK, Europe, Middle East
McGraw-Hill Education
Shoppenhangers Road
Maidenhead
Berkshire, England SL6 2QL
Tel: 44-0-1628-502500
Fax: 44-0-1628-635895
www.mcgraw-hill.co.uk

*Singapore, Malaysia,Thailand, Philippines,
Indonesia, Vietnam, Pacific Rim, Korea*
McGraw-Hill Education
60 Tuas Basin Link
Singapore 638775
Tel: 65-6863-1580
Fax: 65-6862-3354

Australia, New Zealand
Elsevier Australia
Tower 1, 475 Victoria Avenue
Chatswood NSW 2067
Australia
Tel: 0-9422-8553
Fax: 0-9422-8562
www.elsevier.com.au

Customer Service New Zealand
Phone (Free Phone): +64 (0) 800 449 312
Fax (Free Phone): +64 (0) 800 449 318
Email: cservice@mcgraw-hill.co.nz

Brazil
Tecmedd Importadora E Distribuidora
De Livros Ltda.
Avenida Maurílio Biagi, 2850
City Ribeirão, Ribeirão Preto – SP – Brasil
CEP: 14021-000
Tel: 0800 992236
Fax: (16) 3993-9000
E-mail: tecmedd@tecmedd.com.br

India, Bangladesh, Pakistan, Sri Lanka
CBS Publishers & Distributors
4596/1A-11, Darya Ganj
New Delhi-2, India
Tel: 23271632
Fax: 23276712
E-mail: cbspubs@vsnl.com

Contents

Preface

The Manual of Surgical Neonatal Intensive Care addresses the interdisciplinary area of the peri-operative management of newborns with surgical conditions. These babies generally spend less than a day in the operating room, but require days, weeks, or even months of complex pre- and postoperative care that spans medical and surgical areas of expertise. Though many textbooks and manuals address the strictly medical or surgical management of newborns, relatively little has been written about issues that cross medical and surgical specialties. This tends to be working knowledge that is gained by experience. We hope the information in this manual will be useful to both medical and surgical clinicians.

This work is a collaborative effort between the surgical staff at Children's Hospital and the medical staff at Children's Hospital, Beth Israel Deaconess Medical Center, Brigham and Women's Hospital, and hospitals further a field. Its intended audience is surgeons, neonatologists, pediatricians, neonatal nurse practitioners, neonatal nurses, transport clinicians, and any other health care providers expected to render pre- or postoperative care or counseling for newborns with surgical conditions.

Children's Hospital cares for newborns with surgical conditions in both its Neonatal and Pediatric Intensive Care units. We receive babies from local newborn nurseries, our associated Special Care Nurseries, Beth Israel Deaconess Medical Center, and Brigham and Women's Hospital who requires surgery and complex postoperative surgical care, as well as from other referring hospitals across the country and around the world. The contributing authors reflect this web of community and tertiary hospitals.

Where appropriate, chapters follow a standard order: embryology, prenatal diagnosis (treatment), postnatal presentation, postnatal diagnosis, differential diagnosis, pre-operative management, implications for anesthesia, surgical management, postoperative management, and complications/outcomes. In this second edition, we have added several new chapters including one on diagnoses by presenting symptoms and another on gastrointestinal reflux. We have updated all existing chapters and added many illustrations to clarify written descriptions.

We would like to thank all of our contributing authors as well as Drs. Kourembanas and Shamberger for their support. We would also like to thank the nurse practitioners and nurses, fellows and residents, respiratory therapists, nutritionists, and most importantly the babies and their families for all that they have taught us.

Contributors

Stuart B. Bauer, MD

Department of Surgery
Harvard Medical School
Boston, Massachusetts

Elizabeth D. Blume, MD, FACC

Department of Pediatrics
Harvard Medical School
Boston, Massachusetts

Joseph G. Borer, MD

Department of Surgery
Harvard Medical School
Boston, Massachusetts

Athos Bousvaros, MD

Department of Pediatrics
Harvard University
Boston, Massachusetts

Roland Brusseau, MD, FAAP

Department of Anesthesiology
Children's Hospital Boston
Boston, Massachusetts

Y. Avery Ching, MD

Surgical Research Fellow
Department of Surgery
Children's Hospital Boston
Boston, Massachusetts

Bartley G. Cilento Jr, MD, FAAP, FACS

Department of Surgery
Harvard Medical School
Boston, Massachusetts

Melanie Connolly, MSc, RD, CNSD

Department of
Gastroenterology/Nutrition
Children's Hospital Boston
Boston, Massachusetts

David A. Diamond, MD

Department of Surgery
Harvard University
Boston, Massachusetts

Christopher Duggan, MD, MPH

Department of Pediatrics
Children's Hospital
Harvard Medical School
Boston, Massachusetts

Debora Duro, MD, MS

Department of Medicine
Children's Hospital Boston
Boston, Massachusetts

Ellen R. Elias, MD, FAAP

Department of Pediatrics
Unversity of Colorado School of
Medicine
Denver, Colorado

John B. Emans, MD

Department of Orthopaedic
Surgery
Harvard Medical School
Boston, Massachusetts

Neil R. Feins, MD, FAAP, FACS

Department of Surgery
Harvard University
Boston, Massachusetts

Steven J. Fishman, MD, FACS, FAAP

Department of Surgery
Harvard Medical School
Boston, Massachusetts

Francis Fynn-Thompson, MD

Department of Cardiac Surgery
Children's Hospital Boston
Boston, Massachusetts

Laurie J. Glader, MD, FAAP

Department of Pediatrics
Harvard Medical School
Boston, Massachusetts

Michael Glotzbecker, MD

Harvard Combined Orthopaedic
    Residency Program
Boston, Massachusetts

Arin K. Greene, MD, MMSc

Department of Plastic Surgery
Harvard Medical School
Boston, Massachusetts

**Thomas Hamilton, MD,
FACS, FAAP**

Department of Surgery
Children's Hospital Boston
Boston, Massachuetts

Anne R. Hansen, MD, MPH

Department of Pediatrics
Harvard Medical School
Boston, Massachusetts

Charles A. Hergrueter, MD

Department of Surgery
Harvard Medical School
Boston, Massachusetts

John T. Herrin, MBBS, FRACP

Department of Pediatrics
Harvard Medical School
Boston, Massachusetts

Tom Jaksic, MD, PhD

Department of Surgery
Harvard Medical School
Boston, Massachusetts

Monica E. Kleinman, MD

Instructor in Anesthesia for
    Department of Pediatrics
Harvard Medical School
Boston, Massachusetts

Babu V. Koka, MB, BS

Department of Anesthesia
Harvard Medical School
Boston, Massachusetts

Richard S. Lee, MD

Department of Urology
Children's Hospital Boston
Boston, Massachusetts

Sang Lee, MD

Department of Surgery
Beth Israel Deaconess Medical
    Center
Boston, Massachusetts

Craig Lillehei, MD

Department of Surgery
Harvard Medical School
Boston, Massachusetts

**David S.G. Lowinger, MD,
FRACS**

Department of Otolaryngology
Sydney Children's Hospital
Sydney, Australia

**Dorothy M. MacDonald,
BS, RN**

Craniofacial Center at Children's
    Hospital
Boston, Massachusetts

**Joseph R. Madsen, MD,
FACS, FAAP**

Department of Surgery
Harvard Medical School
Boston, Massachusetts

Camilia R. Martin, MD, MS

Department of Pediatrics
Harvard Medical School
Boston, Massachusetts

**Karen R. McAlmon, MD,
FAAP**

Department of Pediatrics
Harvard Medical School
Boston, Massachusetts

Biren P. Modi, MD

Resident
Department of Surgery
Brigham and Women's
    Hospital
Boston, Massachusetts

John B. Mulliken, MD
Department of Surgery
Harvard Medical School
Boston, Massachusetts

Samuel Nurko, MD, MPH
Department of Medicine
Children's Hospital Boston

Laurie A. Ohlms, MD, FACS
Department of Otology and
    Laryngology
Harvard Medical School
Boston, Massachusetts

Konstantinos Papadakis, MD
Department of Surgery
Children's Hospital Boston
Boston, Massachusetts

Corinne C. Pryor, RNC, BA
Senior Staff Nurse
Brigham and Women's Hospital
NICU
Boston, Massachusetts

Mark Puder, MD, PhD
Department of Surgery
Harvard Medical School
Boston, Massachusetts

DeWayne Pursley, MD, MPH
Department of Pediatrics
Harvard Medical School
Boston, Massachusetts

**Sandy Quigley, MS, CPNP,
CWOCN**
Clinical Nurse Specialist in
    Enterostomal Therapy
Children's Hospital
Boston, Massachusetts

Alan B. Retik, MD
Department of Surgery
Harvard Medical School
Boston, Massachusetts

**Steven A. Ringer, MD, PhD,
FAAP**
Department of Pediatrics
Harvard Medical School
Boston, Massachusetts

Anees Siddiqui, MD
Department of Gastroenterology
Children's Hospital Boston
Boston, Massachusetts

**Charles F. Simmons Jr, MD,
FAAP**
Ruth and Harry Roman Chair of
    Neonatology
Cedars-Sinai Medical Center,
    UCLA
Los Angeles, California

Janet S. Soul, MDCM, FRCPC
Department of Neurology
Harvard Medical School
Boston, Massachusetts

Jane E. Stewart, MD
Department of Pediatrics
Beth Israel Deaconess Medical
    Center, Harvard Medical School
Boston, Massachusetts

**Sarah Stewart de Ramirez, MD,
MPH, MSc**
Department of Emergency
    Medicine
Johns Hopkins Hospital
Baltimore, Maryland

Deborah K. Vanderveen, MD
Department of Ophthalmology
Harvard Medical School
Boston, Massachusetts

**Linda J. Van Marter, MD,
MPH, FAAP**
Department of Pediatrics
Harvard Medical School
Boston, Massachusetts

Jay M. Wilson, MD
Department of Surgery
Harvard Medical School
Boston, Massachusetts

ONE

General Considerations

Part 1: Medical Considerations

Anne R. Hansen, MD, MPH

Full-term human gestation is 37 to 42 weeks. Currently, the borderline of viability is approximately 23 to 25 weeks of gestation.

High-Risk Infants

PREMATURITY

Infants born at < 37 weeks of gestation are considered premature. Preterm delivery can be either induced or spontaneous, starting as contractions or premature rupture of membranes. Induced deliveries, whether vaginal or cesarean section, can be for either maternal indications (eg, progressive pregnancy-induced hypertension or cervical incompetence) or fetal indications (eg, distress, infection, poor growth or oligohydramnios).

The etiology of spontaneous preterm labor is infection in some cases, but often it is not known. Risk factors include low socioeconomic status, black race, younger (< 16) or older (> 35 years) maternal age, maternal illness (acute or chronic), multiple gestations, and previous preterm delivery.

Anticipated Complications

Risk is in direct proportion to the degree of prematurity, including the following:

- Neurologic: Intraventricular hemorrhage (IVH), periventricular leukomalacia, retinopathy of prematurity, hearing deficit

- Respiratory: Surfactant deficiency/hyaline membrane disease/respiratory distress syndrome, pneumothorax and other air-leak conditions, pulmonary interstitial emphysema, inadequate respiratory effort or apnea/bradycardia of prematurity, chronic lung disease (CLD)
- Cardiac: Patent ductus arteriosus (PDA), hypotension (secondary to intravascular volume depletion; poor myocardial function and vascular tone; and/or component of adrenal insufficiency)
- Renal/fluid and electrolyte balance: Initially, low glomerular filtration rate (GFR); poor concentrating ability with wasting of free water, electrolytes, and bicarbonates; large insensible losses, result is needed for monitoring of fluids and electrolytes, large total fluid requirement, high level of electrolyte supplementation, sometimes HCO_3 therapy, longer half-life for many medications
- Gastrointestinal (GI): Suck and swallow dyscoordination with requirement for gavage feedings until suck reflex develops at approximately 34 to 36 weeks of gestation, feeding intolerance, necrotizing enterocolitis (NEC), immature hepatic function combined with relative polycythemia resulting in increased risk of hyperbilirubinemia
- Hematologic: Exaggerated and delayed physiologic anemia
- Temperature regulation: Tendency toward hypothermia and temperature instability, with results needed for monitoring, external heat source, generally warming lights or incubator (isolette)

SMALL FOR GESTATIONAL AGE/INTRAUTERINE GROWTH RESTRICTION

Though the terms *small for gestational age* (SGA) and *intrauterine growth restriction* (IUGR) are often used interchangeably, they have two distinct meanings. Fetuses are SGA if they are more than 2 SDs below the mean or < 10% for gestational age. In IUGR, fetuses do not reach their growth potential. A constitutionally small infant who grows steadily along the 5% for gestational age is SGA but not IUGR. A fetus that started growing at the 90% and then drops to the 20% due to maternal hypertension is IUGR but not SGA. Poor growth that starts early in gestation tends to result in symmetric IUGR, in which weight, length, and head circumference (HC) are proportionately small. Poor growth that starts later in gestation generally results in asymmetric IUGR in which the weight is affected most profoundly, the height less so, and the HC is relatively spared. SGA/IUGR status can result from maternal, placental, or fetal factors including the following:

- Maternal: older maternal age (> 40 years), small constitutional size, race, high altitude, medications and/or drugs, malnutrition, chronic disease, any maternal condition resulting in decreased placental blood and oxygen flow (eg, cardiac disease including chronic or gestational hypertension, advanced diabetes, renal disease, hemoglobinopathies including sickle cell, pulmonary disease, collagen vascular disease, antiphospholipid antibodies), uterine anomalies
- Placental: insufficiency resulting from abruption, abnormal implantation, maternal vascular disease (eg, infarction), multiple gestations
- Fetal: familial and/or constitutional, chromosomal, congenital infection (especially rubella and cytomegalovirus), anomalies, and/or syndromes; multiple gestations; some post-term infants

Anticipated Complications

The complications depend on the etiology but can include any of the following: fetal distress, perinatal depression, meconium aspiration, hypoxia, hypothermia, hypoglycemia, polycythemia, hyponatremia, hypocalcemia, pulmonary hemorrhage, and persistent pulmonary hypertension.

LARGE FOR GESTATIONAL AGE

Infants are generally considered to be large for gestational age (LGA) if they are > 2 SDs above the mean or > 90% for their gestational age. LGA status can result from maternal or fetal factors including the following:

- Maternal: Large constitutional size, diabetes before the development of vascular disease (gestational and classes A to C)
- Fetal: Familial and/or constitutional factors, some postterm infants, Beckwith-Wiedemann syndrome, hydrops fetalis

Anticipated Complications

The complications depend on the etiology but can include any of the following: increased rate of cesarean delivery, birth injury (eg, brachial plexus injury), hypoglycemia, polycythemia, and delayed pulmonary maturity.

Fluid, Electrolytes, and Nutrition

Daily fluid and electrolyte requirements depend on gestational and postbirth age (Table 1). After an initially low GFR in the first few days of birth, renal perfusion improves and total fluid and electrolyte requirements tend to increase. A large daily fluid volume is required by infants who have immature renal function or poor skin integrity or who need to remain under an open warmer (vs. an incubator). Infants typically need 3 to 5 mEq/kg/d of sodium, 2 to 3 mEq/kg/d of potassium, and 200 to 500 mg/kg/d of calcium gluconate; however, this varies considerably, especially for infants receiving diuretic therapy.

The initial goal is to achieve a mild degree of dehydration in babies with respiratory disease to minimize risk of pulmonary edema and subsequent CLD. For preterm infants, relative dehydration also decreases the risk of persistent PDA and IVH.

In the first week of life, normally term infants lose approximately 5 to 10% of birth weight and preterm infants lose up to 15% of birth weight. Babies should regain their birth weight by 2 weeks of age.

Once babies are beyond the acute phase of their illness and are recuperating and growing, they most typically receive total fluids of 150 mL/kg/d. Some infants with CLD or congenital heart disease require fluid restriction to avoid pulmonary edema. Other infants with high caloric needs require additional fluids or high–caloric density milk to achieve optimal growth and nutrition.

INTRAVENOUS NUTRITION AND HYDRATION

If an infant cannot be started on enteral feedings, nutrition and hydration need to be maintained intravenously. Intravenous (IV)

TABLE 1   Approximate Total Fluids (mL/kg/d) Required by Birth Weight and Age

	Age (hours)		
Birth Weight (kg)	< 24	24–48	> 48
< 1	100–150	120–160	140–190
1–1.5	80–100	100–120	120–160
> 1.5	60–80	80–120	100–150

fluid with glucose and electrolytes (as opposed to parenteral nutrition [PN]) is administered if it is anticipated that the infant will be receiving enteral feedings within 3 (preterm) to 5 (term) days.

- Glucose concentration is determined to avoid hypoglycemia or hyperglycemia. IV glucose should initially provide 4 to 6 mg/kg/min and then be adjusted to keep the patient euglycemic. For infants, 10% glucose (D10W) is the typical initial IV fluid, but babies requiring more than approximately 150 mL/kg/d may need 5% glucose (D5W) to avoid hyperglycemia. Note that D5W is hypo-osmolar at 252 mOsmol/L compared with 308 mOsmol/L for normal saline and should not be run for more than 24 hours without carefully weighing the risks against the benefits

- IVF with an osmolarity of < 200 mOsmol/L carry an unacceptable risk of hypo-osmolar red blood cell lysis

- Electrolyte supplementation is adjusted based on measurement of serum electrolytes. Choice and concentration of electrolytes vary with the degree of prematurity and chronologic age of the infant, as well as with the total fluid volume being given. D10W with 2 to 3 mEq NaCl/100 mL and 1 to 2 mEq KCl/100 mL is a typical maintenance fluid to run at 150 mL/kg/d. If an infant is hypocalcemic, calcium should be added to the IV fluid, especially if the infant is symptomatic (eg, hypotensive). A typical concentration of calcium gluconate is 100 to 300 g/100 mL in order to provide 200 to 500 mg/kg/d. IV fluids containing calcium should be administered only through a well-functioning IV line, preferably central, to avoid the severe damage caused by infiltration of calcium

PARENTERAL NUTRITION

If it is anticipated that the infant will require IV fluid for longer than 3 (for preterm infants) to 5 (for term infants) days, PN should be started as soon as glucose and electrolyte requirements are stable enough to permit prediction of fluid and electrolyte needs when ordered up to 24 hours in advance. Ordering PN requires a systematic approach, with daily advancement and adjustment. We stock a standard "starter PN" in the pharmacy to give to babies < 1,500 g on the day of admission. We run it at 50 mL/kg/d in order to allow flexibility with the remainder of the total fluids to adjust for the specific glucose and electrolyte needs of that infant.

Fat

Generally use 20% Intralipid (IL). Start with IL calculation to know how much volume to subtract from total fluids to determine volume of non-IL PN.

Start at 1 g/kg/d, advance by 1 g/kg/d until reaching 3 g/kg/d.

Hyperbilirubinemia   In the setting of hyperbilirubinemia, historically clinicians have limited lipids to 1 g/kg/d because of the risk of lipids displacing bilirubin from albumin. More recent research[1] has diminished this theoretical concern, such that the benefits of providing adequate intake of calories and fat to these nutritionally vulnerable infants is generally judged to outweigh the risks.

Lipid Calculation   To calculate daily lipids:
      (_____ g/kg/d) × (patient's weight) = _____ g/d
      (_____ g/d) ÷ (0.2 IL) = _____ mL/d*
      (_____ mL/d) ÷ (24 h/d) = _____ mL/h

* The mL/d of IL must be subtracted from the total daily fluid volume to determine the volume of non-IL PN.

Monitoring Serum Triglycerides (TG)   Serum TG should remain < 200 mg/dL. Measure serum TG at baseline (ideally before first IL infusion begins), while IL dose is being advanced, and when goal IL provision is achieved. If TG > 250 mg/dL and specimen was drawn while IL was infusing, hold IL for 4 hours and repeat TG. If TG persistently > 250 mg/dL despite IL infusion being held for 4 to 24 hours, discuss alternative schedule (eg, 1 to 3 times per week infusion) with nutrition service.

Glucose

- Start at 5 to 8 mg/kg/min. Give minimum of 4 to 5 mg/kg/min to provide adequate glucose to meet basal metabolic requirements.

- Advance glucose concentrations daily as tolerated to provide goal energy needs while maintaining serum glucose in the normal range. If advancing or weaning off IV fluid, do not change glucose provision by > 2 mg/kg/min in a day to avoid hyperglycemia or hypoglycemia.
- Via peripheral IV, best to give 10% or less to avoid sclerosis of vein. Can give up to 12.5% if necessary to maintain serum glucose in normal range, but consider final osmolality of the solution.
- Insulin therapy may be necessary to allow a patient to tolerate the administration of adequate glucose for growth without hyperglycemia.

Glucose Calculation   To calculate glucose administration in mg/kg/min:

$$\frac{(\text{glucose infusion rate}) \times (\% \text{ glucose})}{(144)}$$

Example: patient on 150 mL/kg/d of $D_{12.5}W$:

$$\frac{(150) \times (12.5)}{(144)} = 13 \text{ mg/kg/min}$$

Protein

Start at 1 g/kg/d, advance by 1 g/kg/d until reaching 3 g/kg/d (babies with body weight < 1 kg may need a total of 3.5 g/kg/d protein to achieve optimal growth and nutrition; consult with nutrition service).

Protein Calculation   To calculate daily protein:
(_____ g/kg/d) × (patient's weight) = _____ g/d
(_____ g/d) ÷ (total daily volume of PN) (100) = _____ % amino acids

Total and Ideal Distribution of Daily Calories   Like enteral energy requirements, parenteral caloric intake should be titrated to achieve optimal weight gain (Table 3) and somatic growth. Because of the increased efficiency of parenterally administered calories, as well as the risk of PN liver disease with overfeeding, infants should generally not exceed 80 to 100 kcal/kg/d parenterally. Infants who are AGA and > 28 weeks of gestation need 80 to 90 kcal/kg/d, whereas infants who are SGA of < 28 weeks often need 90 to 100 kcal/kg/d to support optimal weight gain. Calories should be distributed as follows: fat, 30 to 55%; carbohydrates (glucose), 35 to 65%; protein, 7 to 15%.

If the patient is receiving PN peripherally, there is a risk of vein sclerosis, precipitation, or excessive osmolality; therefore, the final osmolality of the solution should be < 900 mOsm, and the following concentrations should not be exceeded:

- Elemental calcium: 30 mg (=1.5 mEq)/100 mL
- Potassium: 4 mEq/100 mL
- Dextrose: 10% with ≤ 3% amino acids; 12.5% with ≤ 2% amino acids

Monitoring Along with monitoring weight gain and somatic growth, infants receiving PN should be monitored biochemically. Weekly, measure serum electrolytes, blood glucose, total and direct bilirubin, ALT, alkaline phosphatase, TG, albumin, prealbumin, calcium, phosphorous, and magnesium. In addition, for infants receiving PN for > 1 month, measure zinc, copper, selenium, aluminum, carnitine, and iron (if not recently transfused)

ENTERAL NUTRITION AND HYDRATION

If the infant has no contraindications to enteral feeding (eg, respiratory distress, hypoxic or ischemic exposure, hypotension, umbilical artery catheter), the infant may be started on enteral feedings. The suck reflex starts at 34 to 36 weeks of gestation; therefore, below this gestational age, infants will initially need to receive enteral feedings via a gavage tube. Premature infants have immature GI tracts and should not immediately receive their full daily volume enterally or milk that has been calorically enhanced. Signs of feeding intolerance include increased volume of gastric aspirates, emesis, abdominal distention, and heme-positive stool (see Chapter 7, "Gastrointestinal Disorders").

Enteral Feeding

Guidelines for initial rates and volume increases for enteral feeding are provided in Table 2.

TABLE 2 Enteral Feeding Guidelines for Premature Infants

Birth Weight (kg)	Initial Rate (mL/kg/d)	Volume Increase (mL/kg/d)
< .8	10	10–20
.8–1	10–20	10–20
1–1.25	20	20–30
1.25–1.5	30	30
1.5–1.8	30–40	30–40
1.8–2.5	40	40–50
> 2.5	50	50

Transition from IV to Enteral Nutrition Fat and protein during transition from IV to enteral nutrition:

- Fat: continue to supply the full 3 g/kg/d of fat parenterally in addition to enteral fat intake in order to offset the decreased caloric density of enteral volume compared with parenteral.
- Protein: IV + PO = 3 to 5 g/kg/d total.

Advancement of Caloric Density Once the infant is tolerating total fluids via the enteral route, the caloric density of milk can be increased by 2 kcal/oz every 24 to 48 hours, as tolerated, until optimal growth is achieved.

Recommendations
- Give first 4 to 6 kcal/oz as concentrated formula if infant is being fed formula, or use 4 kcal/oz as human milk fortifier (HMF) if infant is being fed breast milk.
- Give next 3 to 4 kcal/oz as medium-chain triglycerides (MCTs) or canola oil.
- Give last 2 to 3 kcal by polycose.
- We give supplemental protein to babies < 1.5 kg or < 32 weeks of gestation if they are receiving mostly breast milk. We start the protein when the infant is tolerating a caloric density

of 26 to 30 kcal/oz. We usually give 1 kcal/oz of Beneprotein by adding one-eighth teaspoon to every 25 mL of milk.

- Calcium and PO4 (phosphorous) should be checked 1 week after concentrated formula or HMF is added. It should then be checked every week (HMF) to every other week (concentrated formula). If calcium remains in the normal range, the baby can continue to receive premature formula until due date, 2 kg or discharge home from hospital, whichever comes first.
- Alkaline phosphatase should be checked every week or every other week. If bone density concerns (eg, pathologic fractures noted on radiographs), check PTH and 25-OH Vit. D.

Calories for Optimal Weight Gain   Infants being fed enterally generally need between 110 and 130 kcal/kg/d, provided in 130 to 160 mL/kg/d to achieve optimal weight gain (Table 3). Infants with CLD or other conditions that increase metabolic demand can require up to 150 kcal/kg/d for optimal weight gain. Ideal growth depends on post menstrual age (<http://neonatal .rti.org/dsp-birthcurves.cfm>).

Length   An infant's linear growth should follow a standard growth curve, or cross-up percentiles (not down). Generally, 0.8 to 1.1 cm per week is acceptable for premature infants.

Weight-to-Length Ratio   This should remain > 25%.

TABLE 3   Optimal Weight Gain

Weight or Age	Daily Weight Gain (g)
< 1,800 g	10–20
> 1,800 g to term	20–30
Term to 3 months	20–30
3 to 6 months	15
6 to 9 months	10

Head Circumference   HC should follow standard growth curves. HC growth should be

- 0.5 to 1 cm per week until term,
- 0.5 cm per week from term to 3 months, and
- 0.25 cm per week from 3 to 6 months of age.

Breast Milk, Formula, and Supplemental Vitamins and Minerals   All infants without dietary restrictions should ideally be given breast milk. If breast milk is not available, infants born at < 36 weeks of gestation should be given premature infant formula rather than formula made for term infants. Infants benefit from the additional vitamins and minerals in receive premature formula until due date, 2 kg or discharge home from hospital, whichever comes first.

There are many specialized formulas for babies with dietary restrictions.

- Alimentum, Pregestamil, and Nutramigen are semi-elemental hypoallergenic formulas with hydrolyzed casein as its protein source, not amino acids. Nutramigen is the optimal choice for babies with mild to moderate protein allergy without fat malabsorption.
- The most elemental formulas are Elecare and Neocate. Both have amino acids as protein source. Elecare has 33% MCT, and Neocate has only about 5% MCT as fat source. Babies with severe protein allergies or multiple food allergies should be given Elecare or Neocate. Babies with fat malabsorption short bowel syndrome will be able to absorb the most nutrients from Elecare.

Because the vitamin D content of breast milk is quite low, infants who receive primarily breast milk should be supplemented with vitamin D, 200 IU/d.

Supplemental Iron   Supplemental iron (Fe) should be started when the infant is tolerating 24 kcal/oz milk at full volume. A total of 4 mg/kg/d Fe should be provided routinely to prematurely born infants. If the baby is < 1 kg and/or the hematocrit/retic count is unusually low, a total of 6 mg/kg/d Fe can be given.

- 150 mL/kg/d of formula made for preterm infants generally provides 2 mg/kg/d Fe; therefore, an additional 2 mg/kg/d of supplemental Fe should be given.
- Breast milk has less Fe than formula, although it is thought to be more bioavailable. Infants receiving breast milk should be given 4 mg/kg/d supplemental Fe. HMFs generally contain some Fe and should therefore be subtracted from the total goal to determine the supplemental Fe dose.

Considerations at Discharge   Patients should be discharged home on calorically enhanced formula if weight is < 10% for gestational age, weight is < 2 kg and baby is gaining < 15 g/kg/d, or baby is eating < 130 mL/kg/d.

Reference

1. Rubin M, Naor N, Sirota L, et al. Are bilirubin and plasma lipid profiles of premature infants dependent on the lipid emulsion infused? J Pediatr Gastroenterol Nutr 1995;21:25–30.

Recommended Readings

Cloherty JP, Eichenwald EC, Stark AR. Manual of neonatal care. 5th ed. Philadelphia: Lippincott Williams & Wilkins; 2008.

Part 2: Surgical Considerations

Mark Puder, MD, PhD

The newborn is not simply a small child. Preoperative and post-operative care of newborns require attention to details and collaboration between medical and surgical specialists.

Stabilization and Transport of the Newborn for Surgery

Newborns with problems that require surgery are frequently referred from community hospitals to major centers. It is important that there is a smooth exchange of information between the referring center and the accepting center, including the surgeon and other staff.

REFERRING CENTER

The referring center should

- provide details of the baby's specific problem(s), birth weight, vascular access, medications, and intravenous (IV) infusions.
- copy appropriate records (including baby's and mother's chart) and radiographs to accompany the patient, and
- initiate stabilization and management. Refer to material in this chapter as well as to the detailed recommendations in subsequent chapters for specific diagnoses.

ACCEPTING CENTER

The accepting center should

- provide instructions regarding any specific management recommendations,
- inform the receiving medical providers (neonatologists and surgeons) of the baby's expected problems, condition, vascular access, and specific needs, and
- inform all other relevant staff who will be participating in the baby's care (eg, the neonatologist, radiologist, and anesthesiologist).

PREOPERATIVE PREPARATION OF THE NEWBORN

- Confirm blood type and cross match.
- Complete consent forms for surgery and anesthesia.
- Babies with possible cardiac anomalies should have an electrocardiogram, a chest radiograph, and four limb pressures to facilitate a cardiology evaluation.
- Newborns must receive 1 mg vitamin K intramuscularly to prevent hemorrhagic disease of the newborn. Infants less than 1 kg should receive only 0.5 mg. This is sometimes overlooked during a difficult delivery or resuscitation and can lead to disastrous bleeding complications.

Diseases Requiring Surgery in the Newborn Period

Please also see chapters on specific diseases for full discussion.

TRACHEOESOPHAGEAL FISTULA AND ESOPHAGEAL ATRESIA

- The infant's head should be kept up at a 45° angle. A sump nasogastric tube should be passed through the nose or mouth and be kept on continuous suction to keep the upper pouch empty.
- Bag and mask ventilation is to be avoided if there is a distal tracheoesophageal fistula to prevent gastric distention and further respiratory impairment or gastric perforation.
- Avoid abdominal palpation as this can cause reflux of gastric contents into the lungs via a distal fistula.
- Look for vertebral, anal, cardiac, tracheal, esophageal, renal, and limb anomalies. Though it is not necessary to perform before a transport, a preoperative echocardiogram is required for all of these patients to determine whether there is a right or left aortic arch. This will determine the side of thoracotomy for repair.
- Abdominal distention is a surgical emergency. This can cause cardiac arrest due to pulmonary compression and reflux into the trachea with acute life-threatening pneumonitis.
- A large-bore (14 French [14F]) angiocatheter should be taped to the infant's bed for rapid gastric decompression in case life-threatening distention suddenly develops.

INTESTINAL OBSTRUCTION

The diagnosis and management of intestinal obstruction in infants is different from that in older children. The common causes of obstruction are intestinal atresias, Hirschsprung's disease, meconium ileus, and malrotation.

- Bilious emesis in an infant denotes midgut volvulus until proven otherwise. This is a surgical emergency.
- All infants require an adequate IV and nasogastric tube when intestinal obstruction is suspected.
- Newborn plain radiographs cannot distinguish large from small bowel obstruction because haustral markings are not yet detectable. Only filling the colon with a contrast agent will determine whether dilated loops are colon or small bowel.
- Gastrografin is very hyperosmolar and can cause rapid loss of fluid into the gastrointestinal (GI) tract. This may lead to dehydration and shock. Infants should always have an IV placed and be adequately hydrated prior to a Gastrografin study.

INTESTINAL ATRESIA

Intestinal atresia occurs in decreasing order of frequency as follows: ileum, duodenum, jejunum, colon, and pylorus. A careful antenatal and perinatal history may help to localize the site of atresia. Prenatal ultrasound (U/S) diagnosis of a dilated stomach and or duodenum may be indicative of duodenal atresia. Abdominal distention is seen in most newborns with bowel atresia, although it may be minimal or absent with more proximal atresias. Vomiting usually occurs within the first 48 hours of life. Emesis is bilious except in pyloric atresia.

- Plain radiographs of the abdomen should be obtained in all cases. The double bubble of duodenal atresia is pathognomonic, and no contrast study is indicated. Multiple loops of dilated bowel suggest a distal atresia, necessitating a contrast study.
- A contrast enema is helpful to identify microcolon, which is a highly reliable finding to either diagnose a distal small bowel obstruction or to confirm patency of the colon.
- Up to one-third of children with duodenal atresia have trisomy 21. These children may have complex cardiac anomalies.

All infants with duodenal atresia require a cardiology evaluation prior to surgery.

HIRSCHSPRUNG'S DISEASE

Hirschsprung's disease is also called congenital aganglionic megacolon. It is a frequent cause of neonatal intestinal obstruction. In this disease, there is an absence of ganglion cells that results in a functional obstruction due to ineffective conduction of peristalsis. The aganglionic segment may be limited to the rectosigmoid or extend proximally to involve the entire colon and even up to the stomach. Symptoms are nonspecific and include failure to pass meconium in the first 48 hours of life, episodic abdominal distention, constipation, obstipation, or diarrhea. Diagnosis starts with a contrast enema. Classically, this shows a transition zone at the narrowed rectum with a dilated colon proximally; however, the finding is often absent in infants. If the contrast enema is normal and there is a high suspicion for Hirschsprung's disease, obtain a plain radiograph of the abdomen on the following day. Retained contrast in the colon on this follow-up film is highly suspicious for Hirschsprung's disease.

- A diagnosis of Hirschsprung's disease is confirmed by suction mucosal rectal biopsy or full-thickness rectal biopsy showing an absence of ganglion cells and hypertrophied nerves in the myenteric plexus of the muscularis layer. There is also increased acetylcholinesterase in the aganglionic rectum.
- Initial management of Hirschsprung's disease is with saline rectal irrigations every 6 hours. As long as the infant passes stool with irrigations and the abdomen decompresses appropriately, the infant may be fed ad lib.
- Neonatal primary perineal pull through, with or without laparoscopic assistance, may be performed once the infant is stabilized. We currently avoid colostomy in most cases of Hirschsprung's disease.
- Colostomy may be indicated for enterocolitis or the inability to obtain adequate decompression with irrigation. Long-segment Hirschsprung's disease may also require stoma formation.

MECONIUM ILEUS

Meconium ileus accounts for almost one-third of all obstructions in the small intestine of newborns. It occurs in about 15% of infants with cystic fibrosis. However, 90% of patients with meconium ileus have cystic fibrosis. The incidence of cystic fibrosis in the United States is 1 in 3,000 live births. Males and females are equally affected. It is extremely rare in noncaucasian populations.

- The diagnosis of meconium ileus is suspected in the infant who develops generalized abdominal distention, bilious vomiting, and failure to pass meconium in the first 24 to 48 hours. There is a history of polyhydramnios in 20% of cases. A family history of cystic fibrosis is common.

- The meconium may be palpable as a doughy substance in the dilated loops of distended bowel. The anus and rectum are typically narrow.

- Plain radiographs of the abdomen show bowel loops of variable sizes with a soap-bubble appearance of the bowel contents. Calcifications usually indicate meconium peritonitis, resulting from an intrauterine intestinal perforation. Microcolon is a highly reliable finding for distal bowel obstruction that may be a functional stenosis from inspissated meconium or atresia due to intrauterine volvulus. A contrast enema demonstrates the microcolon with inspissated meconium proximally. A contrast enema is contraindicated if the plain radiograph shows calcification.

- The initial treatment is nonsurgical and begins with a Gastrografin enema. Under fluroscopic control, a 50% solution of Gastrografin and water is infused into the rectum and colon through a catheter. This will usually result in a rapid passage of semiliquid meconium that continues for the next 24 to 48 hours. Follow-up radiographs of kidney, ureter, and bladder (KUBs) at 12 and 24 hours should be obtained to evaluate the progress. Multiple Gastrografin enemas are frequently required. Mucomyst (N-acetylcysteine) can also be used as an enema or by mouth or nasogastric tube to assist in cleaning out the thick meconium (dilute 20% solution to 5% by adding sterile water).

- Surgery is indicated for meconium ileus if the Gastrografin enema fails to relieve the obstruction, there are calcifications in

the abdominal cavity, the infant appears too ill to delay operation, or the diagnosis of meconium ileus is in doubt.

- Infants diagnosed with meconium ileus require a sweat test to
pursue the diagnosis of cystic fibrosis. This test is usually not
practical before surgery because the child must weigh at least 2 kg
and be older than 72 hours. A minimum of 100 mg of sweat is
collected, and a concentration of sodium and chloride above
60 mEq/L is diagnostic. A buccal smear detects cystic fibrosis
with 80 to 90% sensitivity because it looks for only the most
common genetic mutations. Infants with cystic fibrosis should
receive pancreatic enzymes when enteral feedings are begun.

MIDGUT MALROTATION AND VOLVULUS

Midgut malrotation and volvulus are very common causes of
intestinal obstruction in infants and must be considered in every
infant with bilious emesis.

- Clinical findings: The presentation can range from asymptomatic to acutely ill. More than 50% present in the first month
of life, 30% in the first week. Ninety-five percent have vomiting
that becomes bilious. Bloody vomitus suggests bowel necrosis.
Twenty-eight percent have bloody stools. Plain radiographs are
most commonly normal, but they may show either a gasless
abdomen, dilated intestine suggesting small bowel obstruction,
or duodenal obstruction with a double bubble. Unless immediate surgery is necessary, the diagnosis should always be confirmed with an upper GI study to determine the position of
the duodenal-jejunal junction.

- Midgut volvulus is one of the most serious emergencies seen in
the newborn period. Delay in diagnosis can result in loss of the
entire midgut and may be fatal. Sudden onset of bilious emesis is the primary presenting sign. Abdominal distention is
common, but it may be absent. Abdominal tenderness varies.
Rectal examination is usually guaiac positive. Definitive diagnosis requires a contrast study. An upper GI is the preferred study.
With shock or a clear indication for exploration, no studies are
necessary, and the infant should be brought directly to surgery. If
studies are obtained, they should be done expeditiously because
a few hours may be the difference between a totally reversible
condition and loss of the entire midgut and possibly death.

- The treatment is always surgical. A nasogastric tube must be placed, IV hydration started, and the infant transported immediately to the operating room (OR). The surgeon decompresses the volvulus in a counterclockwise fashion. Adhesions are lysed, and the small bowel is placed in the right lower quadrant (RLQ) and the cecum and colon into the left lower quadrant. An appendectomy is performed. Recurrent volvulus occurs in up to 8% of cases.

OMPHALOCELE AND GASTROSCHISIS

- Babies with exposed bowel are at high risk of hypothermia. This is a complication that should be anticipated and avoided by paying close attention to thermoregulation.
- The sac (omphalocele) or exposed intestines (gastroschisis or omphalocele) is immediately covered with an occlusive dressing. The most desirable "dressing" is to place the entire lower half of the infant's body into a Lahey bag (obtained from the OR) to prevent evaporative losses. Coverage with a clear wrap (eg, Saran Wrap) allows inspection of the bowel to monitor for ischemia. Gauze should generally be avoided because it tends to stick to the bowel even if moistened.
- To prevent angulation of the bowel and ischemia, the baby should be placed on his or her side with the bowel supported by towels.
- To prevent further GI distention and aspiration of gastric contents, a nasogastric tube should be placed to continuous suction.
- IV hydration is essential.
- Systemic IV antibiotics (ampicillin and gentamicin) are given to protect the contaminated amnion and viscera. Infection is a devastating problem, especially if a mesh closure is necessary.
- Associated anomalies in infants with omphalocele are common and may include the following types: cardiac (a preoperative echocardiogram is necessary to assess for a cardiac disease or cardiovascular dysfunction), renal (postoperative renal U/S), chromosomal (trisomy 13, 18, 21), Beckwith-Wiedemann syndrome (large tongue, gigantism, hypoglycemia), and rectal (imperforate anus). Gastroschisis is associated with intestinal atresia.

- Immediate surgery is performed with either primary closure of the defect or placement of a Silastic "silo" for gradual reduction. Silo reduction is usually accomplished within 2 weeks.
- If the defect is too large for closure or if there are severe associated abnormalities, omphaloceles may be allowed to epithelialize. Topical agents such as silver nitrate or silver sulfadiazine are applied. Epithelialization takes several weeks and leaves a hernia defect that is repaired at a later date.

NECROTIZING ENTEROCOLITIS

Necrotizing enterocolitis usually occurs in premature and/or low–birth weight infants; 10% of cases are in term infants. Clinical presentation is nonspecific, and radiography is important for diagnosis and to follow the progression of disease. Bowel dilation is the earliest and most common sign. Intramural gas (pneumatosis) confirms the diagnosis. The amount of gas is not related to the severity of disease. Resolution of the gaseous distention is not necessarily related to improvement. Portal venous gas is usually associated with severe disease. Free air is diagnostic of intestinal perforation.

Evaluation and Treatment

- Nothing by mouth (NPO)
- Nasogastric suction
- Broad spectrum antibiotics
- KUB and lateral decubitus radiographs, intitially every 6 to 8 hours
- Serial complete blood count, platelet count, blood pH, and electrolytes

Surgical Indications

- Pneumoperitoneum is an absolute indication for surgery and is best seen on a lateral decubitus radiograph.

Relative Indications

- Abdominal wall cellulitis
- RLQ mass
- Fixed loop of bowel
- Failure to respond to medical therapy

- Persistent thrombocytopenia, acidosis, or hemodynamic instability

Once surgical indications emerge, the baby must be promptly taken to the OR. The critically ill baby with extremely low–birth weight (ie, < 1,000 g) may undergo bedside peritoneal drainage as a temporizing measure or, in some cases, as definitive treatment.

CONGENITAL DIAPHRAGMATIC HERNIA

Congenital diaphragmatic hernia requires specialized medical and surgical care. Despite intensive therapy including extracorporeal membrane oxygenation, mortality continues to be high.

Transport to Treatment Center

- Respiratory: Intubation is required. The peak inspiratory pressure should be just enough to move the chest, in general less than 30 cm H_2O. Avoid muscle relaxation if possible.
- A functional nasogastric tube for suction is essential to prevent gaseous distention of the intestinal contents in the chest.
- Lines: Only peripheral IV lines are necessary for transfer. Umbilical lines and arterial lines can be placed after arrival at the receiving hospital. After transfer, one arterial line (preferably preductal) should be placed, with pulse oximetry in the postductal position.

General Perioperative Fluid Management

NPO ORDERS

Infants may be given clear liquids containing glucose up to 4 hours before surgery. Breast milk is considered a clear fluid unless the infant has received a bowel preparation.

IV FLUIDS

- An infant should not remain without fluid intake for longer than 6 hours. If surgery is delayed, IV fluids should be started preoperatively.

- Patients with fever, vomiting, diarrhea, or undergoing bowel preparation should have IV infusions started the night prior to surgery.

BOWEL PREPARATION FOR GI SURGERY

Elective bowel surgery is often managed with preoperative mechanical bowel preparation (Golytely) followed by oral antibiotics of erythromycin base 50 mg/kg/day plus oral neomycin 50 mg/kg/day divided every 2 to 3 hours for 3 doses on the day before operation. Preoperative IV antibiotics are given 30 minutes prior to incision time (on call to OR).

Golytely is an isotonic solution of polyethylene glycol and electrolytes. The polyethylene glycol has a high molecular weight and is not absorbed in the GI tract. This is used for colon cleaning preoperatively and must be given before midnight. If the effluent is not clear after 4 to 6 hours the dose may be repeated once. Infants under 10 kg should receive maintenance IV fluids during the bowel preparation. Golytely dose: PO/PG 12.5 mL/kg/h × 4 h. When giving PG, it should be through an enteral infusion pump.

DEFICIT THERAPY

- Gastric losses: D_5W 1/2 NS + 20 to 40 mEq KCl/L to replace measured losses
- Distal GI losses: 5% dextrose with Ringer's lactate (D5RL) to replace measured losses
- Third-space losses: D5RL

BODY FLUID COMPOSITIONS

Table 1 provides guidelines regarding the typical composition of body fluids in infants. If more precision is necessary, the actual fluid(s) may be sent for electrolyte analysis.

BLOOD REPLACEMENT

Estimated Blood Volume

The estimated blood volume in humans is as follows:
- Preterm newborn = 90 mL/kg
- Term newborn = 80 mL/kg

ABLE 1 Guidelines Regarding Composition of Body Fluids in fants

Source	Na (mEq/L)	K (mEq/L)	Cl (mEq/L)	HCO_3	pH	Osmolarity
GI tract	70	10 to 15	120	0	1	300
Pancreas	140	5	50 to 100	100	9	300
Bile	130	5	100	40	8	300
Ileostomy	130	15 to 20	120	25 to 30	8	300
Diarrhea	50	35	40	50	alkaline	variable

- Infant = 75 mL/kg
- Toddler = 70 mL/kg
- Adult = 65 mL/kg

Rules of Thumb for Blood Replacement

- 10 mL/kg of packed red blood cells will raise the hematocrit 3 to 4%.
- 1 unit/10 kg of platelets will raise the count by 25,000.
- Use 10 to 15 mL/kg fresh frozen plasma for coagulopathy.
- Use 1 unit/5 kg of cryoprecipitable to replace fibrinogen.

Recommended Readings

Adzick NS, Wilson JM, Caty MG, et al, editors. Boston, Children's Hospital, Department of Surgery, House Officer Manual 2006.

Ashcraft KW, Murphy JP, Sharp RJ, et al. Pediatric surgery. 3rd ed. Philadelphia (PA): WB Saunders; 2000.

Laparotomy versus peritoneal drainage for necrotizing enterocolitis and perforation. N Engl J Med. 2006;354:2225–34.

Part 3: Respiratory Management

Linda J. Van Marter, MD, MPH, and
Anne R. Hansen, MD, MPH

The most appropriate form of respiratory support is largely influenced by the underlying cause of the respiratory failure. Common neonatal causes of hypoxemia and/or respiratory distress or failure include retained fetal lung fluid, pneumonia, surfactant deficiency, extreme pulmonary immaturity (ie, both structural underdevelopment and surfactant deficiency), pulmonary hypertension, pulmonary malformations, and congenital heart disease.

In instances of hypoxemia unaccompanied by significant respiratory failure, supplemental oxygen can be provided using an oxygen hood or nasal cannula. For mild to moderate respiratory distress, minimally invasive continuous positive airway pressure (CPAP) is indicated. When respiratory failure necessitates mechanical support, caregivers must choose among a number of forms of mechanical support, including synchronized intermittent mandatory ventilation (SIMV), newer conventional ventilatory modes such as assist-control (A/C), proportional-assisted ventilation, and neonatal pressure support (NPS) with or without "volume guarantee," and high-frequency oscillatory (HFOV) or jet (HFJV) ventilation. For specific indications, mechanical support is combined with inhaled nitric oxide. Extracorporeal membrane oxygenation (ECMO) is reserved for life-saving therapy among infants failing all other respiratory support technologies.

Oxygen toxicity, barotrauma, and volutrauma (ie, excessive tidal volume) are important mediators of lung injury. Therefore, in providing neonatal respiratory support, the specific technology and respiratory settings are chosen with the aim of providing adequate oxygenation and ventilation with a minimum of lung injury.

Ventilation

Ventilation refers to the adequacy of gas exchange, which is primarily reflected in the elimination of carbon dioxide. Improved ventilation results in a lower Pco_2. The target Pco_2 is determined by the underlying pulmonary disease process and condition of the infant.

- Ventilation is directly proportional to minute ventilation (ie, respiratory rate × tidal volume).
- Among preterm infants with acute respiratory failure, a Pco_2 of 45 to 55 mm Hg is generally considered acceptable because this gentler approach to ventilation reduces the risk of lung injury. A Pco_2 in the 50 to 60 mm Hg range is generally recommended for infants with chronic lung disease. Infants who have chronic lung disease commonly demonstrate renal compensation for persistent respiratory acidosis. The resulting metabolic alkalosis counters the respiratory acidosis associated with the increased Pco_2 and tempers the adverse effects of hypercarbia.
- Among infants with persistent pulmonary hypertension, maintaining normal acid–base balance or mild alkalosis has the beneficial effect of contributing to relaxation of pulmonary vascular resistance. This is accomplished therapeutically both by maintaining adequate ventilation and mild hyperventilation to a target Pco_2 of 35 to 40 mm Hg and, among adequately ventilated infants, partially correcting a metabolic base deficit with sodium bicarbonate (1 to 2 mEq/kg infused over 30 minutes or more).

Oxygenation

Oxygenation refers to oxygen transfer from the inspired gas to the bloodstream. The therapeutic target for oxygenation should be independent of the chosen mode of respiratory support. Among very preterm infants who are at risk of retinopathy of prematurity, the oxygen saturation goal should be 85 to 93%. Because oxygen is a powerful pulmonary vasodilator, among term infants at risk for persistent pulmonary hypertension of the newborn (PPHN), oxygen saturations should be maintained at 97 to 100%.

- Oxygenation can be improved by either increasing the percentage of inspired oxygen or the mean airway pressure (MAP). MAP is directly influenced by peak inspiratory pressure (PIP), positive end expiratory pressure (PEEP), inspiratory time (Ti), and MAP setting (HFOV only).

- An adequate Po_2 is that which provides sufficient oxygen delivery to tissues; among infants, this is generally 60 to 80 mm Hg.
- Oxygen saturation correlates with Po_2, with a steep drop-off at approximately 93%. In newborns, a Po_2 of 60 mm Hg is approximately equivalent to oxygen saturation of 90%; at a Po_2 of ≥ 80 mm Hg the neonate has an oxygen saturation of 100%.
- Fetal hemoglobin has a higher affinity for oxygen than does adult hemoglobin. This shifts the oxyhemoglobin desaturation curve to the left, resulting in a lower Po_2 at a given oxygen saturation than is observed among adults.

Cyanosis is the bluish skin discoloration that often indicates a low blood oxygen level. Visibly detectable cyanosis, however, is not a consistent and reliable marker of hypoxemia. Visible cyanosis is not a direct indicator of Po_2. Rather, it occurs when blood contains ≥ 5 mg/dL of desaturated hemoglobin. This is an important concept to keep in mind when considering newborns whose hemoglobin levels can markedly vary. For example, the newborn with polycythemia will evidence cyanosis at a higher Po_2 than an infant with a normal hemoglobin level, and the anemic infant can be hypoxemic without appearing visibly cyanotic.

Selecting the Mode of Respiratory Support

The goal of respiratory support in the newborn is to maintain adequate gas exchange with the mode that is least likely to damage the developing lung. Options for respiratory support include supplemental oxygen therapy (hood or nasal cannula), CPAP, SIMV, NPS, A/C ventilation, HFOV, and HFJV.

SUPPLEMENTAL OXYGEN THERAPY

In the absence of significant respiratory distress, oxygen saturation monitoring during administration of supplemental oxygen by hood permits assessment of the need for ongoing supplemental oxygen. In the infant requiring a fraction of inspired oxygen (FIO_2) < 0.30, oxygen delivery by low flow nasal cannula (administration of FIO_2 1 at 12 to 250 mL/minute) is appropriate. Both low-flow (mL) and high-flow (L) meters are available for nasal cannula oxygen (NCO_2) delivery. High-flow NCO_2 must be humidified to avoid excessive drying of respiratory passages. One advantage of NCO_2 over hood oxygen is that, if the baby's work of breathing is minimal and he or she is not tachypneic, NCO_2 better enables oral feeding.

- Indications: Transient tachypnea of the newborn (TTN), pneumonia, mild pulmonary edema, and resolving surfactant deficiency
- Adjustments: FIO_2 or nasal cannula flow (mL/min)
- Initial settings: Oxygen (FIO_2) and flow are adjusted to achieve the therapeutic goal.

CPAP

CPAP is a minimally invasive form of respiratory support that provides gentle distending pressure. CPAP can be delivered via specialized nasal prongs by many conventional ventilators as well as "bubble CPAP" in which the pressure is established by submersion of the terminal expiratory limb of the respiratory circuit under the specified number of centimeters of water. Starting CPAP pressures generally are set between 4 and 6 cm H_2O and can be adjusted as needed. CPAP minimizes barotrauma and tracheal colonization associated with intubation and mechanical ventilation and increasingly is becoming the first-line therapy for infants with mild to moderate surfactant deficiency. Early initiation of CPAP has been shown to be more effective than late CPAP in reducing the need for intubation and mechanical ventilation. By minimizing atelectasis and decreasing work of breathing, it is sometimes useful in treating apnea of prematurity.

- Indications: Moderate to severe TTN, mild pneumonia or pulmonary edema, apnea of prematurity, and early, mild, or resolving surfactant deficiency
- Adjustments: FIO_2 and CPAP (cm H_2O)
- Initial settings:
  - CPAP is set at 4 to 6 cm H_2O for respiratory distress and 4 to 5 cm H_2O for apnea. The settings (cm H_2O) can be increased, generally to a maximum of no more than 8 cm H_2O, to achieve better oxygenation.
  - FIO_2 is adjusted as needed to achieve the therapeutic goal.

Some clinicians use high-flow humidified nasal cannula to achieve CPAP; however, this approach has been found to deliver unpredictable levels of CPAP, and therefore, we do not currently recommend this form of CPAP.

SIMV

The most common mechanical support used in the newborn intensive care unit (NICU) is the pressure-limited, time-cycled, continuous-flow ventilator. Modern ventilators offer several support modes, and SIMV is the one we choose most often for the NICU patient population. With SIMV, the ventilator delivers a predetermined number of breaths per minute at the specified settings, and each mechanical breath is synchronized with the patient's inspiration to enhance air exchange. The patient also can generate unassisted breaths.

- Indications: Severe TTN, moderate to severe pneumonia or pulmonary edema, surfactant deficiency, apnea of prematurity, and postoperative recovery
- Adjustments: FIO_2, PEEP, PIP, Ti, and rate
- Adjustable Components
  - FIO_2: Adjust to keep oxygen saturation or PO_2 in the desired range.
  - PEEP: Set at 4 to 6 cm H_2O or higher in the setting of pulmonary edema, pulmonary hemorrhage, or worsening surfactant deficiency accompanied by low lung expansion.
  - PIP: Set to achieve adequate chest wall excursion with the aim of achieving a tidal volume of about 5 to 6 mL/kg per breath.
  - Ti: Setting is guided by the pulmonary time constant of the disease, a measure that is inversely proportional to lung compliance. Low compliance lung diseases, such as surfactant deficiency, have short time constants and thus are best treated with short Tis. Normal compliance entities, such as early meconium aspiration (before secondary surfactant deficiency), or normal lungs have longer time constants. In treating infants with surfactant deficiency or extreme lung immaturity, the Ti is set at 0.3 seconds; among term infants with normal lungs or minimal lung disease and a relatively low respiratory rate (< 25/min), Ti is set at 0.4 seconds. In general, Ti should be set as short as the disease will allow to

minimize lung injury. A prolonged Ti and rapid respiratory rate is associated with a breath-stacking phenomenon accompanied by inadvertent PEEP that can lead to retention of carbon dioxide as well as air trapping that increases the risk of pneumothorax.

- Rate: It is the number of mechanical breaths per minute. After achieving optimal tidal volume, the rate is set to maintain adequate minute ventilation.
- Initial settings: Settings depend on the severity and condition.
  - Average initial settings for surfactant deficiency or homogenous pneumonia are as follows:
    - Ti: 0.3 seconds
    - Rate: 25 to 40/minute
    - PEEP: 4 to 6 cm H_2O
    - PIP: As needed to achieve a peak tidal volume of 5 to 6 mL/kg
    - FIO_2: As needed to keep oxygen saturation at 92 to 96% (85 to 94% for < 32 weeks)
  - Average initial settings for meconium aspiration or patchy pneumonia are as follows:
    - Ti: 0.3 to 0.4 seconds
    - Rate: 25 to 35/minute
    - PEEP: 4 to 6 cm H_2O
    - PIP: As needed to achieve a peak tidal volume of 5 to 6 mL/kg
  - FIO_2: As needed to keep oxygen saturation at 96 to 100%
- Extubation: For a baby on SIMV, extubation is considered when the respiratory rate has been weaned to 15 to 20 breaths per minute, PIP of 17 to 20, and the tidal volumes of spontaneous breaths are similar to those of mechanical breaths. Prior to extubation, consider treating preterm infants with caffeine to avoid apnea and to improve respiratory effort and diaphragmatic excursion.

NPS AND A/C VENTILATION (PATIENT-TRIGGERED VENTILATION)

NPS and A/C ventilation are modes that augment each of the baby's breaths, synchronized with the airflow of the baby's spontaneous inspiration. A minimum back-up rate is specified, beyond which the baby determines the rate at which the support breaths are delivered.

With A-C mode, the baby is augmented to the desired PIP, PEEP, and Ti. NPS permits the baby to terminate the inspiration, thus generating a variable Ti. A-C and NPS modes of ventilation often are used for relatively stable patients in the recuperative phases of their respiratory illness and when acutely ill infants breathe out of phase with SIMV. They are not ideal for infants who have severe or worsening respiratory illness or who have poor respiratory drive.

- Indications: Postoperative recovery and weaning after a prolonged course of mechanical ventilation. Some institutions, including Children's Hospital, Boston, use this mode in preoperative management of congenital diaphragmatic hernia; however, this choice is based on local preference and theoretical benefit, rather than evidence from randomized clinical trials.
- Adjustments: FIO_2, PEEP, pressure support (PS)(PS + PEEP = PIP), and background rate
- Initial settings: Similar to SIMV, with assessments of tidal volumes and adjustment so that TV does not exceed 5 mL/kg.
- Extubation: Extubation generally is successful when the FIO_2 is less than 0.30. Sometimes an initial wean on NPS and a change to SIMV preextubation simplifies the final weaning process. In weaning to extubation on NPS, the back-up rate should be decreased as low as possible and the PS weaned until it delivers ~ 4 mL/kg and the baby appears comfortable and is not tachypneic (often this correlates with a PS of ~ 10).
- Comment: A relatively new approach is mixed mode ventilation in which SIMV and NPS are combined, generally with SIMV at higher settings than supplemental NPS breaths.
- Caution! A hazard with NPS and AC ventilation is that, by stacking breaths, the infant can generate inadvertent PEEP and thereby be receiving very high MAP.

VOLUME GUARANTEE

Some pressure-limited ventilators permit addition of a "volume guarantee" option to a SIMV and patient-triggered ventilatory modes. With this option, a computer algorithm is used to compute variable inspiratory pressures needed to achieve a target tidal volume. The algorithms are based on expired gas volumes that can be made inaccurate by a number of mechanical factors, including leak around the infant's uncuffed endotracheal tube. This mode should not be confused with volume-limited ventilation in which ventilation occurs with a predetermined measured gas volume.

HFOV

Several ventilator models deliver HFOV, a therapy generally reserved for infants who fail conventional mechanical ventilation or require inhaled nitric oxide therapy.

- Indications: Severe lung disease that is unresponsive to other modes of ventilation, pulmonary edema, or hemorrhage. Though inhaled nitric oxide can be given via a conventional ventilator, the combination of HFOV and iNO has been shown to be more effective than either alone in treating infants who have pulmonary hypertension associated with severe parenchymal disease. The use of prophylactic HFOV with the goal of reducing chronic lung disease among extremely preterm infants is controversial and not currently supported by evidence from clinical trials. Although sometimes used to treat infants with pneumothorax or pulmonary interstitial emphysema, this indication also has not been supported by clinical trials.
- Adjustments: FIO_2, MAP, amplitude, and Hertz
- Initial settings:
  MAP: The MAP correlates with oxygenation. Initial MAP is set 2 to 3 cm H_2O higher than that needed on SIMV and may then be increased in increments of 1 to 2 cm H_2O until pulmonary recruitment is accomplished and oxygenation improves. Although the MAP (ie, distending pressure) is greater with HFOV than SIMV, this is modulated by markedly diminished pressure swings (ie, ΔP) at the level of the alveolus. After baseline settings are achieved, MAP should be adjusted according to both oxygenation and chest radiographic appearance. The aim is to expand the lungs so that the diaphragm is slightly flattened (about nine ribs expanded). Data from clinical studies suggest that, for infants with low compliance lung disease (eg, primary or secondary surfactant deficiency), early recruitment with a "high volume" strategy then promptly weaning MAP as tolerated achieves better oxygenation with a minimum of hypocarbia than does a "low volume" approach. In taking this approach, it is important whenever possible to accomplish the MAP wean after

recruitment to minimize the risk of alveolar overdistention or excessive intrapulmonary pressures that impede cardiac function. Lower volume strategies are appropriate for diseases accompanied by air trapping or air leak, such as meconium aspiration, pulmonary interstitial emphysema, or pneumothorax.

Amplitude (ΔP): Amplitude generally correlates with ventilation and the effects of changing it are similar to adjustments of SIMV PIP. Initially, amplitude is adjusted to provide adequate chest vibration (should see gentle vibration of the chest and trunk to the level of the hips). Subsequent adjustments are made in an effort to achieve the target PCO_2.

Frequency (Hertz)(Hz): Often, no adjustments are made in Hz during the course of the baby's HFOV treatment. For most lung disease, Hertz is set at 15 to minimize barotrauma. For inhomogenous lung disease (eg, patchy pneumonia or meconium aspiration), better lung recruitment and ventilation can be seen with reductions in Hertz (6 to 12). Reducing the Hz, however, delivers substantially more power to the lung and markedly increases the risk of barotrauma and volutrauma, especially among the most immature infants.

FIO_2: The FIO_2 is set as needed to maintain target oxygenation.

- Extubation: HFOV can be weaned to CPAP from which the infant is extubated to oxygen or conventional CPAP. More commonly, HFOV support is weaned to a FIO_2 < .30 and MAP < 10 cm H_2O, and the mode is changed to SIMV for the final wean to extubation.
- Comment: Early studies suggested a higher rate of severe intraventricular hemorrhage or periventricular white matter disease among preterm infants treated with HFOV. This association remains controversial but worthy of consideration. These findings may be partially explained by the risk of extreme hyperventilation (PCO_2 < 35 mm Hg) with HFOV treatment. This should be avoided because of potential adverse pulmonary and central nervous system effects of overventilation.

HFJV

Using a somewhat different technology than HFOV, the HFJV mode of high-frequency ventilation combines high frequency and conventional ventilation. It has proven useful in treating the same pulmonary disorders as does HFOV. In addition, it is the single modality proven useful for treating infants with progressive or recurrent pulmonary air leak from processes including pulmonary interstitial emphysema or pneumothorax. Thus HFJV technology has the advantage of potentially combining with background intermittent mandatory ventilation (usually at a low rate). The general HFJV strategy is to begin with combined support and wean as rapidly as possible to the lowest conventional rate that is tolerable (ideally, no conventional breaths).

- Indications: Severe lung disease that is unresponsive to other modes of ventilation, especially those accompanied by pulmonary air leak
- Adjustments: Conventional PIP, PEEP, rate (typically 0 to 8 after transition from SIMV), FIO$_2$, HiFi PIP, HiFi PEEP
- Initial settings:
  1. Set conventional settings as recommended for SIMV.
  2. HFJV, PIP, and PEEP at least 1 cm H$_2$O greater than conventional settings so that jet ventilation is not interrupted by the conventional breaths.
  3. Wean intermittent mandatory ventilation rate as low as can be tolerated.
- Extubation: HFJV support is weaned to a FIO$_2$ < .30 and MAP < 8 cm H$_2$O, then the mode is switched to SIMV for the final preextubation wean.

Supplemental Therapies for Associated Respiratory Conditions

SURFACTANT DEFICIENCY

Exogenous intratracheal surfactant is used to treat pulmonary immaturity (ie, hyaline membrane disease or respiratory distress syndrome) and secondary surfactant deficiency caused by problems including pneumonia or, occasionally, meconium aspiration. Dosage and frequency vary according to the preparation. In general, no more than 48 hours of treatment is given.

PULMONARY HYPERTENSION

Inhaled nitric oxide (iNO) is a valuable therapy for PPHN. In treating PPHN accompanied by pulmonary parenchymal disease, iNO has been shown to be most effective when given with HFOV. When these modalities fail, ECMO (heart–lung bypass) is used.

iNO might have promise as a preventive treatment for chronic lung disease among extremely preterm infants. Early neurological outcomes have varied among studies, however, and reports of 24-month neurodevelopmental follow-up assessments are pending at this time. Currently, iNO is not recommended as standard therapy for preterm infants with surfactant deficiency.

AIRWAY EDEMA

Postextubation airway edema is rare among newborn infants. It can be anticipated prior to extubation by checking for an airleak, which should be detectable at a PIP of 25 cm H_2O for most infants. The infant who has required a prolonged period of intubation (2 to 4 weeks) might benefit from periextubation dexamethasone treatment (three doses of 0.1 mg/kg every 12 h, beginning 8 to 12 h prior to extubation). For postextubation stridor, racemic epinephrine (1:1000) (0.1 mL in 2 mL normal saline by nebulizer) can be useful. Phenylephrine HCl (Neo-Synephrine), diluted to 1/8% (2 to 3 drops every 6 to 8 h for no more than 24 hours), is used to reduce nasopharyngeal edema due to nasotracheal intubation or CPAP.

PAIN/ANXIETY/AGITATION

Intubation and mechanical ventilation are associated with stress and discomfort that many infants might not be able to express. Uncontrolled pain and stress have been shown to adversely affect the developing nervous system. Therefore, except for emergency situations in which the need for immediate intubation is urgent, we recommend premedication for intubation with morphine sulfate 0.1 mg/kg or fentanyl 1 to 2 mcg/kg. During the acute phase of mechanical ventilation, we recommend routine sedation with morphine sulfate 0.1 mg/kg intravenously or fentanyl 1 to 3 mcg/kg every 2 to 4 hours, as needed. Although not recommended for treatment of premature infants, term infants can also be treated concomitantly with an anxiolytic such as midazolam (0.1 mg/kg for premedication and every 8 h, as needed, for agitation).

APNEA/PERIODIC BREATHING

Among preterm infants (especially at or below 32 weeks' gestation), respiratory failure might reflect diminished respiratory drive, and, therefore, when weaning from mechanical support is anticipated, treatment with caffeine or caffeine citrate should be considered.

Recommended Readings

Donn S, Sinha S. Manual of Neonatal Respiratory Care, 2nd edition. Philadelphia: Mosby; 2006.

Goldsmith J, Karotkin E. Assisted Ventilation of the Neonate, 4th edition. Philadelphia: Saunders; 2003.

TABLE 1   Respiratory Support Options

Clinical Presentation	Respiratory Support
Hypoxemia	
Without respiratory distress or severe apnea	Hood oxygen or nasal cannula oxygen (low flow)
With mild respiratory distress and/or moderate apnea	CPAP
With respiratory distress, respiratory failure, or severe apnea	SIMV
Profound hypoxemia	
With respiratory distress	SIMV
With respiratory distress and failure of SIMV	HFOV
With respiratory failure and air leak	HFJV
With respiratory failure and the use of inhaled nitric oxide	HFOV
Postoperative recovery	
With pulmonary parenchymal disease	SIMV or HFOV
Without pulmonary parenchymal disease	SIMV or NPS (A-C)
Congenital cardiopulmonary anomalies	
Diaphragmatic hernia	SIMV or NPS (A-C)
Congenital heart disease	SIMV

A-C = assist-control ventilation; CPAP = continuous positive airway pressure; HFJV = high-frequency jet ventilation; HFOV = highfrequency oscillatory ventilation; NPS = neonatal pressure support; SIMV = synchronized intermittent mandatory ventilation.

TABLE 2 Common Ventilator Adjustments

Mode of Support	Desired Effect	Intervention
Hood or N/C	↓ Pco_2	No change without providing mechanical support
	↑ Po_2	Increase FIO_2 or NC flow
CPAP	↓ Pco_2	If lungs are atelectatic, increase CPAP; If lungs are overdistended, decrease CPAP
	↑ Po_2	↑ FIO_2 or ↑ CPAP (by 1 cm; max of 8 cm H_2O)
SIMV	↓ Pco_2	↑ PIP, ↑ rate consider adding VG, ↓ PEEP, trial A-C or NPS
	↑ Po_2	↑ FIO_2, ↑ PIP, ↓ PEEP, slightly increase inspiratory time
NPS or A-C	↓ Pco_2	↑ PIP (or PS), ↑ background rate
	↑ Po_2	↑ FIO_2, ↑ PIP, ↑ PEEP
HFOV	↓ Pco_2	↑ amplitude, [rarely, ↓ Hz]
	↑ Po_2	↑ FIO_2, ↑ MAP
HFJV*	↓ Pco_2	↑ PIP
	↑ Po_2	↑ FIO_2, ↑ PEEP, ↑ conventional background rate

A-C = assist-control ventilation; CPAP = continuous positive airway pressure; FIO_2 = fraction of inspired oxygen; HFJV = high-frequency jet ventilation; HFOV = high-frequency oscillatory ventilation; IMV = intermittent mandatory ventilation; MAP = mean airway pressure; N/C = nasal cannula; NPS = neonatal pressure support; Pco_2 = partial pressure of carbon dioxide; PEEP = positive end expiratory pressure; PIP = peak inspiratory pressure; Po_2 = partial pressure of oxygen; SIMV = synchronized intermittent mandatory ventilation; VG = volume guarantee. *Exclude pneumothorax before initiating or increasing mechanical ventilation.

Part 4: Differential Diagnoses According to Presenting Symptoms

Anne Hansen, MD, MPH, and
Steven Ringer, MD, PhD

A. Respiratory Distress

Though most etiologies of respiratory distress are treated medically, some respiratory disorders have an underlying etiology that must be surgically repaired.

1. Diaphragmatic hernia/eventration
2. Choanal atresia/stenosis, sinus pyriform stenosis and other airway obstruction
3. Laryngotracheal clefts
4. Tracheal agenesis
5. Esophageal atresia with or without tracheoesophageal fistula (TEF)
6. Congenital lobar emphysema
7. Cystic adenomatoid malformation of the lung or pulmonary sequestration
8. Biliary tracheobronchial communication (extremely rare)

B. Scaphoid Abdomen

1. Diaphragmatic hernia
2. Esophageal atresia without TEF

C. Excessive Mucus and Salivation

1. Esophageal atresia with or without TEF

D. Abdominal Distention

1. Pneumoperitoneum
   a. Primary GI source: necrotizing enterocolitis or localized ischemia of the stomach associated with medications such as indomethacin or steroids, excessive pressure secondary to

obstruction, TEF, or instrumentation (ie, with a nasogastric tube). Perforated stomach is associated with large amounts of free intraabdominal air. Active airleak requires urgent surgical closure. It may be necessary to aspirate air from the abdominal cavity to relieve respiratory distress prior to definitive surgical repair.

b. Secondary to air dissecting into peritoneum from a pulmonary air leak in infants receiving mechanical ventilation. Treatment of pneumoperitoneum transmitted from pulmonary airleak should focus on managing the pulmonary air leak.

2. Intestinal Obstruction
   a. Esophageal atresia with TEF
   b. Obstruction of proximal bowel (eg, complete duodenal atresia) causes rapid distension of the left upper quadrant.
   c. Obstruction of distal bowel causes more generalized distention, varying with location of obstruction.

E. Vomiting

The causes of vomiting can be differentiated by the presence or absence of bile.

1. Bilious emesis is malrotation until proven otherwise.
   a. Intestinal obstruction due to malrotation with or without volvulus, duodenal, jejunal, ileal, or colonic atresias; annular pancreas, Hirschsprung disease, aberrant superior mesenteric artery, pre-duodenal portal vein; peritoneal bands, persistent omphalomesenteric duct, or duodenal duplication.
   b. Decreased motility without intestinal obstruction (see 2c below). Typically, vomiting occurs only once or twice and presents without abdominal distention. This nonsurgical condition is a diagnosis of exclusion.

2. Nonbilious Emesis
   a. Feeding excessive volume
   b. Milk (human or formula) intolerance
   c. Decreased motility
      • antenatal or post natal exposure to $MgSO_4$ or narcotics
      • prematurity

- sepsis with ileus
- central nervous system lesion

d. Lesion above ampulla of Vater
  - Pyloric stenosis
  - Upper duodenal stenosis
  - Annular pancreas (rare)

Failure to Pass Meconium

Can occur in sick and/or premature babies as a result of decreased bowel motility. It also may be the result of the following disorders:

1. Imperforate anus
2. Functional intestinal obstruction, including meconium ileus
3. Hirschsprung's
4. Meconium ileus, meconium plug.

G. Failure to Develop Transitional Stools

Failure to develop transitional stools after the passage of meconium:

1. Volvulus
2. Malrotation

H. Hematemesis or Hematochezia

1. Non surgical conditions: Many patients with hematemesis, and the majority of patients with hematochezia (bloody stools), have a nonsurgical condition. Differential diagnosis includes the following:
   a. Milk intolerance/allergy (usually cow's milk protein allergy)
   b. Instrumentation (eg, nasogastric tube, endotracheal tube)
   c. Swallowed maternal blood: Maternal blood swallowed during labor and delivery or during breast feeding via cracked nipples can be diagnosed by an Apt test performed on blood aspirated from the infant's stomach. Mother's nipples or breast milk can also be assessed
   d. Coagulation disorders including DIC, lack of postnatal Vitamin K injection

2. Surgical Conditions resulting in hematemesis and bloody stool
   a. Necrotizing enterocolitis (most frequent cause of hematemesis and bloody stool in premature infants)
   b. Gastric or duodenal ulcers (due to stress, steroid therapy)
   c. GI obstruction: Late sign, concerning for threatened or necrotic bowel
   d. Volvulus
   e. Intussusception
   f. Polyps, hemangiomas
   g. Meckel's diverticulum
   h. Duplications of the small intestine
   i. Cirsoid aneurysm

I. Abdominal Masses

1. Genitourinary anomalies including distended bladder
2. Hepatosplenomegally: May be confused with other masses; requires medical evaluation.
3. Tumors

J. Birth Trauma

1. Fractured clavicle/humerus
2. Intracranial hemorrhage
3. Lacerated solid organs—liver, spleen
4. Spinal cord transection with quadriplegia

Part 5: Vascular Access

Anne R. Hansen, MD, MPH,
Arin Greene, MD, and Mark Puder, MD, PhD

Epidemiology

The vast majority of patients in an NICU require intravascular access.

Physiology

- Resistance through vascular devices is characterized by Poiseuille's equation as follows:

resistance = 8(viscosity)(catheter length)$/\pi$ (radius^4)

Thus, as the radius of a catheter increases, the resistance through the catheter decreases by the fourth power. A 19% increase in the radius results in a doubling of flow. The resistance through a catheter may also be decreased by decreasing its length.

- Clinically, maximal flow is achieved with catheters and tubing that are short, wide, and contain low-viscosity fluid. Although long central venous catheters (CVCs) are necessary for monitoring and parenteral nutrition, large-bore peripheral catheters are superior for rapid fluid resuscitation.

Sterile Technique

The medical and financial cost of line infections are increasingly recognized and criticized. Line infections are theoretically preventable if meticulous attention is paid to sterile technique both in line placement and maintenance. For peripheral venous and arterial access, we expect the catheter to remain in place for only a few days and therefore consider alcohol to be sufficient for skin sterilization. For vascular access that we expect to remain in place for a longer duration, we sterilize the insertion site with Chloraprep (chlorhexidine and alcohol) due to its superior combination of killing power and duration of action compared to alcohol alone or betadine. Though it is currently only food and drug administration (FDA) approved for use in infants > 2 months of age, in our experience it has been well tolerated in term newborns. Due to the lack of experience with chlorhexidine in preterm babies, we use alcohol for babies < 37 weeks gestation. Because any sterilizing agent burns the skin of extremely preterm infants, we wash the alcohol off with sterile normal saline for babies < 28 weeks gestation.

Peripheral Venous Access

Generally, peripheral intravenous (PIV) access provides the safest and easiest access to the venous circulation; the exception is the emergency placement of an umbilical vein catheter (UVC) in the delivery room. PIV is the access of choice when there is no indication for a CVC. Because of its short catheter length, peripheral venous access is superior to central venous access for volume infusion.

LOCATION

Veins of the hand, forearm, lower leg, and scalp may be used. The most commonly used veins are on the dorsum of the hand. Other sites that can be cannulated include the dorsal surface of the wrist and the basilic veins in the antecubital fold. The external jugular vein is best saved in case a surgically placed central venous line (CVL) is needed.

TECHNIQUE

- The most common method of insertion uses the technique of putting a catheter over a needle. A radiopaque catheter, usually ranging in size from between 22 and 26 gauge, is guided into the vein over the introducer needle.
- Surgical cutdown is indicated after percutaneous attempts at cannulation have failed. This may be performed on any large peripheral vein, most commonly the saphenous, femoral, or antecubital. Vascular cutdown carries a significantly higher risk of infection compared with percutaneous cannulation.

Also, catheters placed using the cutdown technique usually leave a scar.

COMPLICATIONS

- The complications include local infection, sepsis, phlebitis, infiltration with skin injury and/or necrosis, vessel thrombosis, and embolus.
- Treatment of these complications includes removal of the catheter.

Central Venous Access

SIZES

Single lumen: Davol (Broviac or Hickman) 2.7, 4.2, 6.6, and 9.6 French (F)
Double lumen: Davol 7, 9, and 12 F

INDICATIONS

Central venous access is indicated when there is

- An anticipated need for long-term access for the prolonged administration of medications (eg, antibiotics) or fluids (eg, parenteral nutrition),
- Inability to attain peripheral access, and
- Hemodynamic monitoring (rare indication).

LOCATION

The most common sites include the external and internal jugular, facial, cephalic, brachial, saphenous and femoral veins. The ideal tip position for a central line is the junction of the RA and the SVC or IVC.

CATHETER TYPES

- Percutaneous intravenous central catheters (PICCs) have decreased the need for surgically placed central lines. These catheters are placed via a peripheral vein and threaded to a central position. A PICC may last for several weeks.

- Short-term (usually less than 2 weeks), polyethylene (eg, Arrow), nontunneled catheters can be placed percutaneously into the internal jugular, subclavian, and femoral veins using the Seldinger technique. The PICC line may also be used for this purpose.
- For long-term access such as prolonged parenteral nutrition or antibiotic therapy, the Silastic catheters (eg, Broviac or Hickman) are preferable because of their pliability and decreased thrombogenicity. They are usually tunneled subcutaneously along the chest. The catheter is secured to the skin with nonabsorbable sutures at the time of the procedure. Over time, the subcutaneous Dacron cuff secures the catheter independently of the sutures.

POSTOPERATIVE CATHETER CARE

- PICC line dressings do not necessarily need to be changed on a regular basis. The risk of accidentally pulling out the line when pulling off the dressing tape must be weighed against an assessment of the need for cleaning.
- For surgically placed CVLs, the exit site is usually dressed with sterile gauze and Tegaderm. These should be changed using sterile technique. All lines should be secured in a loop to prevent inadvertent removal.
- The size of the catheter and the approximate priming volume should be present in the operative note. This information is important if it becomes necessary to repair or declot a CVL.

COMPLICATIONS

- Early complications of central lines include undesired tip location, perforation of the lung with resulting pneumothorax, perforation of a vein or artery with resulting hemothorax and/or hydrothorax, and perforation of the heart with pericardial tamponade. These complications are usually detected promptly by placing the catheters under fluoroscopic guidance and obtaining immediate postplacement radiographs.
- Technical complications such as vessel injury, pneumothorax, hemothorax, or cardiac complications must be communicated to

and corrected by the surgeon. Treatment may vary from simple observation to placement of a chest tube or thoracotomy.

- Late complications include tunnel or insertion site infections, sepsis, or venous thrombosis including the superior and inferior vena cava, femoral, and subclavian veins.
- Line thrombosis is treated by instilling 1 mL of tissue plasminogen activator (TPA; 5,000 IU per 1 mL vial) using a TB syringe. If aspiration of the clot is not possible in 1 hour, repeat the instillation, and attempt the aspiration again in 8 hours. If the line is refractory to TPA, a volume of 0.1 mL of 0.1 N HCl may be used after consultation with a surgeon. HCl causes severe tissue damage if not placed centrally or if extravasation occurs. HCl is most useful when occlusion is felt to be secondary to precipitation of parenteral nutrition.

Infection

- An infection at the catheter insertion site is defined as purulent drainage from the CVL exit site. Tenderness or erythema along the catheter tunnel also suggests infection. Clinical examination usually establishes the diagnosis. If the insertion site is aspirated, make certain that the aspiration site is thoroughly disinfected. Cultures should be obtained from the catheter site along with peripheral and central blood cultures from each lumen of the CVL (a minimum of 1 mL/bottle). Drainage should always be Gram stained and cultured.
- Central line infection may present with temperature instability, poor perfusion, tachycardia, hypotension, tachypnea, feeding intolerance, or lethargy. Systemic catheter infection is defined as septicemia resulting from an infected intravascular access device. Although the definition is straightforward, the diagnosis is often difficult to make. All infants, and especially preterm infants, are relatively immunocompromised and many also have significant comorbidities that put them at high risk for infections.

Distinguishing catheter-related sepsis from infection elsewhere can be difficult and is often a diagnosis of exclusion. Catheter-tip cultures, one or two peripheral blood cultures, and two blood cultures drawn through the central line should be obtained.

LOCAL THERAPY

- Provide local wound care, including frequent dressing changes.

Systemic Therapy

- Start empiric antibiotic coverage before culture results are available (eg, vancomycin and gentamicin).
- Tailor antibiotic coverage once culture results are available.

INDICATIONS FOR CATHETER REMOVAL

- Persistent local infection after 48 to 72 hours on appropriate antibiotics
- Recurrent positive blood cultures after 2 to 4 days
- Positive culture for fungus (eg, Candida)
- Systemic signs of infection (eg, hypotension)

CENTRAL LINE REMOVAL

- If the line being removed is the patient's only central access and the patient is receiving highly concentrated glucose infusion, it is important that the glucose infusion rate is slowly decreased over the hours to days preceding line removal such that the patient can maintain euglycemia with a glucose concentration of ≤ D12.5W.
- Percutaneous lines can be removed without general or local anesthesia. All intravenous (IV) fluids are discontinued and all ports are capped. The exit site is sterilized. The patient is placed in the supine or Trendelenburg's position, and the catheter is removed. Pressure is held for approximately 5 minutes, and an occlusive dressing is applied.
- Tunneled central lines require local and sometimes general anesthesia for removal. The Dacron cuff must be released from the subcutaneous tissue. This becomes more difficult after approximately 2 weeks. If there is resistance during the removal of a tunneled line, do not continue to pull the line. Inadvertent fracture and dislodgment may occur. A difficult

cuffed-line removal may require additional incisions to dislodge the catheter.
- After the line has been removed, the patient should be observed for 1 hour to evaluate for bleeding or hematoma.

Intraosseous Access

BACKGROUND

- Intraosseous access was first described in 1922 and was used frequently until angiocatheter devices were improved.
- The bone marrow space is a rich, noncollapsible venous network that permits infusion rates similar to IV rates.
- Any substance administered intravenously may also be administered by intraosseous infusion.

INDICATIONS

- Intraosseous access may be used in emergency resuscitative situations until IV access can be obtained.

LOCATION

- The location of choice is the flat, anteromedial surface of the proximal tibia 1 cm inferior and 1 cm medial to the tibial head.
- Secondary sites include the midline of the distal femur 3 cm proximal to the femoral condyles, the distal tibia proximal to the medial malleolus, the anterior superior iliac spine, the lateral malleolus, and the lateral proximal humerus.

TECHNIQUE

- Although any hollow 13- to 18-gauge needle may be used, the most commonly used is a bone marrow needle. The needle is rotated or screwed into the bone with the tip pointing away from the joint space to avoid involvement of the growth plate. Access to the marrow space is felt with a sudden decrease in resistance and confirmed by the aspiration of bone marrow or with successful infusion into the marrow space.
- There are also drills made specifically to insert IO lines with minimal bone injury.

COMPLICATIONS

- Puncturing through back side of bone and accidentally infusing into soft tissue
- Disruption of the growth plate can cause discrepant future bone growth.
- Other potential complications are compartment syndrome, osteomyelitis, skin necrosis, extravasation, and fracture.
- Fat and marrow emboli are extremely rare.

Umbilical Access

BACKGROUND

The umbilical veins and arteries may be accessed for several days after birth, in some cases for up to 2 weeks.

INDICATIONS

- Umbilical artery catheters (UACs) and venous (UVC's) may be used for blood sampling, infusion of some fluids and medications, and monitoring of central arterial and venous pressure.
- Arterial lines are also used for frequent monitoring of arterial blood gases. Blood products, pressors, calcium boluses, and sodium bicarbonate should not be infused through a UAC.
- Venous lines are also used for infusion of pressors and hypertonic solutions. Platelets should not be infused through a UVC. Low venous lines are used for emergency access (especially in the delivery room) and exchange transfusions.

INSERTION TECHNIQUE

- Measure the distance from the shoulder to the umbilical cord (including the length of residual umbilical cord) in cm and calculate the expected depth of catheter insertion in cm:

    UAC: (shoulder to umbilical cord) + 2

    UVC: (shoulder to umbilical cord) $\times$ 2/3

- Sterilize area around cord.
- Tie umbilical cord tape around the base of the cord to control blood flow from the umbilical vessels.

- Using sterile technique, dilate vessel and insert a 3.5 to 5F catheter flushed with heparinized normal saline and attached to a blunt needle and stopcock. Err on the side of placing the catheter in too deeply as it is easier to pull the catheter back than to assure sterility while advancing the catheter more deeply.
- Secure the catheter with a suture through part of the cord and tie around the catheter. Avoid puncturing the catheter or other umbilical vessels with the needle.
- Obtain a radiograph ("babygram") to confirm the position of the catheter tip. Adjust the catheter as indicated. The tip of the UVC should reside in the inferior vena cava, above the diaphragm (ie, above the liver). The UAC should be placed above the celiac artery but below the ductus arteriosus (between T6 and T10). Alternately, the UAC may be placed above the aortic bifurcation or below the inferior mesenteric artery (T3 to T4).
- Tape catheter(s) for added security.

COMPLICATIONS

- Blanching of toes or legs may occur. If this is because of a transient vasospasm, it may resolve with warming of the contralateral leg. If blanching is caused by inadequate distal perfusion, it will persist and the catheter must be removed.
- Other complications include infection, vessel perforation, hemorrhage, renal vein or artery thrombosis, and necrosis of the skin or extremities. All of these complications require prompt removal of the catheter.
- Thrombosis: heparinization of umbilical vessel catheters (1 unit heparin/mL) is important to minimize this risk. If thrombosis occurs, antithrombotic therapy may be needed. Hematology consultation is often useful in making this decision.

REMOVAL TECHNIQUE

Arterial Catheter

UAC should not be left in place for longer than 5 days according to the recommendations of the CDC. In removing the arterial catheter, cut the sutures carefully to avoid cutting the catheter. Pull the catheter back to the 5 cm mark, and leave it in that position for approximately 5 minutes. If it is being transduced, wait until the wave form becomes flat as a functional indicator of vessel constriction. Then, slowly pull the remainder of catheter out over a period of approximately 1 minute to allow for vessel constriction. If bleeding persists after catheter removal, apply pressure to the cord (avoid direct abdominal pressure) until it stops. Remove remaining suture material.

Venous Catheter

UVC should not be left in place for longer than 14 days according to the recommendations of the CDC. Venous catheters are removed as above for arterial catheters except that they need not be held in the 5 cm position before pulling the catheter out over approximately a 1-minute period.

Peripheral Arterial Access

INDICATIONS

- Continuous BP monitoring
- Arterial blood gas measurements (place in right radial artery if preductal values desired)

LOCATION

- The locations of choice are peripheral sites with good collateral flow (eg, radial, posterior tibial, and dorsalis pedis).
- Avoid brachial (because of poor collateral flow) and superficial temporal arteries (because of the risk of cerebral infarcts).

TECHNIQUE

- Always perform Allen's test prior to cannulating a peripheral artery. After releasing pressure on one of the two arteries supplying the limb, the extremity with adequate collateral flow should flush in color in less than 5 seconds.
- Use the smallest catheter possible (usually a 22 or 24 gauge).

- Use a catheter-over-a-needle technique with the bevel of the needle facing up.
- Cannulation may also be achieved using the cutdown technique.

COMPLICATIONS

- Serious complications include infection, obstruction of an artery, skin and/or limb ischemia, and possible limb loss.
- The risk of thrombosis can be reduced by slow continuous infusion with heparin.
- The low risk of retrograde embolization of a clot or air to the cerebral circulation can be further reduced by continuous slow flushing of the catheter.

Recommended Reading

Cloherty JP, Stark AR, editors. Manual of neonatal care. 6th ed. Philadelphia (PA): Lippincott-Raven Publishers; 2008. p. 649–64.

Management of Vascular Access: Venous

	Peripheral IV	UVC	Central Venous Catheter	PICC
Minimum Infusion Rate	1 mL/hr	1 mL/hr	1 mL/hr	1 mL/hr
Can line be "hep-locked"?	Yes, flush with 1 to 2 mL NS q8h and after medication administration	NO	Yes, flush with Heparin 10 U/mL 1 to 2 mL q8h	NO
Does fluid need to be heparinized?	No	Yes, 0.5 units per mL	Yes, 0.5 units per mL	Yes, 0.5 units per mL
What can run through it?	Any saline or dextrose solution (up to D12.5%), any blood product, PN and IL (max PN concentration is PN10/3% AA or PN12.5/2.5%AA, any medication/drip	Any solution, medication, continuous infusion, blood products (except platelets)	Same as for UVC	Any solution, medication, continuous infusion

Continued

Management of Vascular Access: Venous (*Continued*)

	Peripheral IV	UVC	Central Venous Catheter	PICC
Minimum Infusion Rate	1 mL/hr	1 mL/hr	1 mL/hr	1 mL/hr
What can not run through it?	PN more concentrated than noted above, bolus medication if a continuous drip is infusing through the line.	Platelets, a bolus medication if a continuous drip is infusing through the lumen	Same as for UVC	Blood products, a bolus medication if a continuous drip is infusing through the lumen.
Other	Use caution infusing the following through a PIV: dopamine, epinephrine, calcium, potassium, sodium bicarbonate, parenteral nutrition			

PICC = Percutaneously inserted central catheter; UVC = Umbilical venous catheter

Management of Vascular Access: Arterial

	UAC	Peripheral Arterial Line
Minimum Infusion Rate	1 mL/hour	1 mL/hour
Can line be "hep-locked"?	NO	NO
Does fluid need to be heparinized?	Yes, 0.5 units/mL	Yes, 1 unit/mL
What can run through it?	Any saline or dextrose solution, PN, bolus medications (ie, antibiotics)	Saline or 0.45% normal saline
What can't run through it?	Blood products, dopamine, epinephrine, dobutamine, calcium boluses, sodium bicarbonate	Nothing can run through a peripheral arterial line, except the above solutions
Other	Continuous medication infusions should not be administered via a UAC as blood sampling will interfere with constancy of medication administration	

UAC = Umbilical Artery Catheter

TWO

The Fetus

Charles F. Simmons Jr, MD

Advanced fetal diagnostic and imaging studies now facilitate earlier identification of fetal anomalies and fetal pathophysiologic states during early pregnancy. These new maternal–fetal diagnostic and therapeutic capabilities have ushered in a new era of coordinated, multidisciplinary approaches to fetal diagnosis and treatment. In turn, these approaches emphasize not only the fetus as a patient but also the ethical aspects of innovative maternal–fetal treatments and research.

Prenatal Diagnosis

Increasingly, clinicians achieve prenatal rather than postnatal diagnosis of a medically or surgically amenable congenital abnormality. Advances in sophisticated prenatal screening, involving both biochemical and imaging approaches, now make prenatal diagnosis of simple and complex anomalies a common event. Timely and accurate prenatal diagnosis relies upon access to high-quality prenatal care, advanced prenatal diagnostic procedures, and genetic counseling.

BIOMARKER SCREEN

Maternal serum α fetoprotein, unconjugated estriol, and human chorionic gonadotropin screens are readily available in the United States and are recommended for women during their first trimester of prenatal care. The calculation of a woman's risk for carrying an aneuploid fetus relies on age, gestational age, and the specific values for these biochemical tests. As a result of the calculated likelihood of fetal abnormality, additional imaging and genetic evaluation of the fetus may be indicated. In addition, elevated α fetoprotein values may suggest neural tube defects, ventral wall defects such as gastroschisis, or congenital nephrotic syndrome.

CHORIONIC VILLUS SAMPLING

Sampling of the chorion frondosum during the first trimester provides tissue for early genetic and/or biochemical diagnostic testing. This procedure may be performed either transvaginally or transabdominally as early as 8 to 10 weeks' gestation. The tissue obtained may be sent for cytogenetic, molecular genetic, or biochemical analysis. Early chorionic villus sampling (CVS) permits the timely return of diagnostic studies to clinicians and family. The safety and efficacy of early CVS has been established, with a procedure-related morbidity of approximately 0.5%.

AMNIOCENTESIS

Early amniocentesis (before 15 weeks' gestation) is offered in some centers; however, standard amniocentesis is usually performed between 15 and 20 weeks' gestation. Over two decades of safety and efficacy, data support amniocentesis during this second trimester epoch. The transabdominal removal of 20 to 30 mL of amniotic fluid provides a sufficient sample for cytogenetic, biochemical, and/or molecular genetic diagnosis. The procedure-related morbidity of standard amniocentesis approaches 0.5%. Concomitant ultrasound (U/S) imaging provides a comprehensive assessment of organ structure, growth, and development of the fetus.

FETAL BLOOD SAMPLING

Percutaneous sampling of fetal blood can facilitate rapid turnaround of cytogenetic or molecular genetic tests. Fetal transfusion is an early example of fetal therapy, and fetal anemia or thrombocytopenia can be treated through this approach.

PREIMPLANTATION DIAGNOSIS

The combination of assisted reproductive technologies, in vitro fertilization, and preimplantation genetic analysis allows phenotyping of embryos before uterine implantation.

NONINVASIVE FETAL GENETIC ANALYSIS

Genetic analysis of fetal cells or deoxyribonucleic acid in the maternal circulation is a new diagnostic modality being evaluated for molecular genetic analysis or karyotyping of the fetus.

IMAGING

Routine obstetric U/S examinations have led to an increasing frequency of prenatal fetal anomaly diagnosis. These prenatal diagnoses provide an opportunity for prospective discussion and planning of fetal or neonatal diagnosis and intervention. Regular communication amongst the obstetrician, perinatologist, radiologist, neonatologist, pediatric surgeon, and anesthesiologist will optimize outcomes.

Fetal U/S has evolved to include two-dimensional and three-dimensional modalities, with consequent improvements in the resolution and predictive value of diagnoses.

Of note, the combination of U/S assessment of nuchal translucency with biomarker screens increases the predictive value of prenatal screening for aneuploid states including Trisomy 21.

Fetal Doppler Ultrasonography

The ability to investigate fetal blood flow in specific organs, particularly the placenta and umbilical vessels, has added a new means of ascertaining fetal well being, especially during states of reduced fetal growth.

Fetal Echocardiography

Two-dimensional and three-dimensional echocardiography facilitate accurate prenatal diagnosis of many congenital heart lesions.

Fetal Ultrafast Magnetic Resonance Imaging

Rapid-sequence magnetic resonance imaging (MRI) provides high-resolution imaging of fetal development. Of note, MRI of the fetus is of particular value in the differential diagnosis of abnormalities of the central nervous system (CNS) and thoracic lesions.

Specific Fetal Abnormalities

ABNORMALITIES OF AMNIOTIC FLUID VOLUME

Amniotic fluid volume accumulates as a dynamic balance between fetal urine production, fetal lung liquid production, fetal swallowing, and amniotic fluid transfer across the fetal membranes. Disorders of amniotic fluid volume include excessive accumulation (polyhydramnios) and diminished amniotic fluid volume (oligohydramnios).

Polyhydramnios

The accumulation of more than 2 L of amniotic fluid volume during the third trimester is considered abnormal and may reflect abnormal maternal glucose tolerance (either gestational diabetes or preexisting diabetes mellitus), impaired fetal swallowing (such as associated with esophageal atresia, gastrointestinal (GI) tract obstruction, or a neurologic disorder with reduced fetal swallowing), diaphragmatic hernia, or ventral wall defects such as omphalocele or gastroschisis. Newborns with a maternal history of polyhydramnios demonstrate elevated risk of GI tract atresia or obstruction, and therefore, cautious approaches to feeding are recommended, with consideration of GI contrast studies as warranted.

Oligohydramnios

In contrast with polyhydramnios, reduced amniotic fluid volume is observed in cases of uteroplacental insufficiency and fetal growth restriction, instances of premature rupture of fetal membranes (PROM), and reduced fetal urine output secondary to renal agenesis or dysplasia (often associated with Potter's sequence of craniofacial abnormalities and pulmonary hypoplasia). A newborn with a history of oligohydramnios should be considered at increased risk of reduced glomerular filtration rate (GFR), although oligohydramnios is most frequently due to uteroplacental insufficiency or unrecognized PROM.

MECONIUM PERITONITIS

Meconium peritonitis is often a sequel of fetal intestinal perforation. It is manifested by abdominal calcifications or discrete punctate echodensities visualized using U/S. Ascites may develop due to meconium peritonitis, and these, in turn, are a result of one of the following:

- Meconium ileus with perforation
- Intestinal atresia with perforation
- Intestinal malrotation with in utero volvulus

Meconium peritonitis can create exuberant adhesions and secondary extrinsic intestinal obstruction, leading to abdominal distention and bilious vomiting after birth.

FETAL ASCITES

Fetal ascites may develop as an isolated disorder or may present with more generalized edema, a state termed "hydrops." Primary fetal ascites can result from the following conditions:

- Obstructive uropathy, which is most often the result of posterior urethral valves
- Meconium peritonitis
- Fetal anemia from hemolytic disease, marrow suppression secondary to parvovirus infection, or hemoglobinopathy, such as α thalassemia
- Congestive heart failure (CHF) due to tachyarrhythmia, bradyarrhythmia, or structural heart disease, especially right-sided lesions
- Chylous ascites due to lymphatic obstruction or anomaly
- Hepatic synthetic failure or hepatic vascular obstruction

HYDROPS

Hydrops may result from a multitude of etiologies, including the following:

- Fetal anemia from hemolytic disease, marrow suppression secondary to parvovirus infection, or hemoglobinopathy, such as α thalassemia
- CHF failure due to tachyarrhythmia, bradyarrhythmia, or structural heart disease, especially right-sided lesions
- Chylous ascites due to lymphatic obstruction or anomaly
- Hepatic failure or hepatic vascular obstruction
- Congenital viral infection (parvovirus, cytomegalovirus), bacterial infection (syphilis), or parasitic infection (toxoplasmosis)

Maternal–Fetal Medical and Surgical Therapy

Invasive fetal therapy was developed more than 30 years ago and involved in utero fetal transfusion for fetal anemia due to severe hemolytic disease. Over the past two decades, additional innovative therapies and research have emerged designed to medically and surgically treat fetal abnormalities.

PRENATAL MEDICAL THERAPIES

Some prenatal medical therapies include the following:

- Fetal transfusion for fetal anemia and hydrops
- Antiarrhythmic agents (eg, digoxin) for fetal tachyarrhythmias
- Glucocorticoid therapy for fetal 21-hydroxylase deficiency
- Glucocorticoid therapy for pulmonary surfactant deficiency
- Glucocorticoid therapy for autoimmune fetal heart block
- Vitamin B_{12} or biotin for methylmalonic acidemia or multiple carboxylase deficiency

PRENATAL MATERNAL–FETAL SURGICAL INTERVENTIONS

Prenatal maternal–fetal surgical interventions continue to be proposed and evaluated. There is an increasing cohort of infants who are survivors of innovative approaches to fetal correction of fetal anomalies. Research performed by multidisciplinary teams in centers of excellence will further define those disorders and approaches amenable to fetal therapies.

RECOMMENDATIONS

In general, maternal–fetal surgery can be recommended for those fetal disorders in which

- the maternal morbidity and mortality is low,
- the natural history and pathophysiology of the fetal disorder is well understood,
- prenatal diagnosis and stratification for fetal risk is accurate, and
- in utero open or endoscopic surgery has been proven safe and effective, first in animal models and subsequently in infants at risk with the disorder.

DIAGNOSTIC IMAGING

Diagnostic imaging defines anatomy and subsequently the prognosis associated with prenatal strategies. As already noted, these studies may include:

- ultrasonography and
- MRI.

SURGICAL APPROACHES

Open Fetal Surgery

Open fetal surgery, which involves open hysterotomy and fetal surgery, was the first surgical approach to correct fetal anomalies. After open hysterotomy, the incidence of preterm labor is high, which limits the potential of this approach. Open fetal myelomeningocoele surgery is currently in the process of evaluation in a multicenter clinical trial.

Minimally Invasive Maternal–Fetal Surgery

The recognition that preterm labor remains a significant morbidity of invasive hysterotomy has led to the development of endoscopic approaches to fetal treatment when applicable as outlined in more detail below.

SPECIFIC FETAL DISORDERS

Twin-Twin Transfusion

- Twin-twin transfusion complicates up to 15% of monochorionic twin pregnancies.
- Laser therapy of communicating fetal vessels is the recommended therapy for severe twin-twin transfusion syndrome diagnosed between 16 and 26 weeks gestation to treat manifestations of fetal CHF.
- Safe approaches exist to threat all stages of severity (Quintero staging system) as well as treatment of cases with anterior placenta.
- Complications of fetal therapy include preterm rupture of membranes and preterm delivery.
- Survivors of TTTS sometimes exhibit CNS lesions consistent with in utero thromboembolic events.

In addition, fetal umbilical cord ligation, selective recipient twin phlebotomy, and serial amniodrainage have all been used to reduce the adverse consequences of the shunt between affected fetuses.

Cystic Adenomatoid Malformation

Isolated cystic adenomatoid malformation (CAM) with fetal hydrops at an early gestational age may be an indication for possible fetal intervention. In contrast, most fetuses without hydrops survive until birth and experience either spontaneous involution or undergo postnatal resection of the CAM. Fetal lobe resection can reverse hydrops and allow sufficient lung development and subsequent meaningful neonatal recovery. Of note, maternal mirror syndrome, sometimes encountered in concert with fetal hydrops and placentomegaly, is a life-threatening maternal syndrome characterized by hypertension, proteinuria, pulmonary edema, and peripheral edema. Because this condition may not improve with fetal intervention, it is a relative contraindication to maternal–fetal surgery.

Congenital Diaphragmatic Hernia

The prognosis of prenatally diagnosed congenital diaphragmatic hernia (CDH) depends on the following factors: the presence of polyhydramnios, gestational age at diagnosis, the presence of liver herniation, the presence of concomitant anomalies, and the lung to thorax or lung to biparietal diameter ratio. Prenatal surgical interventions for CDH that have been considered include the following: open fetal surgical repair, open surgical tracheal occlusion, endoscopic external tracheal occlusion, and endoscopic endoluminal tracheal occlusion. Poor outcomes have been observed with fetal surgery in cases of liver herniation and left CDH; this is believed to be secondary to abnormal fetal circulation ensuing from the surgical manipulation of the liver. Studies in fetal animal models suggest that fetal tracheal occlusion stimulates fetal lung growth and reduces fetal lung hypoplasia. Fetal tracheal occlusion has been achieved by open fetal surgery and by endoscopic tracheal clip or plug placement. Because of the subsequent birth of a newborn with upper airway obstruction, the ex utero intrapartum treatment, or ex utero intrapartum treatment (EXIT) procedure, was developed: following hysterotomy, the exteriorized fetus continues placental gas exchange via the umbilical cord, or extracorporeal membrane oxygenation (ECMO) is instituted, whereas the fetal tracheal clip is removed, and the upper airway repaired. The indications for fetal CDH interventions continue to be investigated and remain to be defined.

Fetal Neck Mass

Critical airway obstruction in a fetus due to severe goiter, bronchogenic cyst, or cervical teratoma can be assessed during an EXIT procedure, and appropriate treatment can be instituted with the fetus transitioned from placental to pulmonary or ECMO gas exchange as warranted.

Sacrococcygeal Teratoma

Teratomas are the most frequent form of tumor in the fetus and newborn. Although they can develop in the neck region, the retroperitoneum, or the germ cells of the ovaries, most teratomas present in the sacrococcygeal region. Most teratomas are benign; however, some are malignant. Large sacrococcygeal teratomas can lead to in utero fetal CHF and fetal hydrops. Thus, innovative approaches have been evaluated, including fetal intervention, preterm delivery, early perinatal surgery, and ECMO support as warranted. Sacrococcygeal teratomas diagnosed before 30 weeks' gestation have a high likelihood of fetal hydrops, and without intervention, they will result in death in utero. These tumors are often sufficiently large to warrant cesarean delivery, and they can present thermoregulation challenges as well as lead to the development of serious coagulopathy. There have been isolated reports of fetal resection of sacrococcygeal teratoma, with subsequent resolution of fetal hydrops over 1 or 2 weeks. Radiofrequency ablation and laser ablation of arterial blood supply to the tumor has also been achieved.

Obstructive Uropathy

Bilateral fetal hydronephrosis with oligohydramnios can be detected while there remains significant preservation of fetal glomerular filtration. Under these conditions, the fetus can potentially benefit from the placement of a drainage catheter in the bladder or fetal laser treatment of posterior urethral valves. In contrast, unilateral hydronephrosis or bilateral hydronephrosis with adequate amniotic fluid volume or bilateral hydronephrosis with severe impairment of the GFR warrant continued observation without prenatal urinary tract treatment or diversion. Percutaneous U/S-guided vesicoamniotic shunting (VAS) is recommended in selected fetuses with obstructive uropathy. VAS should currently be offered only to patients with a normal karyotype, without sonographic or biochemical evidence of renal cystic dysplasia, and lack of major associated anomalies.

Hydrocephalus

Although hydrocephalus was a logical early candidate disorder for fetal intervention with ventriculoamniotic shunting, prenatal treatment of hydrocephalus is discouraged because minimal improvement in postnatal outcome has been observed despite significant maternal and fetal morbidity.

Myelomeningocele

The maternal and fetal risks and benefits of in utero surgical approaches to myelomeningocele are yet to be systematically evaluated. Currently, a clinical trial is under way that will evaluate in utero treatment of fetal myelomeningocele at several fetal therapy centers in the United States. The results of this trial will help refine the risk-benefit analysis of this innovative therapy. It is possible that improvement in either the motor function of the lower extremities or the natural history of hydrocephalus due to Arnold-Chiari malformation may be observed. As of 2007, approximately 400 fetal operations have been performed for myelomeningocele world wide. Despite this large experience, the technique remains of unproven benefit. Preliminary results suggest that fetal surgery results in reversal of hindbrain herniation (the Chiari II malformation), a decrease in shunt-dependent hydrocephalus, and possibly improvement in leg function. Clinical trial results are awaited to distinguish selection bias and changing management. A randomized prospective trial (the MOMS trial) is currently being conducted through 2009 by three centers in the United States.

Cardiac Valvular Stenosis

Critical pulmonary or aortic stenosis may benefit from fetal intervention. Recent studies suggest that maternal transabdominal intrauterine fetal catheterization via the fetal left ventricle can be performed in selected fetuses with severe aortic stenosis. After delivery, improvement in left ventricular function has been observed compared with untreated fetuses. Prenatal decompression of the left atrium via atrial septoplasty or ortic valvuloplasty may be associated with greater hospital survival. The effects of fetal intervention on lung function and long-term survival require further study.

PERIOPERATIVE MANAGEMENT OF THE FETUS

After appropriate selection of mothers and fetuses as candidates for intervention, maternal anesthesia is administered, favoring halothane anesthesia because of its myometrial relaxant properties. In addition, judicious use of nitric oxide donors, such as intravenous nitroglycerin, has been reported to reduce the incidence of perioperative myometrial contractions. Control of uteroplacental blood flow is ensured through monitoring of maternal central venous pressure and oxygen saturation in an appropriate intensive care facility. Fetal electrocardiogram and uterine activity are continuously monitored.

PERIOPERATIVE MANAGEMENT OF THE MOTHER

Myometrial relaxation is achieved with halothane anesthesia, judicious use of indomethacin, which may constrict fetal ductus arteriosus and betamimetic agents and/or magnesium sulfate. Furthermore, attention must be devoted to possible postoperative maternal pulmonary edema, persistent postoperative amniotic fluid leak, and progressive separation of amnion and chorion. Chorioamniotic separation can lead to amniotic band syndrome or later PROM. Maintenance of maternal cardiac output and uteroplacental blood flow must be balanced against risk of maternal pulmonary edema. Vigorous maternal diuresis reduces the risk of postoperative pulmonary edema.

LABOR AND DELIVERY

Following convalesence, the mother and fetus are followed by fetal monitoring and frequent U/S assessments until the onset of preterm or term labor.

Preterm Labor

After preterm fetal intervention, preterm labor may ensue before 36 weeks' gestation. Tocolysis is attempted, if appropriate, until fetal lung maturity can be demonstrated, using antenatal glucocorticoid therapy as indicated.

Cesarean Delivery

Cesarean delivery is indicated in all cases of fetal intervention involving hysterotomy. Less invasive fetal endoscopic surgical therapies may offer the possibility of vaginal delivery because uterine integrity is less threatened by minimally invasive surgical approaches.

ECMO

Perinatal cardiopulmonary support via ECMO has proven critical for the survival of many infants with previous lethal disorders. Although this mode of gas exchange and cardiac support can provide a bridge to postnatal stabilization, it is difficult to predict the extent to which pulmonary gas exchange is impaired by the fetal abnormality before removal of the uteroplacental circulation. Appropriate selection of candidates remains a priority.

Recommended Readings

Bellotti M, Rognoni G, de Gasperi C, et al. Controlled fetal blood-letting of the recipient twin as a new method for the treatment of severe twin-twin transfusion syndrome: preliminary results. Ultrasound Obstet Gynecol 2001;18:666–8.

Cochrane DD, Irwin B, Chambers K. Clinical outcomes that fetal surgery for myelomeningocele needs to achieve. Eur J Pediatr Surg 2001;11 Suppl 1:S18–S20.

Fauza DO, Barnewolt C, Brown SD, Jennings RW. Ultrasound-guided fetal tracheal occlusion. J Pediatr Surg 2002;37:300–2.

Graf JL, Albanese CT, Jennings RW, et al. Successful fetal sacrococcygeal teratoma resection in a hydropic fetus. J Pediatr Surg 2000;35:1489–91.

Holmes N, Harrison MR, Baskin LS. Fetal surgery for posterior urethral valves: long-term postnatal outcomes. Pediatrics 2001;108:E7.

Kunisaki SM, Fauza DO, Barnewolt CE, et al. Ex utero intrapartum treatment with placement on extracorporeal membrane oxygenation for fetal thoracic masses. J Pediatr Surg 2007; 42:420–5.

Liang CC, Cheng PJ, Lin CJ, et al. Outcome of prenatally diagnosed fetal hydronephrosis. J Reprod Med 2002;47:27–32.

Makino Y, Kobayashi H, Kyono K, et al. Clinical results of fetal obstructive uropathy treated by vesicoamniotic shunting. Urology 2000;55:118–22.

Paek BW, Jennings RW, Harrison MR, et al. Radiofrequency ablation of human fetal sacrococcygeal teratoma. Am J Obstet Gynecol 2001;184:503–7.

Quintero RA. Fetal obstructive uropathy. Clin Obstet Gynecol 2005;48:923–41.

Rosen MA. Anesthesia for fetal procedures and surgery [review]. Yonsei Med J 2001;42:669–80.

Stevens GH, Schoot BC, Smets MJ, et al. The ex utero intrapartum treatment (EXIT) procedure in fetal neck masses: a case report and review of the literature. Eur J Obstet Gynecol Reprod Biol 2002;100:246–50.

Sutton LN, Sun P, Adzick NS. Fetal neurosurgery. Neurosurgery 2001;48:124–44.

Sutton LN. Fetal surgery for neural tube defects. Best Pract Res Clin Obstet Gynaecol 2007;20

Vida VL, Bacha EA, Larrazabal A, et al. Hypoplastic left heart syndrome with intact or highly restrictive atrial septum: surgical experience from a single center. Ann Thorac Surg 2007;84:581–5.

Wilson JM, DiFiore JW, Peters CA. Experimental fetal tracheal ligation prevents the pulmonary hypoplasia associated with fetal nephrectomy: possible application for congenital diaphragmatic hernia. J Pediatr Surg 1993;28:1433–9.

THREE

Otolaryngology, Head and Neck Surgery

Part 1: Laryngeal and Tracheal Anomalies

David S.G. Lowinger, MD, FRACS, and
Laurie A. Ohlms, MD, FACS

Embryology of the Larynx

Initial development of the larynx and trachea occurs in the fourth week of gestation. A laryngotracheal groove forms in the ventral floor of the primitive pharynx deepening to form a diverticulum. Invaginations of the wall produce a tracheoesophageal septum separating the laryngotracheal tube from the esophagus.

The larynx forms from the endodermal lining at the cranial end of the laryngotracheal tube and the surrounding fourth and sixth arch mesenchyme:

a. Arytenoid swellings develop on either side of the laryngotracheal groove forming a T-shaped lumen.
b. The walls of the lumen oppose. The lumen is occluded with an epithelial lamina.
c. At the tenth week of gestation, recanalization of the laryngeal lumen is accompanied by mucosal proliferation, condensation of the laryngeal cartilages, and development of intrinsic laryngeal muscles.
d. In a 4-month fetus, the larynx is at the level of the fourth cervical vertebra. By term, it has descended caudally toward the level of C6.

Morphology of the Neonatal Larynx

- The most prominent surface landmarks of the anterior neck are the hyoid bone and the anterior cricoid arch. The thyroid cartilage is flat and broad. The hyoid overlaps the thyroid cartilage notch. The cricothyroid membrane is short.
- Compared with the adult larynx, the proportion of the vocal cord, that is, cartilaginous is greater. The arytenoid cartilages are bulkier. The posterior lamina of the cricoid cartilage is thicker. The narrowest region of the upper airway is at the subglottis rather than at the vocal folds.
- The epiglottis is long and narrow, and it may be omega shaped. Its tip may reach the soft palate with which it interlocks during suckling allowing the neonate to breathe nasally while feeding.

Laryngomalacia

DEFINITION

Malacia is derived from Greek meaning morbid softening. Laryngomalacia is a structural weakness of the supraglottic tissues allowing collapse into the glottic introitus on inspiration (Figure 1).

EMBRYOLOGY

The neonatal larynx differs from that of an older child or adult:

- The larynx is proportionally smaller, and the arytenoids and aryepiglottic folds are relatively larger.
- The epiglottis is narrower and longer.
- The preepiglottic and paraglottic spaces contain a greater amount of connective tissue.
- The laryngeal tissues are generally softer and more flaccid with poor neuromuscular tone.
- It is proposed that laryngomalacia is an exaggeration of these immature characteristics resulting in symptomatic airway collapse.

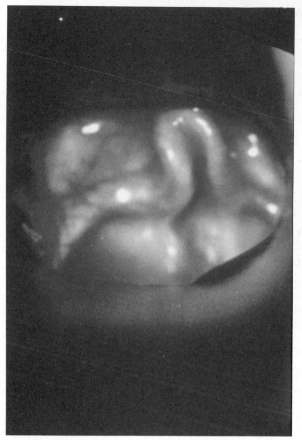

Figure 1   Endoscopic view of supraglottic collapse in a child with laryngomalacia.

PHYSIOLOGY

The supraglottic collapse and resulting stridor occur due to the effects of Bernoulli's principle and the Venturi effect. Bernoulli's principle states that the faster air flows through a tube, the less the pressure is exerted against the walls of the tube. The Venturi effect is that when the walls of the tube are flaccid, the low pressure draws them in. In a neonate, fast airflow generated by inspiration through a soft narrowed larynx causes the supraglottic tissues to collapse inward causing turbulent airflow producing audible stridor and in some cases obstruction.

CLASSIFICATION

A descriptive classification (mild, moderate, and severe) is used, depending on the degree that the short aryepiglottic folds restrict the supraglottis and the amount of loose redundant supraglottic tissue.

INCIDENCE

- The most common cause of inspiratory stridor in infants.
- Accounts for 50 to 75% of congenital laryngeal anomalies.
- May present at birth or usually within the first 2 months.
- Signs tend to peak at 6 to 12 months of age.
- The ratio of males to females is 2:1.
- No increased incidence in preterm neonates.

CLINICAL FEATURES

- Breathing: Stridor is worse with crying, with high respiratory rate, and while feeding. Although this may improve when sleeping or in prone position, up to 25% of patients suffer from obstructive sleep apnea (OSA). Cyanotic and severe apneic episodes are uncommon.
- Feeding: There may be obstruction when sucking, dyscoordinated swallowing, and a high incidence of gastroesophageal reflux.
- Growth and development: Failure to thrive due to increased work of breathing and feeding difficulties.
- Vocalizing/Cry: These are usually unaffected.

DIFFERENTIAL DIAGNOSIS

- Other supraglottic pathology: papillomatosis, infective supraglottitis, and neoplasms
- Nasal or oropharyngeal anomalies causing obstruction tend to produce a stertorous rather than stridulous sound.

- Vocal fold anomalies tend to affect the cry and vocalizing as well.
- Subglottic/tracheal pathology tend to produce biphasic stridor.
- Up to 30% of infants have a synchronous airway abnormality associated with laryngomalacia. Therefore, other pathology must be ruled out before concluding a diagnosis of laryngomalacia alone.

ASSESSMENT

- Complete examination of head and neck including the nose, nasopharynx, and oropharynx.
- Awake laryngoscopy with a flexible nasopharyngoscope.
- Laryngomalacia is severe or atypical requires a formal rigid diagnostic laryngoscopy and bronchoscopy.

IMAGING

- Chest x-ray exclude mediastinal/tracheal/pulmonary pathology.
- Lateral airway x-ray of little benefit.

OTHER

- Monitoring of O_2 saturation.
- pH probe may be indicated if significant reflux is suspected.

MANAGEMENT

- Watchful waiting: The majority of patients can be managed conservatively. During this period, it is important to monitor weight gain and avoid upper respiratory infections. A pediatrician and otolaryngologist should regularly assess the patient.
- Nonoperative intervention in an intensive care unit (ICU) setting, and continuous positive airway pressure (CPAP) may be effective as a temporizing measure. Significant gastroesophageal reflux is treated with medical therapy. If sucking is problematic, nasogastric feeding may be required to ensure adequate weight gain.
- Surgery: Only 5 to 10% of patients with laryngomalacia come to surgery.

INDICATIONS FOR SURGERY

- Severe airway obstruction with cyanotic episodes, OSA, or right heart failure
- Failure to thrive
- Concurrent medical/surgical problems exacerbated by the sequelae of laryngomalacia
- Family/social concerns (eg, inability to closely monitor infant at home)

SURGICAL MANAGEMENT

- Diagnostic laryngoscopy and bronchoscopy: The larynx is closely examined, and other airway pathology is excluded.
- Laser or sharp supraglottoplasty: This procedure involves using the laser or microsurgical instruments to divide tight aryepiglottic folds or to excise redundant tissue in the supraglottis.
- Tracheotomy: It is rarely performed for laryngomalacia. It may be required for patients who have not improved with supraglottoplasty or who have concurrent airway/pulmonary anomalies.

PREOPERATIVE ISSUES

- Ensure that the patient is otherwise fit for operating room (OR). Particularly, pulmonary status should be optimized.
- Any bleeding diathesis must be corrected.
- Parental consent for a diagnostic laryngobronchoscopy and supraglottoplasty with or without the laser.

ANESTHETIC ISSUES

- As for any diagnostic laryngoscopy on a neonate, appropriate OR temperature, full anesthetic monitoring, and an experienced anesthetist are required.
- The anesthetic involves an inhalation induction with maintenance of spontaneous ventilation. Muscle relaxants are not used. Intravenous access is obtained, and equipment for intubation is on hand.
- If laser is to be used, a laser-safe endotracheal tube (ETT) or jet ventilation may be used.

POSTOPERATIVE MANAGEMENT

- Following supraglottoplasty, improvement is usually immediately noticeable with resolution of the stridor and obstruction.
- In the immediate postoperative period, prophylactic antibiotics and intravenous steroids to reduce edema may be prescribed. The patient receives humidified room air or oxygen and may receive antireflux medications.
- Record and assess weight gain.

SURGICAL COMPLICATIONS/OUTCOME

- For those who require surgery, laryngoplasty has a 70 to 80% success rate. A few patients may require a repeat procedure.
- Supraglottoplasty carries a low morbidity and should not adversely affect the voice.

COMPLICATIONS

Intraoperative: bruising of lips and gums, bleeding, and laser burns
Short term: bleeding, edema, airway obstruction, and infection
Long term: recurrence and scarring

OUTCOME

Although the stridor may worsen up to 6 to 12 months of age, most infants will develop normally with watchful waiting and will outgrow their laryngomalacia by 18 to 24 months with no long-term sequelae.

Laryngeal Web

DEFINITION

A laryngeal anomaly in which a membranous remnant stenoses the glottic aperture (Figure 2).

EMBRYOLOGY

In laryngeal development, an epithelial lamina bridges the vocal folds. At the tenth week, this lamina involutes opening the glottic lumen. Failure of complete involution leaves a congenital web.

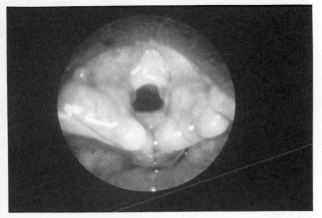

Figure 2 Endoscopic view of laryngeal web.

Acquired webs may form due to granulation and fibrosis when 2 adjacent mucosal surfaces are traumatized. This usually occurs at the anterior commissure of the larynx following intubation or instrumentation of this region.

INCIDENCE

- Uncommon
- Common sites are anterior glottic > post glottic > subglottic.
- 30% are associated with another airway anomaly.

CLASSIFICATION

It may be described by location, extent, and thickness.

CLINICAL FEATURES

- Respiratory distress, especially if causing severe stenosis of the larynx
- Stridor (may be surprisingly minimal if an anterior web)
- Weak or absent cry

DIAGNOSIS

- Suspect if neonate is born with breathing difficulties that worsen on exertion and a weak or an absent cry.
- Suspect if an older baby has been hoarse from birth and has had recurrent croup.
- Webs can usually be seen on awake flexible laryngoscopy in the ICU. Direct laryngoscopy under anesthesia will be required to detect small webs, to determine the thickness and subglottic extent, and to exclude associated anomalies.

DIFFERENTIAL DIAGNOSIS

- Other anatomical and neuromuscular laryngeal anomalies, especially vocal cord palsy
- Subglottic stenosis

ASSESSMENT/DIAGNOSIS

- Suspect if neonate has breathing and crying difficulties from birth.
- Full examination of the head and neck, ears, nose, and throat. Assess for other airway anomalies.
- Complete pediatric examination.
- A laryngeal web will often be readily diagnosed on flexible laryngoscopy; however, direct laryngoscopy under anesthesia will be required for complete assessment of the extent of the web and management.

IMAGING

- Chest x-ray
- Lateral and posteroanterior (PA) film may demonstrate the web.
- Imaging does not replace diagnostic laryngoscopy.

MANAGEMENT

The urgency of treatment depends on the severity of symptoms; an extensive obstructing web may require immediate tracheotomy. Most smaller webs are assessed and simply treated in the first few days of life. Diagnostic laryngoscopy determines the thickness of the web and any associated anomalies of the larynx, trachea, and esophagus allowing surgical options to be discussed and planned.

INDICATIONS FOR SURGERY

- A symptomatic web

SURGICAL MANAGEMENT

The aim of surgical intervention is to remove the web attaining an adequate airway while preserving phonation.

- Endoscopic division: A thin anterior glottic web may be divided by sharp instrument incision or laser. The neonate is instantly improved and the cry normalized.
- Open repair: A thick, extensive, or recurrent web may require a laryngofissure approach with formal excision of the web. A laryngotracheal reconstruction with a cartilage graft may be necessary to ensure an adequate lumen. A keel or stent is usually placed for a few weeks, and the airway is secured with a temporary tracheotomy.
- Tracheotomy may be required to ensure airway patency in an acutely obstructing web at birth or as a temporary measure until formal reconstruction takes place.

PREOPERATIVE ISSUES

- These neonates are often referred from a neonatal ICU (NICU) and will require short-term postoperative NICU monitoring.
- Ensure that the patient is otherwise fit for operation.
- Any bleeding diathesis must be corrected.
- Agreement with the intensivist, anesthetist, otolaryngologist, and parents of the child with regard to the planned airway procedure and any significant comorbidity.
- Parental consent for a diagnostic laryngoscopy, bronchoscopy, and esophagoscopy with an understanding that a small web will be divided. Further consent for reconstructive procedures would be sought as necessary.
- In the OR, a range of bronchoscopes, esophagoscopes, telescopes, and ETTs should be available.
- In acute cases or extensive webs a tracheotomy tray should be on standby.

ANESTHETIC ISSUES

- As for any diagnostic laryngoscopy on a neonate, appropriate OR temperature, full anesthetic monitoring, and an experienced anesthetist are required.
- Close cooperation is required between the anesthetist and the otolaryngologist.
- Until the web is assessed and/or divided, the airway should be considered partially obstructed with both expiration and assisted inspiration impeded. The neonate should, therefore, maintain spontaneous respiration. No muscle relaxant should be used. A gaseous agent is preferred for induction and maintenance of anesthesia.
- A thick, extensive web may impede the passage of an ETT. A range of small diameter tubes should be available.

POSTOPERATIVE MANAGEMENT

- For extubated/decannulated patients, maintenance of hydration, nutrition, and humidification
- For those who return from surgery intubated or with a tracheotomy, appropriate sedation and tube care are required. Most patients who underwent an open procedure and had a keel or stent placed will require close supervision until removal. In the immediate postoperative period, antireflux treatment, prophylactic antibiotics, and intravenous steroids may be prescribed.

SURGICAL COMPLICATIONS/OUTCOME

- Intraoperative: Bleeding, damage to neurovascular structures, edema, and airway obstruction requiring tracheotomy, complications of laser surgery if used.
- Short term: Infection, granulation, and scarring
- Long term: Failure of the repair, reformation of the web, voice changes, and airway problems requiring revision surgery

OUTCOME

- An isolated thin anterior web is simply diagnosed and treated. Following division of the web, the neonate is usually immediately improved.

- Extensive webs may be life threatening at birth. Often a tracheotomy is required with a staged open repair later. Using current reconstructive techniques, we aim to achieve an adequate airway with an optimum voice.

Laryngotracheal Cleft

DEFINITION

A laryngeal anomaly characterized by a midline deficiency in the posterior larynx that may extend to the tracheoesophageal wall (Figure 3).

EMBRYOLOGY

An incomplete fusion of the posterior lamina of the cricoid and the tracheoesophageal septum.

INCIDENCE

- Uncommon
- May be isolated, familial (autosomal dominant), or a part of a syndrome (eg, vertebral, anal, cardiac, tracheal, esophageal, renal, and limb, Pallister-Hall, Opritz-Frias syndromes).

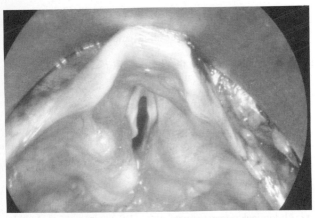

Figure 3 Endoscopic view of laryngotracheal cleft.

- May be associated with cleft lip and palate, subglottic and tracheal stenosis, tracheoesophageal fistula (TEF), cardiac abnormalities, and anomalies of the gastrointestinal and genitourinary tracts.

CLASSIFICATION

The Benjamin-Inglis classification is in common usage.

- Type I: limited to the supraglottis
- Type II: includes a partial cleft of the cricoid cartilage
- Type III: includes a complete cleft of the posterior cricoid lamina and may extend down toward the thoracic inlet
- Type IV: laryngotracheoesophageal cleft

CLINICAL FEATURES

- Swallowing difficulties: cough, aspiration, persistent or recurrent pneumonia, and failure to thrive
- Stridor/weak cry

DIFFERENTIAL DIAGNOSIS

- Other anatomical and neuromuscular laryngeal anomalies, especially vocal cord palsy

ASSESSMENT/DIAGNOSIS

- Suspect if neonate has breathing and swallowing difficulties from birth.
- Full examination of the head and neck, especially nasal patency, oropharynx, and anterior neck.
- Complete pulmonary examination.
- Examine for other syndromic features.
- A laryngeal cleft may be seen on flexible laryngoscopy; however, direct laryngoscopy under anesthesia will be required to detect subtle clefts, to determine subglottic extent, and to exclude associated anomalies.

IMAGING

- Chest x-ray: recurrent/persistent lower respiratory tract infection
- Abdominal x-ray: features of a TEF (large stomach bubble, dilated loops of bowel)

- Modified contrast swallow: demonstrate laryngeal penetration and/or aspiration
- Imaging does not replace diagnostic laryngoscopy.

MANAGEMENT

- Depends on the severity of symptoms associated with the cleft such as the degree of aspiration, breathing, and feeding difficulties.
- Management may be influenced by associated or syndromal anomalies.
- Diagnostic laryngoscopy should determine the type of cleft and any associated anomalies of the larynx, trachea, and esophagus.

CONSERVATIVE TREATMENT

- In consultation with a pediatrician, speech therapist, and dietician
- Trial of thickened oral feeds and postural feeding. If required, tube or gastric feeding
- Antireflux medications
- Monitor for declining pulmonary function and inadequate weight gain

SURGICAL TREATMENT

- Endoscopic repair: clefts type I and II.
- Open repair: cleft type III and IV and recurrent cleft type I and II. The technique used is an anterior laryngofissure approach with direct repair using local tissue flaps.
- An extensive cleft may require a lateral pharyngoesophagotomy approach and even a thoracotomy.
- Gastric feeding tube placement is a useful adjunct in managing extensive clefts.
- Tracheotomy (long term) is uncommonly required to ensure airway patency and minimize bronchial soiling.

INDICATIONS FOR SURGERY

- Airway compromise requiring support
- Deteriorating pulmonary function due to aspiration
- Recurrent/persistent pneumonia
- Inability to achieve adequate weight gain with conservative measures Poor cry/voice

SURGICAL MANAGEMENT

The aim of surgical intervention is to restore the primary laryngeal function of airway protection.

- Endoscopic repair: This procedure is performed through a laryngoscope using delicate endolaryngeal instruments. Initially, the mucosa lining the opposing sides of the cleft is incised then rotated and sutured to close the defect.
- Open repair with anterior laryngofissure: The laryngofissure approach involves a transverse neck incision and dissection onto the cricoid and thyroid cartilages. These are then incised in the midline affording excellent exposure of the posterior glottis, enabling repair of the cleft. Stents are not routinely required.
- Open repair with lateral pharyngoesophagotomy: Approaching via a left neck incision, the pharynx, hypopharynx, and upper esophagus are exposed. This dissection may be made easier by initially placing a bougie in the esophagus. The repair is performed through a vertical pharyngeal incision. A thoracotomy may be required for clefts that extend below the thoracic inlet.
- Following the above repair procedures, in order to allow swelling to subside, the neonate be returned to the ICU intubated or with a tracheotomy for a few days.
- Long-term tracheotomy: If repair procedures are contraindicated or have failed a long-term tracheotomy may be required.

PREOPERATIVE ISSUES

- Ensure that the patient is otherwise fit for operation.
- Any bleeding diathesis must be corrected.
- A combined conference with the intensivist, otolaryngologist, cardiothoracic surgeon, and parents of the child to discuss the neonate's ventilation requirements and any comorbidity prior to definitive airway surgery.
- Parental consent for a diagnostic laryngoscopy, bronchoscopy, and esophagoscopy initially with further consent for reconstructive procedures as indicated.
- In the OR, a range of bronchoscopes, esophagoscopes, telescopes, and ETTs should be available.

ANESTHETIC ISSUES

- As for any diagnostic laryngoscopy on a neonate, appropriate OR temperature, full anesthetic monitoring, and an experienced anesthetist are required.
- As these patients may have aspiration pneumonia, review by a pulmonary physician and appropriate measures to maximize pulmonary function are indicated.
- Patients with associated syndromes require cardiac assessment.

POSTOPERATIVE MANAGEMENT

- For extubated/decannulated patients, maintenance of hydration, nutrition, and humidification
- For those who return from surgery intubated or with a tracheotomy, ensure appropriate sedation and tube care. Most patients may be extubated within a few days once the laryngeal edema has subsided.
- In the immediate postoperative period, antireflux treatment, prophylactic antibiotics, and intravenous steroids may be prescribed.

SURGICAL COMPLICATIONS/OUTCOME

- Intraoperative: bleeding, damage to neurovascular structures, inadequate tissue for repair, and excessive tension on the repair
- Short term: breakdown of the repair, infection, and bleeding
- Long term: failure of the repair, dysphagia, and voice changes

OUTCOME

- A shallow cleft in an otherwise normal neonate may be asymptomatic or require little intervention.
- Deeper clefts, however, may cause marked morbidity and mortality.
- Significant intrathoracic involvement portends a poor prognosis.
- Clefts involving the larynx alone have a better outlook especially with current surgical repair techniques.

Unilateral Vocal Fold Palsy

DEFINITION

Immobility of one vocal fold due to a neurological deficit.

ETIOLOGY

- Neuropraxia due to vagus nerve stretching or compression during birth
- Congenital cardiovascular anomaly
- Iatrogenic: neck/mediastinal/thoracic surgery
- Idiopathic
- Neoplasm of the skull base/neck/mediastinum
- Congenital central nervous system deficit

INCIDENCE

- Second most common neonatal laryngeal pathology after laryngomalacia.
- Left vocal fold more commonly involved due to longer course of left recurrent laryngeal nerve.
- Peripheral etiology is more common than central etiology.

CLINICAL FEATURES

- Weak, breathy cry
- May have aspiration and feeding problems
- May have stridor

DIAGNOSIS

- Suspect if neonate is born with primarily phonatory and swallowing difficulties.
- A vocal fold palsy is best seen on awake flexible laryngoscopy, when the neonate cries.
- Direct laryngoscopy under anesthesia will be required to confirm the diagnosis especially to exclude a mechanical fixation of the vocal fold (eg, with a web or an arytenoid joint problem) and to exclude other airway anomalies.

DIFFERENTIAL DIAGNOSIS

- Other primary laryngeal anomalies (eg, laryngomalacia, webs, cysts, clefts, and papilloma)
- Obstructing lesions of the supralaryngeal airway, subglottis, and trachea

ASSESSMENT/DIAGNOSIS

- Suspect if neonate has a weak cry and feeding difficulties.
- Full examination of the head and neck.
- Complete pulmonary examination for signs of aspiration.
- Examine for other cranial nerve palsies.
- Complete neurological assessment.
- An immobile vocal fold may be seen on flexible laryngoscopy; however, direct laryngoscopy under anesthesia will be required for the reasons outlined above.

IMAGING

- Computed tomography (CT)/magnetic resonance imaging (MRI) of the brain as well as the skull base, neck, and chest (ie, along the course of the nerve)
- Chest x-ray: recurrent/persistent lower respiratory tract infection. Cardiac imaging, as indicated

MANAGEMENT

Depends on the severity of symptoms associated with the palsy such as the degree of aspiration, breathing, and feeding difficulties. In the neonate, strong phonation is a secondary concern. Management may be influenced by associated or syndromal anomalies.

Diagnostic laryngoscopy should determine the glottic gap (distance between the medial edge of the vocal folds), the degree of compensatory movement by the contralateral side, and any associated anomalies of the larynx, trachea, and esophagus.

CONSERVATIVE TREATMENT

- In consultation with a pediatrician, speech therapist, and dietician
- Trial of thickened oral feeds and postural feeding. If required, tube or gastric feeding

- Antireflux medications
- Monitor for declining pulmonary function and pneumonia
- Ensure adequate weight gain

SURGICAL TREATMENT

- Resection of any lesion or vessel impinging upon the nerve
- Gastric feeding tube placement if required to maintain weight gain
- Tracheotomy (long term) is rarely required to ensure airway patency and minimize pulmonary soiling.
- If cry/voice remains hoarse, vocal fold medialization may be performed in early childhood.

INDICATIONS FOR SURGERY

- Presence of a resectable lesion or vessel impinging upon the nerve
- Airway compromise requiring support
- Deteriorating pulmonary function due to aspiration
- Recurrent/persistent pneumonia
- Inability to achieve adequate weight gain with conservative measures
- Poor cry/voice continuing into childhood

SURGICAL MANAGEMENT

The aims of surgical intervention are initially to restore the primary laryngeal function of airway protection and to ensure adequate nutrition and weight gain. Later, phonation may be enhanced by a vocal fold medialization procedure.

- Tracheotomy: If significant aspiration occurs or conservative measures have failed, a long-term tracheotomy may be required.
- Vocal fold medialization: Usually, performed later in childhood. It involves an external approach to the larynx, creation of a window in the thyroid cartilage, and placement of a silastic or hydroxyapatite implant to push paralyzed cord to the midline.

PREOPERATIVE ISSUES

- Ensure that the patient is otherwise fit for operation.
- Any bleeding diathesis must be corrected.

- A combined conference with the intensivist, otolaryngologist, and parents of the child to discuss the neonate's ventilation requirements and any comorbidity prior to definitive airway surgery.
- Parental consent for a diagnostic laryngoscopy, bronchoscopy, and esophagoscopy initially.
- In the OR a range of bronchoscopes, esophagoscopes, telescopes, and ETTs should be available.

ANESTHETIC ISSUES

- As for any diagnostic laryngoscopy on a neonate, appropriate OR temperature, full anesthetic monitoring, and an experienced anesthetist are required.
- As these patients may have aspiration pneumonia, review by a pulmonary physician and appropriate measures to maximize pulmonary function are indicated.
- Patients with associated syndromes require cardiac assessment.

POSTOPERATIVE MANAGEMENT

- For extubated/decannulated patients, maintenance of hydration, nutrition, and humidification
- For those who return from surgery intubated or with a tracheotomy, appropriate sedation and tube care are required.

SURGICAL COMPLICATIONS

- The most common complication of diagnostic laryngoscopy is oropharyngeal bruising from the passage of instruments.
- On occasion, diagnosis of vocal fold hypomobility may be subtle. Repeat flexible and/or rigid laryngoscopy may be required to confirm the diagnosis.

OUTCOME

- 90% of unilateral vocal fold palsies spontaneously recover within 6 to 12 months.

Bilateral Vocal Fold Palsy

DEFINITION

Immobility of both vocal folds due to a neurological deficit.

ETIOLOGY

- Congenital central nervous system deficit (eg, Arnold-Chiari malformation, hydrocephalus)
- Neuropraxia due to vagus nerve stretching or compression during birth
- Idiopathic
- Iatrogenic (uncommon at this age)

INCIDENCE

- Less common than unilateral palsy.
- Second most common cause of infantile stridor (most common is laryngomalacia).
- Central etiology is more common than peripheral etiology.
- A high vagus lesion may also cause a loss of laryngeal sensation.

CLINICAL FEATURES

- Stridor, airway obstruction
- May have aspiration and feeding problems.
- Cry is often normal.

DIAGNOSIS

- Suspect if neonate is born with fixed upper airway obstruction.
- Vocal fold palsy is best seen on awake flexible laryngoscopy when the neonate tries to breath and cry. Direct laryngoscopy under anaesthetic will be required to confirm the diagnosis, to exclude a mechanical fixation of the vocal folds (eg, with an anterior or interarytenoid web or bilateral arytenoid dislocations), and to exclude other airway anomalies.

DIFFERENTIAL DIAGNOSIS

- Other structural and neuromuscular anomalies of the larynx involve the vocal folds (eg, laryngomalacia, webs, cysts, clefts, and papilloma)
- Subglottic stenosis
- Tracheal stenosis, complete rings

ASSESSMENT/DIAGNOSIS

- Suspect if neonate has stridor with or without a normal cry and feeding difficulties.
- Full examination of the head and neck.
- Examine for other cranial nerve palsies.
- Complete neurological assessment including fundoscopy for hydrocephalus.
- Immobility of the vocal fold may be seen on flexible laryngoscopy; however, direct laryngoscopy under anesthesia will be required for the reasons outlined above.

IMAGING

- CT/MRI of the brain is of paramount importance.
- Imaging of the skull base, neck, and chest (ie, along the course of the vagus nerves)
- Chest x-ray: recurrent/persistent lower respiratory tract infection

MANAGEMENT

- These patients require close observation in a NICU setting.
- Intervention depends on the degree of airway obstruction associated with the palsy. This is best determined by clinical observation for respiratory distress during feeding, crying, and sleep. Aspiration and feeding difficulties are also important.
- Management may be influenced by associated intracranial, neurological, or syndromal anomalies.
- In an acute obstruction, intubation may be required while clinical, neurological, and imaging assessments are obtained.
- Diagnostic laryngoscopy confirms the diagnosis, excludes a mechanical cause for vocal immobility, and determines any other anomalies of the larynx, trachea, and esophagus.

CONSERVATIVE TREATMENT

- Initially, in an ICU setting in consultation with the intensivist, pediatrician, speech therapist, and dietician
- Humidification of inspired air, supplemental oxygen, CPAP, and intubation

- Close monitoring of weight gain in setting of increased work of breathing and possible feeding difficulties postural feeding. If required, tube or gastric feeding
- Antireflux medications
- Monitor for declining pulmonary function, aspiration, and pneumonia
- Once stable, able to be discharged
- Utilization of an apnea monitoring at home, parents trained to recognize impending obstruction
- Close contact with and access to pediatrician, otolaryngologist, and hospital

SURGICAL TREATMENT

- Correct any treatable neurological cause (eg, placement of a ventricular shunt to manage hydrocephalus and Arnold-Chiari malformation)
- Tracheotomy: if conservative measures fail
- Gastric feeding tube placement: if required to maintain weight gain
- If the palsy does not spontaneously resolve with time, procedures to lateralize one of the vocal folds may be performed. These include a cordotomy, arytenoidectomy, or arytenoidopexy.

INDICATIONS FOR SURGERY

- Neurosurgery: treatable anomaly identified
- Tracheotomy: airway compromise requiring ongoing support and failure of conservative measures
- Deteriorating pulmonary function due to aspiration
- Inability to achieve adequate weight gain with conservative measures

SURGICAL MANAGEMENT

The aim of surgical airway intervention (tracheotomy) is initially to overcome the airway obstruction to ensure adequate ventilation and oxygen delivery. This also allows feeding, weight gain, and eventually discharge home. Later, if spontaneous recovery of movement does not occur, more permanent vocal fold lateralization procedures may be considered, so that the patient may be decannulated. Such procedures improve the airway but may adversely affect phonation.

- Tracheotomy: If significant aspiration or conservative measures have failed, a long-term tracheotomy may be required.
- Vocal fold lateralization: Involves a transoral or external approach to the larynx. It is usually performed later in childhood. A cordotomy involves incising one of the vocal folds with the laser. This may be combined with rotation or removal of an arytenoid cartilage to increase the lumen of the posterior glottis.

PREOPERATIVE ISSUES

- Ensure that the neonate is otherwise fit for operation.
- Any bleeding diathesis must be corrected.
- Discussion with the intensivist, otolaryngologist, neurologist, and parents of the child to discuss the findings of the neurological investigations, the neonate's respiratory requirements, and any associated anomalies prior to definitive airway surgery.
- Parental consent for a diagnostic laryngoscopy, bronchoscopy, and esophagoscopy initially. A tracheotomy is considered as indicated above.
- In the OR, a range of bronchoscopes, esophagoscopes, telescopes, and ETTs should be available.

ANESTHETIC ISSUES

- As for any diagnostic laryngoscopy on a neonate, appropriate OR temperature, full anesthetic monitoring, and an experienced anesthetist are required.
- Appropriate neurology, cardiac, and pulmonary consultations are obtained.
- Close cooperation is required between the anesthetist and the otolaryngologist.
- Until the larynx and the distal airway have been evaluated the airway should be considered partially obstructed with both expiration and assisted inspiration impeded. The neonate should, therefore, maintain spontaneous respiration. No muscle relaxant should be used. A gaseous agent is preferred for induction and maintenance of anesthesia.
- Intubation will quickly overcome the airway obstruction associated with a bilateral vocal fold palsy.

POSTOPERATIVE MANAGEMENT

- An NICU setting for close observation.
- For extubated/decannulated patients, close monitoring of respiratory effort and oxygen saturation and maintenance of hydration, nutrition, and humidification.
- For those who return from surgery intubated or with a tracheotomy, appropriate sedation and tube care are required.
- Tracheotomy care instruction for the parents.

SURGICAL COMPLICATIONS

- Tracheotomy: See below.
- Vocal fold lateralization procedures may adversely effect phonation and glottic continence.

OUTCOME

50 to 70% of bilateral vocal fold palsies spontaneously recover within 5 years. Recovery at even up to 11 years has been reported. Prognosis depends on the causative factors with neurological paralysis more likely to resolve than idiopathic.

Subglottic Stenosis

DEFINITION

The subglottis is the region between the vocal folds and the first tracheal ring. It is completely encircled by the cricoid cartilage. In the neonate, this is the narrowest part of the upper airway. A full-term infant usually has a subglottic diameter of 5 mm.

Subglottic stenosis is defined as a subglottic narrowing resulting in symptomatic airway obstruction (Figure 4). It may be arbitrarily defined as a subglottic diameter of < 4 mm in a term infant or < 3 mm in a premature neonate.

EMBRYOLOGY

Congenital subglottic stenosis may be due to anomalous development of the cricoid cartilage or arrested development of the conus elasticus.

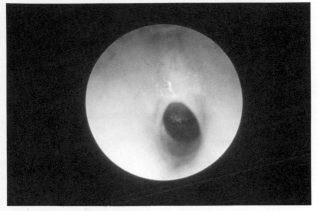

Figure 4 Endoscopic view of subglottic stenosis.

INCIDENCE

- Stenosis of the upper airway is rare; however, the subglottis is the most common region affected. Current incidence is up to 2% of neonates admitted to a neonatal ICU.
- This condition is most common in infancy and is most often of iatrogenic cause with up to 90% caused by endotracheal intubation.

CLASSIFICATION

a. Congenital: Hard-cricoid cartilage anomaly, trapped first tracheal ring. Soft-mucosal or submucosal hyperplasia/fibrosis
b. Acquired: Iatrogenic, traumatic, infective, neoplastic, granulomatous, and idiopathic

GRADING

Direct laryngoscopy is required to grade subglottic stenosis. The degree of occlusion of the lumen is recorded:

- <70%
- 70 to 90%

- >90%
- Complete occlusion

CLINICAL FEATURES

Depend on the degree of subglottic narrowing. In the NICU setting, it may present as follows:

- Stridor: usually biphasic, fixed
- Respiratory distress: due to airway obstruction
- Failed intubation
- Failed extubation
- Atypical croup

DIFFERENTIAL DIAGNOSIS

- Laryngeal pathology tends to effect the cry/voice/swallowing.
- Tracheal pathology includes complete rings and TEF.

ASSESSMENT

- Complete examination of head and neck including the nose, nasopharynx, and oropharynx.
- Awake laryngoscopy with a flexible nasopharyngoscope.
- To adequately assess suspected subglottic stenosis, direct laryngoscopy and bronchoscopy, under general anesthesia, are usually required.

IMAGING

- PA and lateral airway x-rays may demonstrate the subglottic narrowing.
- Chest X-ray to exclude pulmonary pathology

MANAGEMENT

- Depends on the severity of the stenosis, pulmonary function, and any associated anomalies.
- Diagnostic laryngobronchoscopy should determine the nature and grade of stenosis and any associated anomalies of the larynx, trachea, and vocal folds.
- Conservative treatment: A soft, mild stenosis may respond to careful management in an ICU setting of hydration,

intravenous steroids, and humidified air. Racemic epinephrine may also be used. If the patient deteriorates, intubation and surgical management are indicated.

- Surgical treatment: tracheotomy, anterior cricoid split, laryngotracheoplasty, and cricotracheal resection

INDICATIONS FOR SURGERY

- Airway obstruction not responding to conservative treatment
- Significant associated anomalies

SURGICAL MANAGEMENT

The aim of surgical intervention is to provide an adequate, secure, stable airway.

- Diagnostic laryngoscopy and bronchoscopy using rigid telescopes are indicated as the primary diagnostic procedure. The otolaryngologist is most vigilant to use extreme caution when examining the subglottis to avoid edema and worsening constriction.
- Tracheotomy enables the removal of ETTs allowing subglottic edema to settle. This is usually used as a temporary measure until the stenosis resolves, the patient outgrows the stenosis, or a laryngotracheoplasty is performed.

When considering the following procedures, a stable pulmonary status is most important. The aim of repairing the stenosis is to avoid the need for long-term intubation or tracheotomy. Declining pulmonary function requiring ventilation would compromise this repair.

- Anterior cricoid split: This procedure has been used as an alternative to tracheotomy in neonates with both congenital and acquired subglottic stenosis who have adequate pulmonary function to allow extubation. The patient is intubated. A transverse skin incision is made over the cricoid cartilage. The upper trachea, anterior cricoid, and thyroid cartilage are exposed. A vertical midline incision is made splitting the cricoid, upper 2 tracheal rings, and lower one-third of the thyroid cartilage. The cricoid springs open expanding the subglottic diameter. The wound is loosely closed over a nonsuction drain. The patient is returned to the ICU and remains intubated for approximately

1 week. Antibiotics are usually prescribed. Corticosteroids may be given prior to extubation, and the patient must be closely monitored to ensure airway patency.

- Laryngotracheoplasty (or laryngotracheal reconstruction [LTR]): This procedure is useful for patients with ongoing subglottic stenosis and for those who required primary tracheotomy. The operation is performed under general anesthesia. A transverse skin incision is made at the level of the cricoid cartilage. The anterior cricoid, thyroid cartilage, and trachea are exposed and divided in the midline. A cartilage graft is harvested from costal, thyroid, or auricular cartilage. It is shaped and sutured into the anterior and/or posterior cricoid ring thereby increasing the diameter of the subglottis. This may be performed as a single-stage procedure with a transnasal ETT sited for a week. Otherwise, a temporary tracheotomy is formed, and an intraluminal stent is placed. The stent is removed in the OR after around 2 weeks, and the patient is decannulated. Either way, the neck wound is closed over a nonsuction drain, and the patient is monitored in the ICU. The patient is prescribed prophylactic antibiotics.
- Cricoid resection with thyrotracheal reconstruction: This procedure is uncommonly required for severe fixed stenosis of the subglottis that is not amenable to the above procedures. The principle involves total resection of the stenotic segment of the subglottis followed by direct approximation of the trachea to the thyroid cartilage. Adequate length is obtained by releasing the suprahyoid strap muscles. To avoid tension on the anastomosis in the recovery period, the chin may be sutured to the chest for a week. Once healed the tracheotomy may be removed.

PREOPERATIVE ISSUES

- Ensure that the patient is otherwise fit for OR. Particularly, pulmonary status should be optimized.
- Single-stage laryngotracheal reconstruction has a greater chance of successful outcome if the child weighs more than 4 kg.
- Any bleeding diathesis must be corrected.
- Perioperative hydration, humidification, and steroids may be required.

- A combined conference with the intensivist, otolaryngologist, and parents of the child to discuss the neonate's ventilation requirements and comorbidity prior to definitive airway surgery
- Parental consent for a diagnostic laryngobronchoscopy and tracheotomy with further consent for reconstructive procedures as indicated.
- In the OR, a range of bronchoscopes, telescopes, and ETTs should be available and the tracheotomy tray on standby.

ANESTHETIC ISSUES

- As for any diagnostic laryngoscopy on a neonate, appropriate OR temperature, full anesthetic monitoring, and an experienced anesthetist are required.
- The anesthetic for the diagnostic laryngoscopy involves an inhalation induction with maintenance of spontaneous ventilation. Muscle relaxants are not used. Intravenous access is obtained, and equipment for intubation is on hand.
- If intubation is necessary, the smallest size tube is used.
- Vigilance for gas trapping and pneumothorax with supported ventilation.
- Vigilance for postobstructive pulmonary edema if recent onset stenosis

POSTOPERATIVE MANAGEMENT

- ICU setting required for most patients.
- For extubated/decannulated patients, maintenance of hydration and humidification
- Tracheotomy care, as indicated.
- For anterior cricoid split and LTR patients, care with the ETT, minimizing movement of the tube and avoiding accidental extubation. This may require the infant to be sedated for days. The depth of sedation and muscle relaxation should be discussed with the surgeon.
- In the immediate postoperative period, prophylactic antibiotics and intravenous steroids to reduce edema may be prescribed.

SURGICAL COMPLICATIONS/OUTCOME

A careful diagnostic laryngoscopy should not worsen subglottic stenosis.

COMPLICATIONS

Intraoperative: bleeding, neurovascular damage
Short term: bleeding, edema, infection, loss of the airway if accidental decannulation, wound dehiscence, if graft donor site problems, graft necrosis, granulation tissue
Long term: recurrence of stenosis, scarring, tracheocutaneous fistula

OUTCOME

Whether congenital or acquired, subglottic stenosis in a neonate is a challenge to treat. The aim of management is to ensure an adequate airway while maintaining normal phonation and glottic competence. Success of surgical management is enhanced by careful ICU support in the perioperative period.

Tracheomalacia

DEFINITION

Collapse of the trachea causing symptomatic obstruction of the lumen especially on expiration and coughing.

ETIOLOGY

Primary (or intrinsic): congenitally absent, soft, or immature tracheal cartilage
Secondary (or extrinsic): weakness of the tracheal wall due to prolonged intubation, iatrogenic trauma, or extrinsic compression by a vascular structure, mediastinal mass or abscess, or cardiac hypertrophy

INCIDENCE

- Rare
- Secondary is more prevalent than primary
- May be associated with laryngomalacia
- 10 to 20% of patients with a TEF have tracheomalacia

CLINICAL FEATURES

- Upper airway obstruction, worse with activity/feeding/crying/if unwell
- Expiratory stridor
- Brassy cough
- Cyanotic spells especially while feeding
- Recurrent lower respiratory tract infections
- Cry is usually normal

DIAGNOSIS

- Suspect if upper airway obstruction which is worse on exertion associated with an expiratory stridor.

DIFFERENTIAL DIAGNOSIS

- Subglottic stenosis (usually biphasic stridor)
- Tracheal stenosis, complete rings
- Infectious tracheitis (patient is usually febrile, unwell)
- Gastroesophageal reflux, TEF, cleft
- An airway foreign body
- Pulmonary pathology

ASSESSMENT/DIAGNOSIS

- Suspect if neonate has intermittent airway obstruction, cough, and stridor but a normal cry.
- Full examination of the head and neck.
- Complete pulmonary examination.
- Complete cardiovascular examination.
- Diagnostic laryngoscopy, bronchoscopy, and esophagoscopy under general anesthesia are required to make the diagnosis. The trachea appears collapsed and flattened on expiration, with an increase in the normal ratio of lateral to anteroposterior lumen diameter (normally 4:1).

IMAGING

- Chest x-ray: recurrent/persistent lower respiratory tract infection
- Chest CT identify extrinsic mediastinal mass, anomalous vessels
- Lateral and PA airway x-ray may identify other tracheal or subglottic anomalies.

- Contrast swallow: if a TEF or cleft is suspected
- Cardiovascular imaging (echo/MRI) as indicated
- Imaging does not replace diagnostic bronchoscopy

MANAGEMENT

- Intervention depends on the degree of airway obstruction associated with the tracheomalacia. This is best determined by clinical observation for respiratory distress during feeding and crying. Management may be influenced by associated airway, esophageal, or syndromal anomalies.
- Cyanotic or dying spells are a strong indication for intervention.
- In an acute obstruction, intubation may be required.
- Diagnostic laryngoscopy confirms the diagnosis, suggests whether the problem is extrinsic or intrinsic to the trachea, and determines other important anomalies of the larynx, trachea, and esophagus.

CONSERVATIVE TREATMENT

- An ICU setting may be required during diagnosis and assessment and following intervention.
- Airway support options include humidification, supplemental oxygen, CPAP, and intubation.
- Close monitoring of weight gain due to increased work of breathing and possible feeding difficulties. Postural feeding (antireflux positioning), tube, or gastric feeding if required.
- Antireflux medications, mucolytics
- Monitor for worsening obstruction and declining oxygen saturation.
- Once stable, able to be discharged.
- Utilization of an apnea monitoring at home, parents trained to recognize impending obstruction, and close contact with and access to pediatrician, otolaryngologist, and hospital.

SURGICAL TREATMENT

- Correct any treatable extrinsic compression
- Aortopexy to correct vascular compression
- Tracheotomy: if conservative measures fail

- Stent placement: current developments in devices and techniques are making endoluminal stenting an increasingly viable option
- Gastric feeding tube placement if required to maintain weight gain

INDICATIONS FOR SURGERY

- Identification of resectable extrinsic lesion
- Cyanotic or dying spells
- Aortopexy: obstruction not responding to conservative treatment and compressive anomalous vessel identified
- Tracheotomy: airway compromise requiring ongoing support, failure of conservative measures
- Endoluminal stent: as above

SURGICAL MANAGEMENT

The aim of surgical airway intervention is initially to overcome the airway obstruction to ensure adequate oxygen delivery. With time, the patient may outgrow an intrinsic weakness of the trachea and may be decannulated.

- Tracheotomy: See below for details.
- Aortopexy: Performed by cardiothoracic surgeons. It involves a median sternotomy and suturing of the aorta to the back of the sternum pulling the anterior tracheal wall forward.
- Segmental resection and reconstruction: Otolaryngologist in combination with a cardiothoracic surgeon.
- Tracheal stents: Metallic or silicone, placed via bronchoscope or catheter.

PREOPERATIVE ISSUES

- Ensure that the patient is otherwise fit for operation.
- Any bleeding diathesis must be corrected.
- Parental consent for a diagnostic laryngoscopy, bronchoscopy, and esophagoscopy initially. A tracheotomy is considered as indicated above.
- In the OR, a range of bronchoscopes, esophagoscopes, telescopes, and ETTs should be available.

ANESTHETIC ISSUES

- As for any diagnostic laryngoscopy on a neonate, appropriate OR temperature, full anesthetic monitoring, and an experienced anesthetist are required.
- Appropriate neurology, cardiac, and pulmonary consultations are obtained.
- Close cooperation is required between the anesthetist and the otolaryngologist.
- Until the larynx and the distal airway have been evaluated, the airway should be considered partially obstructed with both expiration and assisted inspiration impeded. The neonate should, therefore, maintain spontaneous respiration.
- No muscle relaxant should be used. A gaseous agent is preferred for induction and maintenance of anesthesia.
- Intubation will usually improve the airway obstruction associated with tracheomalacia.

POSTOPERATIVE MANAGEMENT

- An NICU setting for close observation.
- For extubated/decannulated patients, close monitoring of respiratory effort and oxygen saturation and maintenance of hydration, nutrition, and humidification
- For those who return from surgery intubated or with a new tracheotomy, appropriate sedation and tube care
- Tracheotomy care instructions for the parents.

SURGICAL COMPLICATIONS

- Tracheotomy: See below.
- Aortopexy.

OUTCOME

Long-term outcome depends on the severity of tracheal collapse and the management of any causative pathology. Most cases of mild tracheomalacia will become asymptomatic with growth and development of the neonate. Severe cases may require surgical intervention with multidisciplinary care.

Tracheotomy

DEFINITION

A procedure in which a neck incision is made, the trachea is exposed, incised and cannulated to establish a surgical airway (Figure 5).

INDICATIONS

- Upper airway obstruction
- Requirement for long-term ventilatory support
- Prevention of aspiration and pulmonary soiling
- Access for tracheal toilet

TRACHEOTOMY VERSUS PROLONGED INTUBATION

Advantages

- Less glottic and subglottic trauma
- More comfortable: patient able to be awake, move around, and usually take oral feeds
- Airway more secure
- Neonate better able to be transferred to ward or home

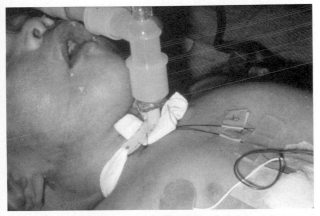

Figure 5 Tracheotomy tube in place.

Disadvantages

- Risks (as below) of a surgical procedure
- External incision: neck skin scar

Overall

- A term neonate may be intubated for over 3 weeks before consideration of a tracheotomy is required. Preterm infants may be intubated until they approach their due date before tracheostomy is considered. It is prudent, however, for an otolaryngologist to monitor for airway trauma in cases requiring prolonged intubation.
- For neonates requiring prolonged intubation for subglottic stenosis, an alternate procedure to a tracheotomy, such as a cricoid split, may be indicated (as above).

ANESTHETIC ISSUES

- Procedure performed in a fully equipped OR.
- Close communication with otolaryngologist regarding anesthetic techniques for diagnostic laryngoscopy/ bronchoscopy, usually initially spontaneous ventilation, no muscle relaxants, gaseous anaesthetic, and atropine to minimize bradycardia.
- For tracheotomy, it is preferable to secure the airway with an ETT or ventilating bronchoscope prior to any neck incision.

SURGICAL MANAGEMENT

- All neonates planned to undergo a tracheotomy must initially have a diagnostic laryngoscopy and bronchoscopy to determine current airway pathology.

TECHNICAL DETAILS FOR TRACHEOTOMY IN NEONATES

- Trachea initially secured with an ETT or ventilating bronchoscope
- Neonate positioned with shoulder roll and head ring
- Vertical or horizontal neck incision
- Removal of subcutaneous fat

- Thyroid isthmus may be cauterized or suture ligated
- Vertical incision through second and third tracheal rings
- Determine appropriate tube diameter (sized according to internal diameter) and length
- Once tube is placed ensure good bilateral air entry. If concerned, one may check the position of tube with flexible or rigid bronchoscopy.

POSTOPERATIVE MANAGEMENT

- Neonates require intensive care monitoring in the postoperative period.
- A chest x-ray is performed as soon as the patient arrives to exclude pneumothorax/pneumomediastinum and confirm position of the tube.
- Close monitoring of pulmonary function and oxygen saturation is required.
- Humidification and gentle suctioning of secretions keeps the tube clean.
- Appropriate sedation and tube care, for the first week, ensures that accidental dislodgment does not occur while the tract is healing.
- The tube is changed after 5 to 7 days. The sedation may then be weaned as the healed tract allows easier replacement of an accidentally dislodged tube.

COMPLICATIONS

Early

- Intraoperative difficulties: loss of airway, damage to adnexal structures in the neck, and anesthetic problems/relations
- Hemorrhage: sites include skin edge, thyroid gland, and minor and major neck vessels.
- Pneumothorax and pneumomediastinum: damage to lung apex (extends into root of neck in neonates), excessive positive pressure ventilation, creation of false passage, and partial dislodgment of tube
- Loss of airway: accidental decannulation, misplaced tube, and obstruction of tube or bronchi
- Infection: local cellulitis warrants intravenous antibiotics

Late

- Granulation tissue may be at the stoma or at the tip.
- Suprastomal collapse: Due to pressure on the rings above the tube. Increased risk with lower age of neonate and duration of intubation.
- Subglottic stenosis: Due to collapse or granulation tissue.
- Erosion: Rarely erosion of the tracheal wall may occur due to pressure necrosis. This may cause a tracheoesophageal or tracheovascular fistula.
- Tracheocutaneous fistula: Once the tube is removed, a persistence of the tract to the skin surface may need to be surgically resected and closed.
- Speech delay: A concern with long-term tracheotomy over the age of 1 year. Patients should be evaluated and followed by a speech and language pathologist.
- All patients with a tracheotomy must attend regular review with their otolaryngologist to assess for features of a late complication, adjust tube size with age, and assess for readiness for decannulation.
- Babies discharged home with tracheotomies have an increased mortality rate compared with babies matched by gestational age without tracheotomies. Cause of death may be occlusion of the tube, pneumonia, or fistula formation.

Decannulation

- Once the underlying pathology has resolved and the patient deemed fit for decannulation, a diagnostic laryngoscopy and bronchoscopy should be performed to assess and manage suprastomal collapse, granulation tissue, and other airway anomalies.
- In neonates, as there is little room around the tube, trial occlusion of the tube is not appropriate. Complete decannulation, early in the day, in the OR or ICU is performed. The neonate is closely monitored for signs of impending airway obstruction.

REASONS FOR FAILED DECANNULATION

- Suprastomal collapse
- Tracheal granulation tissue

- Laryngomalacia/tracheomalacia
- Laryngeal anomaly such as vocal fold immobility, scar, web, or aspiration
- Subglottic stenosis
- Ongoing neurological deficit
- Poor pulmonary function

Recommended Readings

Benjamin B, Inglis A. Minor congenital laryngeal clefts: diagnosis and classification. Ann Otol Rhinol Laryngol 1989; 98:417–20.

Cummings CW, Fredrickson JM, Harker LA, et al, editors. Otolaryngology head and neck surgery. St Louis (MO): Mosby; 1998.

Daya H, Hosni A, Bejar-Solar I, et al. Pediatric vocal fold paralysis: a long-term retrospective study. Arch Otolaryngol Head Neck Surg 2000;126:21–5.

Healy GB. Common problems in paediatric otolaryngology. Chicago (IL):Year Book Medical Pub; 1990.

Myer CM III, Cotton RT, Shott SR, editors. The pediatric airway. Philadelphia (PA): Lippincort; 1995.

Myer CM III, Cotton RT, Holmes DK, et al. Laryngeal and laryngotracheoesophageal clefts: role of early surgical repair. Ann Otol Rhinol Laryngol 1990;99:98–104.

Mc Queen CT, Shapiro NL, Leighton S, et al. Single stage laryngotracheal reconstruction: the Great Ormond Street experience and guidelines for patient selection. Arch Otolaryngol Head Neck Surg 1999;125:320–2.

Walner DL, Loewen MS, Kimura RE. Neonatal subglottic stenosis-incidence and trends. Laryngoscope 2001;111:48–51.

Wetmore RF, Muntz HR, Mc Gill TJ, editors. Pediatric otolaryngology. New York: Thieme; 2000.

Part 2: Nasal Anomalies

David S.G. Lowinger, MD, FRACS, and Laurie A. Ohlms, MD

Choanal Atresia and Stenosis

DEFINITION

Choanal atresia occurs when the posterior nasal choana is completely obstructed. Choanal stenosis is defined as narrowing of the choana.

EMBRYOLOGY

During the fourth to twelfth week of gestation, the nose develops as neural crest cells migrate from their origin in the dorsal neural folds. Altered migration of these neural crest cells prevents thinning of the nasobuccal membrane, resulting in choanal atresia.

INCIDENCE

- Choanal atresia: 1 of every 5,000 to 7,000 live births
- Females to males: 2:1
- 90% bony, 10% membranous
- Usually unilateral, may be bilateral
- Associated congenital anomalies occur in 50% of patients with choanal atresia, such as CHARGE association: colobomas, cardiac defects, genitourinary anomalies, mental retardation, and hearing loss

CLINICAL FEATURES

- Neonates are preferential nasal breathers, thus nasal obstruction results in significant airway and feeding difficulties.

Bilateral Choanal Atresia

- Cyclical cyanotic episodes, relieved by crying
- Respiratory distress/desaturation
- Difficulty with feeding

Unilateral Choanal Atresia

- Unilateral rhinorrhea in the older infant

DIFFERENTIAL DIAGNOSIS

- Nasal pathology: pyriform aperture stenosis, nasolacrimal duct cysts, nasal mass, septal deviation
- Other upper airway pathology: laryngomalacia, tracheoesophageal fistula

ASSESSMENT

- Complete head and neck examination.
- Decongest nose and pass No. 6 French soft catheter into nasal cavity.
- Flexible fiberoptic examination of the nasal cavity

IMAGING

- Axial computed tomography (CT) scan (Figure 6) nose and paranasal sinuses

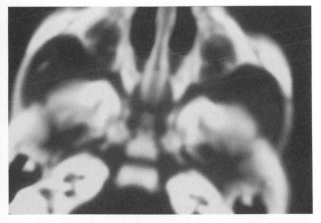

Figure 6 Axial computed tomography scan of a child with bilateral choanal atresia.

MANAGEMENT

- Depends on the severity of stenosis and presence of bilateral atresia
- Oropharyngeal airway or McGovern nipple will initially stent the airway
- Gavage feeding may be necessary while awaiting surgical repair
- The patient with CHARGE association may require tracheotomy with planned atresia repair when the child is older and other issues are stabilized.
- Unilateral atresia: usually no airway obstruction, elective repair

SURGICAL MANAGEMENT

- Surgical approach depends on the degree of stenosis, bony or membranous.
- Transnasal endoscopic repair: the atretic plate is removed using telescopes and a small drill.
- Transpalatal repair: intraoral incisions through the palate allow direct visualization and repair.

PREOPERATIVE ISSUES

- Ensure that the patient is otherwise fit for general anesthesia.
- Any bleeding diathesis must be corrected.
- Perioperative hydration, humidification, and steroids may be required.
- A combined conference with the intensivist, otolaryngologist, and parents of the child to discuss the management plan and to obtain informed consent.

ANESTHETIC ISSUES

- Intravenous (IV) access is obtained. Blood is usually not required.
- Bronchoscopy equipment should be on hand in the event of a difficult intubation.

POSTOPERATIVE MANAGEMENT

- ICU setting is required.
- Patients are usually extubated, with a nasal stent fashioned from an endotracheal tube sutured to the nasal septum.

- Stent care: regular irrigation and suctioning. Teach parents stent care as stents may be in place for 2 to 6 weeks.
- Prophylactic antibiotics to cover nasal flora while stents are in place.

SURGICAL COMPLICATIONS

- Displacement of the stent
- Alar or septal necrosis from stent irritation
- Recurrent choanal stenosis
- Changes in mid-face growth

OUTCOME

- Many patients return to the operating room for stent removal and dilatation.
- Long-term follow-up is essential as restenosis is common.

Congenital Nasal Pyriform Aperture Stenosis

DEFINITION

As neonates are obligate nasal breathers, nasal obstruction results in airway compromise and feeding difficulties. Congenital nasal pyriform aperture stenosis (CNPAS) is present when such symptoms arise in the neonate due to a narrowing of the anterior nasal bony inlet. The nasal bones and the nasal processes of the maxilla bound this region. It is a relatively new diagnosis first described in 1988.

EMBRYOLOGY

Currently, it is thought to be due to excessive thickness of the bone of the nasal process of the maxilla on each side, no illustration for this point.

INCIDENCE

- Rare
- Usually an isolated finding. May be associated with a large, single central incisor and with anterior pituitary anomalies.

CLINICAL FEATURES

Depend on the degree of narrowing of the nasal aperture. In the neonatal intensive care unit setting, it may present as:

- Cyclical cyanotic episodes relieved by crying
- Respiratory distress/desaturation
- Difficulty with feeding
- Failure to thrive

DIFFERENTIAL DIAGNOSIS

- Nasal pathology: bilateral choanal stenosis, septal deviation/hematoma, nasal mass, nasal bone fracture, and nasopharyngeal mass
- Other upper airway pathology including oropharyngeal masses, base of tongue anomalies, and above laryngeal and tracheal anomalies as well as tracheoesophageal fistula

ASSESSMENT

- Complete examination of head and neck including the nose, nasopharynx, and oropharynx.
- Telescopic examination of the nasal cavity and nasopharynx
- Awake, flexible laryngoscopy
- Findings: Anterior rhinoscopy demonstrates a bony narrowing of the anterior nasal passages. Often the flexible nasopharyngoscope cannot be inserted beyond this area. If this is the case, the nasopharynx and larynx may be examined by passing the scope through the mouth.

IMAGING

- CT scan of the nose and paranasal sinuses in axial and coronal planes with both bone and soft tissue windows (Figure 7).
- The CT field may be widened to include the anterior pituitary and the dental roots of the incisors.
- Lateral airways view and chest x-ray exclude other anomalies.

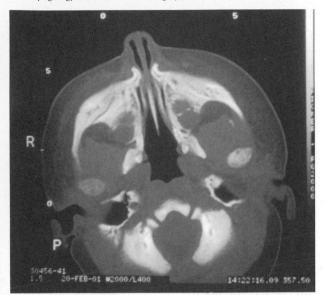

Figure 7   Axial computed tomography scan of a child with congenital nasal pyriform aperture stenosis.

MANAGEMENT

- Depends on the severity of the stenosis and the resulting clinical manifestations
- Conservative treatment: careful management, in an ICU setting of topical decongestants, and humidified air. A oropharyngeal airway or McGovern nipple may both stent the airway and allow feeding. If the patient deteriorates, intubation may be required and surgical management is indicated.
- Surgical treatment: repair of the CNPAS, tracheotomy (rarely required)

INDICATIONS FOR SURGERY

Airway obstruction and/or poor feeding not responding to conservative treatment

SURGICAL MANAGEMENT

The aim of surgical intervention is to improve the diameter of the nasal passages providing an adequate, secure airway.

- Initially, once anesthesia is induced, a careful examination of the nasal cavity is performed. Diagnostic laryngoscopy and bronchoscopy may also be done to exclude other anomalies of the airway.
- Repair of CNPAS: The bony margins of the nasal aperture may be approached via a transnasal or sublabial route. Due to the small size of the nasal vestibule of neonates, the sublabial technique is most often preferred. A sublabial incision is made. The periosteum is elevated from the floor of the nose with care to avoid damaging the tooth buds. The lateral nasal wall is exposed, and the overgrowth of the maxillary nasal processes drilled down. A nasal stent is usually placed and secured. It may remain for 1 to 4 weeks.
- Tracheotomy: This is seldom required. It may be employed as a temporary measure if safe intubation and ventilation cannot be maintained and access to the repair operation is delayed.

PREOPERATIVE ISSUES

- Ensure that the patient is otherwise fit for OR. Particularly, pulmonary status should be optimized.
- Any bleeding diathesis must be corrected.
- Perioperative hydration, humidification, and steroids may be required.
- A combined conference with the intensivist, otolaryngologist, and parents of the child to discuss the management plan. Parental consent for a diagnostic nasendoscopy and laryngobronchoscopy as well as the repair of the CNPAS.

ANESTHETIC ISSUES

- IV access is obtained. Blood is not usually required.
- Once a diagnostic laryngobronchoscopy has been completed, oral intubation occurs.

POSTOPERATIVE MANAGEMENT

- ICU setting is required.
- Patients are usually extubated with a nasal stent made of a 3.5-mm endotracheal tube in place.
- Maintenance of hydration and air humidification.
- Oral intake may commence 24 hours following the sublabial incision. Gentle oral care should be provided for the first week.
- Stent care: regular irrigation and cleaning. Ensure that there is no pressure from the stent on the nasal alar. Teach the parents stent care.
- Depending on the surgeon, postoperative prophylactic topical or oral antibiotics and IV steroids to reduce edema may be prescribed.
- Monitoring of airway and feeding status prior to discharge to ward.

SURGICAL COMPLICATIONS

A careful diagnostic laryngoscopy should not worsen subglottic stenosis.

COMPLICATIONS

Intraoperative: bleeding, trauma to lips, gums, and nasal alar.
Short term: bleeding, edema, infection, and loss of nasal airway if accidental removal of stents, dislodgement of stent, wound dehiscence and fistula, epiphora, nasolacrimal duct problems
Long term: recurrence of stenosis, scarring, tooth bud damage, changes in mid-face growth

OUTCOME

Repair of CNPAS is usually successful with immediate resolution of symptoms. Ongoing follow-up is required after removal of the stent to ensure that complications and restenosis do not occur and the patient continues to thrive. As with other airway procedures, success of surgical management is enhanced by careful ICU monitoring and support in the perioperative period.

Recommended Readings

Brown OE, Myer CM, Manning SC. Congenital nasal aperture stenosis. Laryngoscope 1989;99:86–91.

Crockett DM, Healy GB, McGill TJ, et al. Computed tomography in the evaluation of choanal atresia in infants and children. Laryngoscope 1987;97:174–83.

Ey EH, Han RB, Juan WK. Bony inlet stenosis as a cause of nasal airway obstruction. Radiology 1988;168:477–79.

Goldberg D, Flax-Goldberg R, Joachims HZ, Peled N. Congenital nasal pyriform aperture stenosis-Diagnostic quiz case. Arch Otolaryngol Head Neck Surg 2000;126:94–6.

Josephson GD, Vickery CL, Giles WC, et al. Transnasal endoscopic repair of congenital choanal atresia. Arch Otolaryngol Head Neck Surg 1998;124:537–40.

FOUR

Cleft Lip/Palate and Robin Sequence

John B. Mulliken, MD, and
Dorothy M. MacDonald, BS, RN

Embryology

Cleft lip/palate results from a failure of normal orofacial development during the 6th to 12th weeks of embryonic life. The nose first appears as medial and lateral swellings in the lower portion of the frontonasal process. During the 6th to 7th weeks, the advancing maxillary processes (upper portions of the first pharyngeal arch) fuse with the medial nasal prominences, whereas the latter merge with one another. Thus, the cleft between maxillary processes and medial nasal prominences is lost and the upper lip is formed. This process results in the *primary palate* that is composed of 3 parts: labial or philtral component; central segment, the future anterior dental arch containing the four maxillary incisor teeth; and triangular palatal element that extends from the alveolar ridge to the incisive foramen. Any alteration in this process can cause unilateral or bilateral labial cleft, including a defect in the alveolar ridge and nasal deformity. The embryologic term for this malformation is cleft of the primary palate.

Cleft of the *secondary palate* (hard and soft palate, posterior to the incisive foramen) occurs between 8 and 12 weeks of embryonic life. The palate forms by a shelf-like outgrowth from each maxillary process. These vertical shelves "horizontalize" (over 24 hours) during the 7th week and begin to fuse with the premaxillary segment and with each other, joining in the midline from anterior-to-posterior. The soft palate and uvula form by merging a mesenchymal outgrowth below ectoderm. A cleft palate is caused by either a reduction in size of the maxillary shelves, failure of horizontalization, or a disturbance in the cellular process of fusion and merging.

Incidence

Cleft lip, with or without cleft palate (CL/P), occurs in approximately 1 in 1,000 caucasian births (range 700 to 1300). The frequency in American Indians is the highest of any ethnic group (3.6 in 1,000 births). The birth prevalence in Asians is 1.7 to 2 per 1000. The lowest incidence is in black infants (0.3 per 1,000 births). CL/P is more common in males, more so if the cleft is severe. Ninety percent of cleft lips are unilateral and two-thirds are on the left side. In a unilateral cleft lip, complete and incomplete forms are about equally common. Unilateral complete cleft lip and cleft alveolus occurs with an intact secondary palate in approximately 10% of patients. The types of bilateral cleft lip are: 50% symmetrical complete; 25% symmetrical incomplete; and 25% asymmetrical (complete on one side and incomplete on the other).

The incidence of isolated cleft palate (CP) is much lower than CL/P, approximately 1:2,500 births in both white and black populations. Females are affected almost twice as commonly as males. Perhaps this is related to the finding that the palatal shelves fuse approximately 1 week later in females as compared to males. CP with cleft lip is more likely to be associated with other congenital anomalies (13 to 50%) than cleft lip/palate (7 to 13%).

Prenatal Diagnosis

Several retrospective studies of parental attitudes have documented a preference to know prenatally the diagnosis of a cleft lip. This provides the opportunity for counseling and psychological preparation. Ultrasonic diagnosis of cleft lip/palate is increasingly common. CL/P can be identified as early as 13 to 16 weeks of gestation by transvaginal sonography. In experienced hands, transabdominal ultrasonic detection is possible by 16 weeks, and discovery is expected by 24 weeks of gestation. Nevertheless, the published detection rates range from 20 to 30%. This discrepancy is attributed to the fact that assessment of the fetal lip/nose is usually not included in standard sonography for gestational age and detection of fetal malformations. By targeted examination in tertiary centers, the accuracy of prenatal diagnosis of CL/P is 50 to 75%. Three-dimensional ultrasonography increases accuracy and minimizes false-positive findings. False-positive identification of a nasolabial cleft is extremely rare. Overdiagnosis of the severity of the defect sometimes occurs. Visualization of a CP by either 2- or 3-dimensional ultrasonography is difficult.

Prenatal magnetic resonance imaging (MRI), available in some large referral centers, provides accurate detection of a labial cleft and measurement of alveolar cleft width. MRI also can accurately reveal whether or not there is a cleft of the secondary palate and even an isolated CP.

Postnatal Presentation

The plan for dental and surgical management is determined by the type and extent of the labiopalatal cleft. Differentiation between a unilateral and bilateral labial cleft is obvious. The term *incomplete* denotes that the labial cleft does not extend through the nostril floor; the term *complete* signifies that it does. The old eponym "Simonart band" to designate a tiny strip of tissue at the top of the labial cleft is incorrect and should be abandoned. The neonatologist should be aware of a subtle form of cleft lip called a microform, which comprises about 10% of unilateral incomplete forms. In a microform, there is a minor nasal deformity, a notching of the vermilion-cutaneous line, and a flattened or grooved philtral line. A microform on the contralateral side of a more major cleft lip is often overlooked. Whenever there is a cleft lip, the alveolar ridge should be examined for possible involvement. The common phenotypic variations of cleft lip are illustrated in Figure 1.

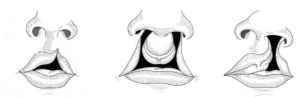

Figure 1   Types of cleft lip: (Left) Unilateral incomplete; (Center) Unilateral complete; (Right) Bilateral complete.

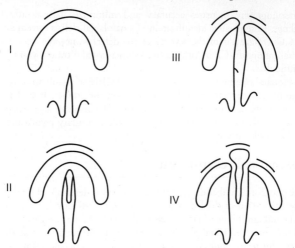

Figure 2 Veau classification: I cleft soft palate; II complete cleft secondary palate; III unilateral complete cleft lip/palate; and IV. bilateral complete cleft lip/palate.

Cleft of the secondary palate occurs in 2 major forms: soft palate only, which may extend into the posterior hard palate; and complete defect of the soft/hard palate, which is either unilateral or bilateral. The type and extent of palatal clefting is designated by the Veau classification (Figure 2).

Associated Anomalies

Every newborn with CL/P or CP should be assessed for the possibility of other craniofacial and extracraniofacial anomalies. There is a long list of well-recognized syndromes associated with CL/P and CP. Cleft lip/palate centers report that up to 30% of affected children have other anomalies. These congenital anomalies tend to be under-diagnosed at birth or in the neonatal period, especially in those infants with a less severe expression of a genetic disorder.

- Bilateral cleft lip/palate is a common finding in various trisomies, particularly involving chromosome 13, deletions (such as 4p-, Wolf-Hirschhorn syndrome), and duplications.
- About 5% of CL/P cases are genetic in origin. Van der Woude syndrome is the most common autosomal dominant disorder associated with clefting, either CL/P or CP. Nevertheless, only about 1% of syndromic cleft infants have this condition. Van der Woude syndrome is characterized by paramedian "pits"(sinuses) of the lower lip. A similar orofacial phenotype occurs in popliteal pterygium syndrome. The gene for these allelic syndromes is interferon regulatory factor 6 (IRF6). It is estimated that 15% of sporadic cases of CL/P involve variations in IRF6.
- About 12% of patients with complete CL/P have nasolabial premaxillary hypoplasia, known as "binderoid" facies.
- Cardiac anomalies occur in approximately 8% of CP infants, either by chance or as part of a syndrome.

Nevertheless, most cases of CL/P occur as isolated (sporadic) anomalies, ie, they are non-syndromic. (Figure 3).

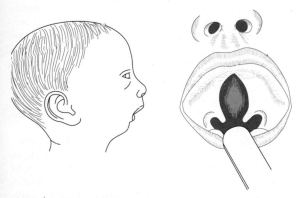

Figure 3 (Left) Infant with Robin sequence. (Right) Intraoral view of U-shaped cleft palate.

A small lower jaw is easily detected on prenatal ultrasonography. The possibility of *Robin sequence* (RS) should be considered in any infant born with an isolated CP. RS is a postnatal (not a prenatal) diagnostic term that denotes mandibular micrognathia/retrognathia, glossoptosis, and respiratory and feeding problems. Usually, there is a CP but this is not an obligatory finding for RS. Mandibular micrognathia refers to size, retrognathia to position. Most RS infants are either micro- or retrognathic but not both. The palatal cleft usually extends to the incisive foramen and often is U-shaped in RS in contrast to a V-configuration in common CP.

Pathogenically, RS can be envisioned as either malformational (caused by intrinsic mandibular hypoplasia) or deformational (caused by extrinsic mandibular constraint) Another useful binary designation for RS is nonsyndromic versus syndromic. There are over 30 known syndromes associated with RS.

Stickler syndrome is the most common cause of syndromic RS, accounting for 30 to 40% of cases. This autosomal dominant disorder often first comes to the attention of the family after birth of a child with CP or RS. There are at least 3 known collagen mutations that cause Stickler syndrome: COL2A1, COL11A1, and COL11A2. The infant with Stickler syndrome is floppy (marfanoid) with hypermobile joints. Other phenotypic features include prominent eyes, high-grade myopia, flat midface, depressed nasal bridge, minor epicanthal folds, long philtrum, and sensorineural deafness. These findings can target genes for mutational analysis. For example, COL2A1 is the most abundant collagen in the vitreous, and Stickler syndrome with severe myopia is more likely. COL11A1 mutations are more likely with ophthalmologic signs and major hearing loss. COL11A2 is the more likely mutation in patient without ocular finding who otherwise has typical Stickler features.

Velocardiofacial syndrome (VCFS) is the second most common cause of syndromic RS (15 to 17%). The mandible in VCFS is normal in size but retrognathic in position because of an obtuse cranial base angle (platybasia). Cardiac anomalies occur in approximately 50% of VCFS infants: the most common are tetralogy of Fallot with pulmonary atresia, truncus arteriosus, right-sided aortic arch, and interrupted aortic arch (Type B). The physical findings are subtle and include narrow palpebral fissures, relatively broad nasal bridge, and downturned oral commissures. Usually, the secondary palate is intact, but there can be a submucous cleft palate, overt or occult. Laryngeal webbing is pathognomic for VCFS but occurs in only 10% of patients.

Babies with VCFS often have a poor suck (generalized hypotonia) and feeding problems, including gastroesophageal reflux. Molecular diagnosis is made by fluorescent in situ hybridization; most VCFS patients have a microdeletion on chromosome 22q11. DiGeorge sequence, that is, immune deficiency and abnormal calcium homeostasis are part of deletion 22q11. Only 10% of VCFS infants have DiGeorge sequence, whereas 90% of infants with DiGeorge sequence have VCFS.

Preoperative Management

CLEFT LIP/PALATE

The neonate with an orofacial anomaly must be able to breathe and suckle. An infant with a cleft lip/palate usually breathes well; feeding is the major issue. The mother should be encouraged to breast-feed if the labial cleft is incomplete, and there is an intact secondary palate or only a cleft soft palate. This becomes easier once the milk starts to flow, but it is not always successful. The newborn with a complete labiopalatal cleft needs special attention. The mother should not be given false hope that she will be able to breast-feed. There are many traditional devices to aid in feeding; the best is the Haberman (Medela®). Parents quickly learn to use the Haberman feeder after instructed by a nurse trained in these techniques. The weight of the baby should be checked weekly; sometimes calories need to be increased. The mother should try to use a breast pump to extract milk for feeding. Pumping for 5 minutes, then stopping, massaging, and reattaching delivers more of the hind milk that contains more calories in fat.

Preoperative orthopedic manipulation of the maxillary segments is generally used for the infant with a complete CL/P, which is unilateral or bilateral. There are 2 strategies. Active dentofacial orthopedics involves construction of a device that is pinned to the maxillary palatal shelves. The maxillary segments are aligned by activating a turnscrew, and the premaxilla is retruded by tightening elastic chains. Passive dentofacial orthopedics involves the placement of a removal appliance that is gradually trimmed so as to mold the alveolar segments into a better position. The passive method requires external compression on the premaxilla, either by an elastic band or by tape to the cheeks. A surgical alternative is a preliminary labial closure called a lip adhesion.

ROBIN SEQUENCE

A few days after birth, the severity of RS can be clinically graded using the following scale:

- Grade I: eats and breathes well with supine positioning
- Grade II: breathes well but obstructs when fed by mouth
- Grade III: cannot breathe or eat without obstruction and desaturation

Infants in the Grade III group manifest periods of cyanosis, usually with substernal and intercostal constrictions. Feeding through a nasogastric tube (NGT) is only a temporizing measure for these infants. Long-term use of gavage results in oral aversion; it may take months before the child will eat normally. Nevertheless, this is the best method of feeding in the short term. Some infants need surgical placement of a gastrostomy or percutaneous endoscopic gastrostomy.

Initially, the airway may be controlled by a nasopharyngeal tube. The infant should be monitored with a pulse oximeter and placed in the lateral position with the head of the bed slightly raised. A pacifier (non-orthodontic) can be used to keep the tongue forward.

Operative intervention is necessary for the infant with RS who desaturates despite all attempts at positioning or who cannot be fed orally (many Grade II and all Grade III). The options include: gastrostomy, tongue-lip adhesion, mandibular distraction, and tracheostomy. Many infants with RS have ankyloglossia; however, the tongue-tie should not be severed until the child is older and when the airway is secure.

Anesthesia

It is important to distinguish whether an infant has an associated syndrome. Intubation is more likely to be difficult in an infant with syndromic cleft lip/palate.

There is a hierarchy of difficulty in intubation even with non-syndromic infants. The procumbent premaxilla in an infant with bilateral complete cleft lip interferes with alignment of the airway during laryngoscopy. Infants with a left unilateral complete cleft lip are more difficult to intubate than a right-sided cleft because the laryngoscope blade falls into the cleft.

Intubation can be daunting in a neonate with RS because the larynx is positioned cephalad under the base of the tongue. There is very little space into which to displace the tongue, and the larynx remains anterior to the laryngoscope blade making it difficult to visualize the aditus. For this reason, the infant should be intubated by the anesthesiologist who has the most experience in airway management in babies with craniofacial anomalies, particularly RS. Often fiberoptic endoscopic intubation is needed. An otorhinolaryngologist should be present for the initial intubation of an infant with RS. Not only may this specialist assist in intubation, it is critical that the airway be assessed for other causes of obstruction, such as anomalies of the epiglottis and laryngomalacia. Most babies with RS have gastroesophageal reflux that requires appropriate management.

Surgical Management

CLEFT LIP/PALATE

Surgical protocols differ among centers. In general, a cleft lip is repaired along with closure of the alveolar cleft and correction of the nasal deformity, around 3 to 6 months of age. The technical details for nasolabial repair vary depending on the severity and extent of the cleft. Preoperative dentofacial orthopedics is used for both the unilateral and bilateral complete deformity and on the complete side for a bilateral asymmetric cleft lip. Incomplete unilateral and bilateral CL is usually repaired in a single stage, along with closure of the alveolar ridge, at 3 to 6 months. In our unit, a lip-nasal adhesion is the first operative step for an infant with a unilateral complete cleft lip or for the complete side of a bilateral asymmetrical cleft lip. The second stage repair is scheduled about 3 months later. In other centers, unilateral nasolabial repair is accomplished in a single stage. Palatoplasty is undertaken at 8 to 10 months of age; the entire palate is closed in

1 operation. Some centers practice staged palatal closure: first the soft palate and later the hard palate. There is increasing evidence that staged palatal closure results in inferior speech outcome and without any benefit to facial growth.

Normal speech becomes increasingly unlikely if palatal repair is delayed beyond 1 year of age.

ROBIN SEQUENCE

Tongue-lip adhesion, with or without a feeding gastrostomy, is the first step in the management of the airway in an infant with Grade II or III RS. After nasotracheal intubation, a guy suture is placed through the tip of the tongue, a T-shaped incision is marked on the undersurface of the tongue, and a mirror-image incision on the lingual side at the midline of the lower lip. Holding the tongue forward, the genioglossus is stripped from the inner surface of the mandible. A circummandibular suture is placed to hold the tongue in a procumbent position. The muscle and mucosa of the tongue are apposed to the corresponding layers of the lower lip. The infant often can be extubated postoperatively, depending on the status of the airway. The infant returns to the ICU with a tongue suture in place. The tongue and lip are separated at the time of palatal closure.

Tongue-lip adhesion is effective for most infants with nonsyndromic RS and syndromic RS. Tracheostomy is only indicated if the tongue-lip adhesion fails to control the airway or if there are other issues in the lower airway or other complicating problems, such as intracranial bleeding, pulmonary edema, pneumonia, or congestive heart failure. In some centers, mandibular distraction is offered as an alternative to tracheostomy for the infant with syndromic RS and a hypoplastic mandible that would not be expected to exhibit catch-up growth.

Postoperative Management

CLEFT LIP/PALATE

The suture line must be protected and kept clean after both lip-nasal adhesion and definitive nasolabial repair. At completion of the nasolabial closure, a U-shaped metal bar, called a Logan bow, is taped to the cheeks. This bow was once used to diminish tension on the labial repair. The Logan bow is now used to protect the healing lip and to hold a sponge that is soaked in iced saline for the first 24 hours. The moistened sponge absorbs serosanguinous ooze from the suture line and minimizes swelling. After 24 hours, the suture line is recoated with antibiotic ointment, for the next 3 days. Usually, the infant is discharged on the second postoperative day. Thereafter, topical antibiotic ointment is discontinued, and the lip is cleansed daily with soap and water. The sutures are removed on postoperative day 4 to 5 (under a short general anesthetic). A Steri-Strip is placed over the healing lip and changed as needed for 6 weeks postoperatively.

Upon completion of palatal repair, a gauze pack, soaked in balsam of Peru, is sutured to each side of the alveolar ridge. This pack holds the mucoperiosteal palatal flaps to the bony shelves and minimizes pain and bleeding. This pack is removed prior to discharge from hospital, usually on postoperative day 2. Nevertheless, many cleft centers to not use a postoperative palatal pack.

ROBIN SEQUENCE

The infant with RS returns to the ICU following the tongue-lip adhesion. The intraoperatively placed tongue suture can be used to pull the tongue anteriorly if the infant develops breathing difficulty because of lingual swelling. A nasopharyngeal airway is also useful. Oral secretions are thick and copious for the first 48 hours postoperatively. Gentle suctioning is needed, and the nasal passages should also be suctioned. Prone positioning facilitates drainage of the oral secretions and helps posture the tongue forward.

The sutured junction of the advanced tongue and lower lip must be kept clean, using 1/4 strength hydrogen peroxide and a thin coating of vaseline-based antibiotic ointment. The oral mucosa should be cleansed several times per day with moistened cotton-tipped swabs. After 3 days, peroxide cleansing is stopped, and vaseline ointment is used to keep crusts from forming on the suture line.

The infant is fed through a NGT or the gastrostomy within 24 hours postoperatively. Oral feedings are withheld until 10 days postoperatively and are initiated slowly with liquid by a dropper. The Haberman feeder can be tried 3 weeks after the tongue-lip adhesion, initially for no more than 20 minutes per feeding, gradually increasing the time coincident with the gain in tensile strength. Feeding via NGT or gastrostomy continues until the infant can take sufficient volume by mouth.

The infant should be monitored for 8 to 12 weeks postoperatively with a pulse oximeter. Respiratory precautions are also needed during this time. During the initial postoperative phase, adjustment of the caloric intake may be necessary to insure healing.

Tongue-lip adhesion advances the tongue and also seems to potentiate narrowing of the palatal gap. The U-shaped CP narrows sufficiently so that palatoplasty can be accomplished at the usual time, that is, about 8 to 10 months. The lower incisors begin to erupt about the time of palatoplasty and sometimes are seen as the tongue-lip adhesion is taken down. Every infant with a history of RS should be observed in the ICU post palatal repair, whether or not a preliminary tongue-lip adhesion was necessary.

Complications/Outcome

CLEFT LIP

Immediate complications after repair of cleft lip are rare. Ecchymosis can cause superficial epithelial loss at the tip of flaps. In the weeks postoperatively, a tiny abscess can appear caused by infection around a dermal suture or blocked adnexal gland. This pustule should be evacuated and, if present, the intradermal suture should be removed. If there is local cellulitis, oral antibiotics should be given. A Steri-Strip® is placed across the lip and changed as necessary for 6 weeks. In some infants, the labial scar thickens and pulls the lip upward. Digital massage of the labial scar is helpful, and application of a sunscreen (block) is mandatory. In time, the scar softens and matures as the lip descends. Normal formation of scar can also distort the nostril for several months, but nostril shape usually improves in time.

CLEFT PALATE

Postoperative bleeding is rare after palatoplasty; infection is not a problem. Once the immediate potential for airway obstruction is passed, there are only minor issues relating to sleep and feeding.

The incidence of palatal fistula (usually located at the junction of the hard/soft palate) should be less than 3%.

Periodic assessment of children with repaired cleft lip/palate is the obligation of every cleft lip/palate team. These children are seen every 6 to 12 months in an interdisciplinary clinic. Speech, hearing, dentition, and facial growth, are evaluated yearly throughout childhood and adolescence.

Nasolabial revisions are commonly done prior to attending school or at the time of bone grafting the alveolar cleft (around 9 to 11 years of age). Although an indirect measure of outcome, auditing the number and types of nasolabial revisions is important so the surgeon can make necessary adjustments in the technique of primary repair.

In the past, judgement of appearance was, by necessity, qualitative usually based on a rating scale using photographs and graded by a blinded panel. Anthropometry (the direct measurement of the nasolabial features) is a quantitative method; these measurements can be compared to the dimensions of normal age- and sex-matched children. New technologies for indirect anthropometry, such as laser scanning and 3-dimensional photogrammetry, will soon become more widely used for outcome assessment of appearance.

The critical determinant of outcome after palatoplasty is whether or not the child has velopharyngeal insufficiency (VPI). This judgement is primarily subjective, which is based on the keen ear of an experienced speech pathologist. The incidence of VPI depends on the severity of the cleft deformity and the skill and experience of the surgeon. The published rate of VPI is used to be around 20%; now many centers are reporting less than 10% VPI. A child with bilateral complete cleft lip/palate is more likely to develop VPI than a child with unilateral cleft lip or an isolated cleft palate. There are 2 effective surgical procedures (pharyngeal flap and sphincter pharyngoplasty) for correction of VPI. These operations are usually performed around 5 to 6 years of age.

Midfacial hypoplasia is long-term problem that, like speech, correlates with severity of the initial deformity. The frequency of maxillary anterior and vertical deficiency is around 25 to 40% in unilateral complete CL/P and 2 fold higher in bilateral complete CL/P. Patients with cleft lip only, without cleft palate, almost never have maxillary undergrowth. Midfacial retrusion can be corrected by combined orthodontic and orthognathic surgical techniques. The standard procedure is maxillary advancement (Le Fort I osteotomy). Usually, this correction is undertaken in adolescence after completion of growth. There are indications and techniques for earlier maxillary advancement in a child with severe retrusion.

ROBIN SEQUENCE

There is concern if a child with RS exhibits VPI because a secondary procedure, either pharyngeal flap or sphincter pharyngoplasty, can potentially cause obstructive sleep apnea. Sometimes the VPI can be managed by palatal elongation and reposition of the palatal musculature.

There is confusion in the medical literature as to the potential for growth of the underdeveloped mandible. For the nonsyndromic RS child, there is typically early catch-up growth and a nearly normal upper/lower jaw relationship is expected. Mandibular growth potential differs depending on the particular syndrome. For example, in the most common associated disorder, Stickler syndrome, mandibular growth is nearly normal. In contrast, a patient who has Treacher Collins syndrome or bilateral hemifacial microsomia, the mandible will remain hypoplastic; elongation, orthognathic procedures, and augmentation are usually necessary.

References

1. Cohen MM Jr. Etiology and pathogenesis of orofacial clefting. Oral Maxillofac Surg Clin North Am 2000;12:379–97.
2. Cohen MM Jr. Robin sequences and complexes: causal heterogeneity and pathogenetic/phenotypic variability. Am J Med Genet 1999;84:311–5.
3. Marrinan EM, LaBrie RA, Mulliken JB. Velopharyngeal function in nonsyndromic cleft palate: relevance of surgical technique, age at repair, and cleft type. Cleft Palate Craniofac J 1998;35:95–100.
4. Mulliken JB, Martinez-Peréz D. The principle of rotation-advancement for repair of unilateral complete cleft lip and nasal deformity: technical variations and analysis of results. Plast Reconstr Surg 1999;104:1247–60.

5. Mulliken JB. Primary repair of bilateral cleft lip and nasal deformity. Plast Reconstr Surg 2001;108:181–94.
6. Nargozian CD. The difficut airway in the pediatric patient with a craniofacial anomaly. Anesthesiol Clin North America 1998;16:839–52.
7. Smith AS, Estroff JA, Barnewolt C, Mulliken JB, Levine D. Prenatal diagnosis of cleft lip and palate using MRI. AJR Am J Roentgenol 2004;183:229–35.

FIVE

Cardiovascular Disorders

Part 1: Patent Ductus Arteriosus

Elizabeth D. Blume, MD, and
Francis Fynn-Thompson, MD

Embryology

The ductus arteriosus is a normal physiological structure. It connects the main pulmonary artery to the aorta, allowing for the necessary right-to-left shunting needed during normal fetal circulation. It is formed from the distal portion of the sixth aortic arch, usually on the left side connecting to the left pulmonary artery. If the aortic arch is on the right, the ductus may also be on the right and connect to the right pulmonary artery. The normal diameter of the ductus arteriosus at birth is 10 mm.

Incidence

- The incidence of patent ductus arteriosus (PDA) depends on the age of the patient.

  Overall in term infants: 1 in 2,000 live births
  Overall in preterm infants: 8 in 1,000 live births
  Incidence of PDA in infants less than 1,750 g: 45%
  Incidence of PDA in infants less than 1,200 g: 80%

- Increased incidence of PDA is associated with family history, meconium aspiration secondary to low partial pressure of oxygen (PaO_2), rubella, and high altitude (up to a 30 times greater risk with lower PaO_2).

Prenatal Diagnosis and Prenatal Issues

- Normal prenatal structure
- Normally, the ductus arteriosus closes in the first day of life, secondary to loss of maternal prostaglandin (PGE) and increase in PaO_2.
- Premature infants have a decreased ability to metabolize PGE in their lungs; therefore, they are at an increased risk of having persistently high PGE levels.

Postnatal Clinical Presentation

- The presentation of PDA depends on ductal size and the magnitude of the shunt, as well as the gestational age.
- In the premature infant, the myocardium contains more water, less contractile mass, and less sympathetic innervation. The ventricles are less distensible than at term. Therefore, with a smaller shunt, distention of the left ventricle (LV) produces higher LV end-diastolic pressure and pulmonary venous congestion.
- Overperfusion of the lungs secondary to decreasing pulmonary vascular resistance is exacerbated by exogenous surfactant.
- Underperfusion of the gut and kidneys secondary to redistribution of cardiac output away from the descending aorta towards the lungs (diastolic steal) increases the risk of necrotizing enterocolitis (NEC) and renal dysfunction.

Clinical Examination

The clinical examination depends on the magnitude of the shunt and the condition of the lungs when PDA presents.

WITHOUT INITIAL LUNG DISEASE

- Classically, a continuous murmur is present. In premature infants, the murmur can be systolic and "rocky" sounding with a loud pulmonic component of the second heart sound (P_2).
- Wide pulse pressure (due particularly to lowered diastolic component)
- Bounding peripheral pulses, palpable palmar pulse

- Pulmonary edema
- Eventual ventricular failure with tachycardia and tachypnea

WITH LUNG DISEASE

The most common presentation of PDA is acute decompensation in ventilatory status in a patient who is recovering from respiratory distress syndrome.

Diagnosis

- The clinical examination can be helpful if the shunt is large.
- The chest radiograph, although it can be normal, may show cardiomegaly, left atrial and LV enlargement, and increased pulmonary blood flow if the shunt is large.
- The electrocardiogram can be normal, but it may reveal left atrial enlargement and biventricular hypertrophy.
- Obtain an echocardiogram to exclude associated heart disease. Coarctation is difficult to assess in the presence of a large PDA.
- Assess the size of the shunt and ventricular function.

Differential Diagnosis

- Worsening lung disease
- Other cardiac shunt lesions that increase pulmonary blood flow

Preoperative Management

- Nothing by mouth
- Fluid restriction
- Consider diuretics
- If pressors are needed, avoid agents that increase systemic afterload, such as epinephrine and dopamine, because of the resulting increase in left to right shunt.
- Prostaglandin inhibitors, such as indomethacin and ibuprofen, can close approximately 80% of PDAs. The effectiveness of these agents is inversely proportional to gestational age and day of life. Indomethacin has been the traditional treatment for medical closure of PDA's, whereas ibuprofen is a relatively new

option that theoretically is equally efficacious but causes less impairment of renal perfusion.

Indications for Surgery

Surgery for PDA is usually indicated (1) after medical failure (often defined as two or three courses of indomethacin), or (2) if there is a contraindication to indomethacin including renal dysfunction, coagulopathy, thrombocytopenia, and/or NEC, or (3) if there is a severe decline in clinical status and/or the presence of shock.

Anesthesia

Surgery can be performed in the neonatal intensive care unit or in the operating room for the premature infant and newborn. To facilitate surgery, infants on high-frequency ventilators should be given a trial of conventional ventilation. Often hand ventilation for transport and the entire duration of the surgery is required.

Surgical Management

- Left posterolateral thoracotomy (fourth intercostal space) approach. The approach to the PDA can be transpleural or extrapleural. To facilitate exposure, gentle retraction of the lung is required. This may need to be intermittent to allow for adequate ventilation. In infants less than 1,500 g, a single metal clip can be used to interrupt the PDA.
- Video-assisted thoracoscopic ligation is used occasionally in full-term infants and frequently in larger children.
- Consider median sternotomy in critically ill neonates unable to wean from high-frequency ventilation, although this is rarely required.
- The left recurrent laryngeal nerve should be identified and preserved.
- Systemic blood pressure (BP) of the upper and lower extremities should be monitored during ligation for appropriate response and to rule out impingement on the descending aorta.

- Placement of a chest tube is optional; it serves to drain residual air or fluid. The presence of residual air can be interpreted as a pneumothorax in an infant with tenuous ventilatory requirements.
  1. Place the tip of the chest tube posteriorly, toward the apex of the left pleural space.
  2. Set the chest tube to 10 cm H_2O suction.
  3. Discontinue using the chest tube when (1) the lung is fully expanded, (2) there is no air leak, and (3) there is minimal fluid output, typically within 24 to 48 hours, if there are no further indications.
  4. Obtain a chest radiograph following removal of the chest tube to rule out pneumothorax.
  5. If there is persistent drainage, suspect chylothorax.

Postoperative Management

- Obtain a radiograph of the chest to assess the position of the endotracheal tube and chest tube and to rule out pneumothorax, atelectasis, and/or effusion.
- Assess BP of the four extremities to rule out impingement on the descending aorta.
- If the patient was on furosemide preoperatively, it is usually helpful to continue at a dose of 1 mg/kg for 24 to 48 hours postoperatively.
- Hypotension is usually responsive to volume expansion. This may be seen in patients with long-standing (> 5 days), large PDAs and left to right shunting. These previously volume-loaded left ventricles may need temporary volume expansion to maintain cardiac output in the first 24 to 48 hours postoperatively.

Complications and Outcome

- Procedural mortality for PDA at most centers approaches 0%. The risks increase in severely premature infants who have multisystem organ failure.
- There may be intraoperative bleeding from ductal disruption, which can be lethal. Delayed hemorrhage is rare.

- Impingement on the aorta should be suspected if BP of the upper extremity is higher than BP of the lower extremity. Aortic occlusion following PDA ligation has been reported.
- Occlusion of the left pulmonary artery can occur, and it is difficult to diagnose. An echocardiogram can be useful in making the diagnosis.
- There is an incidence of approximately 3 to 5% of recurrent laryngeal nerve palsy with paralysis of the left vocal cord. It should be suspected if there is persistent postextubation stridor or feeding difficulties.
- Chylothorax
- Atelectasis
- Residual shunt from incomplete ligation or recanalization of ductus
- Pneumothorax

Recommended Readings

Frank Sellke, Scott Swanson, Pedro J. del Nido. Sabiston & Spencer Surgery of the Chest, 7th Ed. Elsevier; 2005.

Keane and Fyler "Patent Ductus Arteriosus" Chapter 35 in Nadas' Pediatric Cardiology. Eds. Keane, Lock, Fyler. Elsevier; 2006.

Drayton, Skidmore. Ductus arteriosus blood flow during the first 48 hrs of life. Arch Dis Child 62:1030, 1987

Gross RE, Hubbard JP. Surgical ligation of a patent ductus arteriosus. Report of the first successful case. JAMA 112:729. 1939.

Part 2: Vascular Rings

Elizabeth D. Blume, MD, and
Francis Fynn-Thompson, MD

Embryology

The formation of the normal aortic arch is a process of fusion and segmental resorption of the paired first to sixth branchial arches with the paired dorsal aorta. The paired aorta are present by the 21st day of gestation. Each arch corresponds to a branchial pouch derived from the embryonic foregut. An understanding of the normal and abnormal development of the mediastinal great vessels will aid in the understanding of vascular rings and pulmonary artery sling pathology but is beyond our scope here.

Definition

A vascular ring is an aortic arch anomaly in which the trachea and the esophagus are completely surrounded by vascular structures. These vessels need not be patent.

Classification

The following is a classification of the most common types of vascular rings in order of incidence. Most vascular rings consist of a dominant right aortic arch (right and left arch refers to which bronchus is crossed by the arch, not which side of the midline).

- Double aortic arch has two arches: anterior leftward arch and posterior rightward arch; right arch usually dominant.
- Right aortic arch, aberrant left subclavian, left ligamentum
- Right aortic arch, mirror-image branching, retroesophageal ligamentum
- Left aortic arch, mirror-image branching

Postnatal Presentation

The symptoms of a vascular ring depend on how tightly the ring encircles both the trachea and the esophagus.

- Respiratory signs and symptoms include stridor, unilateral air-trapping on chest radiograph. Respiratory distress is rare, but can occur.
- Feeding difficulties
- Asymptomatic

Diagnosis

- Barium swallow may reveal a posterior indentation of the esophagus, which is diagnostic. The type of lesion can often be ascertained by the "angle" of the indentation.
- An echocardiogram should be obtained to rule out intracardiac anomalies (although they are rare); sometimes, it is difficult to see the atretic portions of the ring.
- A computed tomographic (CT) scan and/or magnetic resonance imaging (MRI) is important for the precise diagnosis of vascular rings. These studies are particularly important with double arch, to rule out coarctation and determine which is the dominant vessel. They can be useful in patients with longer segment tracheal stenosis, when planning for tracheal reconstruction.
- Bronchoscopy is helpful if tracheal stenosis is suspected.
- Angiography is rarely needed except in cases of double arch and if a CT or MRI is not available, to rule out internal "web-like" coarctation.

Differential Diagnosis

Stridor in the newborn is secondary to obstruction at the following anatomic sites:

- Nasal: Choanal atresia (relieved with crying), edema, tumor
- Oral: Retrognathia and/or micrognathia, glossoptosis, lymphatic malformations, tongue cysts
- Laryngeal: Postintubation airway edema, laryngeal malacia, vocal cord paralysis, subglottic stenosis, hemangioma, laryngeal web, cleft, or cyst

- Tracheal: Tracheomalacia; tracheal web (see Chapter 6, "Respiratory Disorders").

Preoperative Management

If respiratory and/or dysphagic symptoms are present, surgical division is indicated.

- Obtain a chest radiograph to help determine arch sidedness and to rule out air trapping.
- Obtain an echocardiogram for arch anatomy and to rule out other structural heart disease.
- Obtain a contrast chest CT or MRI to precisely define the arch anatomy and help with operative planning.
- Maximize the nutritional status.
- Commence chest physiotherapy to decrease the risks of infection.
- Pulmonary infection is not always a contraindication to surgery because division of the ring will aid in clearing the infection.

Anesthesia

- Use pulse oximetry on each hand and foot to assess temporary occlusion of the arch and confirm the anatomy.
- Blood pressure cuffs should be put on each arm and a leg. There should be no gradient with occlusion of the "nondominant" arch.

Surgery

- An incision is made on the side of the ligamentum component of the vascular ring or the nondominant aortic arch.
- Of vascular rings, 95% are approached via left thoracotomy.
- The child is placed in full right lateral decubitus position, and the chest is entered at the fourth intercostal space.
- Video-assisted thoracoscopic or robotic-assisted ligation in older children in whom nonpatency of nondominant arch has been established by preoperative imaging studies.
- Following the release of the vascular ring, it is important to mobilize the esophagus from the associated fibrous adhesions.

Postoperative Management

- Feeding difficulties should resolve quickly.
- Respiratory symptoms often persist because tracheomalacia is common in patients with vascular rings. Stridor may persist for months.

Complications and Outcome

Mortality risk is 5% with most deaths in the earlier eras and in the presence of intracardiac or severe tracheal anomalies.

Pulmonary Artery Slings

The left pulmonary artery arises from the right pulmonary artery and passes leftward between the esophagus and the trachea. The ligamentum courses from the main pulmonary artery to the aorta, effectively creating a ring around the trachea but not the esophagus. This is called a pulmonary artery sling.

- Of pulmonary artery slings, 50% also have complete tracheal rings.
- A barium swallow will show the anterior indentation of the esophagus.
- There is a high incidence of long-segment stenosis with pulmonary artery sling. Therefore, a full assessment is needed of the trachea including a CT scan, MRI, and/or bronchography, and/or angiography.

Surgery

Surgery for this condition depends on the extent of tracheal involvement. Surgery involves the following:

- Division and reimplantation of the left pulmonary artery (LPA)
- Tracheal resection and anastomosis with relocation of the LPA
- Long-segment tracheal reconstruction with reimplantation of the LPA

Recommended Readings

Powell and Mandell "Vascular Rings and Slings" Chapter 54 in
    Nadas' Pediatric Cardiology. Eds. Keane, Lock, and Fyler.
    Elsevier; 2006.

Larsen WJ. Human Embryology. New York: Churchill
    Livingstone, 1997.

Gross RE. Surgical relief for tracheal obstruction from a vascular
    ring. N Engl J Med 233:586, 1945.

Frank Sellke, Scott Swanson, Pedro del Nido Sabiston & Spencer
    'Surgery of the chest' 7th Ed; 2005.

Part 3: Vascular Anomalies

Arin K. Greene, MD, MMSc, and
Steven J. Fishman, MD, FACS, FAAP

Vascular anomalies are disorders of blood vessels that usually present during childhood. These lesions affect all parts of the vasculature: capillaries, veins, arteries, or lymphatics. Although benign, vascular anomalies can cause local destruction and systemic morbidity. To optimize outcomes, patients with problematic lesions should be referred to an interdisciplinary Vascular Anomalies Center.

Vascular anomalies are broadly divided into two groups: tumors or malformations (Table 1). Tumors have proliferating endothelium, whereas malformations show normal endothelial turnover. Malformations are caused by errors in vasculogenesis and are further classified into slow-flow or high-flow lesions. Diagnostic confusion is common in this field because (1) different vascular anomalies often look similar and (2) many practitioners incorrectly label lesions by their descriptive rather than by their histological names (Table 2).

Embryology

- The etiopathogenesis of newborn vascular tumors has not yet been elucidated. However, evidence suggests that hemangioma might result from a somatic mutation in an endothelial progenitor cell derived from or common to the microvillous endothelium of the fetal portion of the placenta.
- Errors in smooth muscle signaling cause vascular malformations. Vascular endothelium differentiates from mesoderm in early gestation, and smooth muscle associates with branching endothelial tubes. Errors in vascular morphogenesis of various channel types can result in capillary, venous, lymphatic, or arterial malformations. Although familial vascular malformations exist, most are sporadic.

Incidence

- Hemangiomas occur in 4 to 10% of full-term Caucasian newborns. They are present more commonly in premature and

TABLE 1   Current Biological Classification of Vascular Anomalies

Tumors	Malformations		
	Slow Flow	Fast Flow	
Infantile Hemangioma	Capillary (CM)	Arterial Malformation (AM)	
Rapidly Involuting Congenital Hemangioma (RICH)	Venous (VM)	Arteriovenous Fistula (AVF)	
Non-involuting Congenital Hemangioma (NICH)			
Kaposiform Hemangioendothelioma (KHE)	Lymphatic (LM)	Arteriovenous Malformation (AVM)	
Pyogenic Granuloma	Klippel Trenaunay (CLVM)	Parkes Weber (CLAVM)	

TABLE 2 Commonly Used Incorrect Descriptions of Vascular Anomalies

	Tumors		Malformations	
Correct Biological Name	Incorrect Description	Correct Biological Name	Incorrect Description
Hemangioma	"Capillary hemangioma," "Strawberry hemangioma"	Capillary (CM)	"Port wine stain" "Hemangioma"
Kaposiform hemangioendothelioma (KHE)	"Hemangioma"	Venous (VM)	"Cavernous hemangioma"
Pyogenic granuloma	"Lobular capillary hemangioma"	Lymphatic (LM)	"Lymphangioma" "Cystic hygroma"

light-skinned infants. They occur about three times more commonly in girls than boys.
- Vascular malformations occur in approximately 0.5 to 1% of the population. Capillary malformation is most common followed by venous and lymphatic malformations.

Prenatal Diagnosis and Treatment

- Vascular malformations, in particular those causing bony or soft tissue overgrowth, occasionally can be seen on antenatal ultrasound.
- Antenatal therapy is not indicated. Labor and delivery generally do not require alteration. However, extremely large soft tissue lesions may be best delivered by Cesarean section to prevent dystocia. Large cervicofacial malformations can obstruct the upper airway, leading to asphyxiation at delivery. Use of the ex utero intrapartum treatment procedure with intubation or tracheostomy prior to cutting the umbilical cord may be necessary.
- Commonly seen antenatal "cystic hygromas" are better termed posterior nuchal translucencies. These often are associated with lethal chromosomal abnormalities. They must be distinguished from true lymphatic malformations, which, if cervical, are typically anterior and are not associated with chromosomal aberrations. It is essential to differentiate these lesions during antenatal counseling, especially if termination of pregnancy is being considered.
- Infantile hemangioma is not visualized antenatally because it becomes apparent after birth. However, congenital hemangiomas, which are fully grown at birth, may be appreciated in utero.

Postnatal Presentation: Tumors

- Infantile hemangioma, the most common vascular anomaly, may appear as a pale, pink stain at birth. It typically becomes obvious 2 weeks postnatally, as the lesion begins to proliferate. Superficial hemangioma appears red, whereas deeper lesions may be noted later as a blue mass visualized through the skin

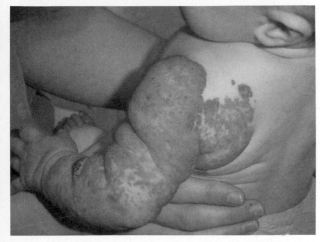

Figure 1 8-month-old female infant with an infantile hemangioma of the left upper extremity.

(Figure 1). A large hemangioma of the liver may present with hepatomegaly, anemia, abdominal compartment syndrome, high-output cardiac failure, or hypothyroidism (due to the expression of a deiodinase that inactivates thyroid hormone).

- Congenital hemangioma is an uncommon type of hemangioma that is fully grown at birth. This tumor may undergo rapid regression over the first year of life (rapidly involuting congenital hemangioma [RICH]) or not involute at all (noninvoluting congenital hemangioma [NICH]).

- Kaposiform hemangioendothelioma (KHE) is a vascular tumor that often is confused with hemangioma. Unlike hemangioma, KHE typically is flat, reddish-purple, present at birth, and usually affects the trunk or extremities. It does not completely regress and can cause Kasabach-Merritt phenomenon (KMP): profound thrombocytopenia (< 10,000 mm³), petechiae, and bleeding.

Postnatal Presentation: Malformations

- Capillary malformation (CM) is macular and can be difficult to distinguish from fading macular stain of infancy (stork-bite

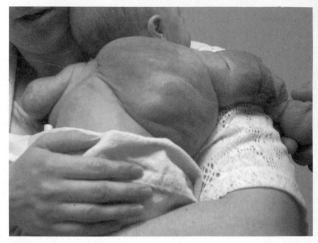

Figure 2 3-month-old female infant with a macrocystic lymphatic malformation of posterior trunk.

or angel kiss). CM may cause soft-tissue or bony overgrowth. When located in the trigeminal nerve distribution (V1 or V2) the child may have Sturge-Weber syndrome. As a result, the patient should have an ophthalmologic examination for glaucoma and an magnetic resonance imaging (MRI) to assess for brain abnormalities.

- Lymphatic malformation (LM) may affect any location as a soft, bulky mass with a bluish hue through the overlying skin (Figure 2). However, it most commonly affects the cervical, facial, supraclavicular, or axillary regions. Cervical involvement should prompt evaluation for extension into the mediastinum. LM may not be obvious at birth and can present later in childhood when symptomatic. Intralesional bleeding and infection are the most common complications. Treatment strategy is based on whether the LM is macrocystic, microcystic, or combined.

- Venous malformation (VM) appears as a purplish, soft, compressible, soft tissue mass that is usually noted at birth and does not change significantly over time (Figure 3). VM of the head and neck may cause significant distortion or airway compromise. Extremity lesions may lead to pathologic fracture or

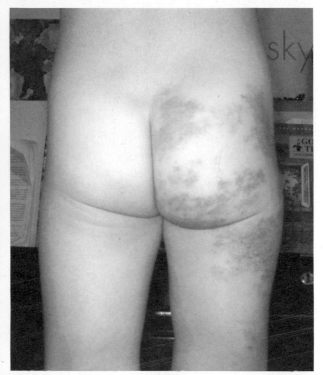

Figure 3 4-year-old female child with a venous malformation of the buttock.

hemarthrosis and degenerative arthritis. A large VM can develop thrombosis leading to pulmonary embolism. Gastrointestinal VM can cause bleeding and anemia. Stagnation within the VM stimulates a localized intravascular coagulopathy and painful phlebothromboses.

- Arteriovenous malformation (AVM) usually is not visible in the neonatal period. The exception is Parkes-Weber syndrome, which is a capillary-lymphatic-arteriovenous malformation with limb overgrowth. AVM is warm and pulsatile and can cause high-output cardiac failure (Figure 4). Severe cases

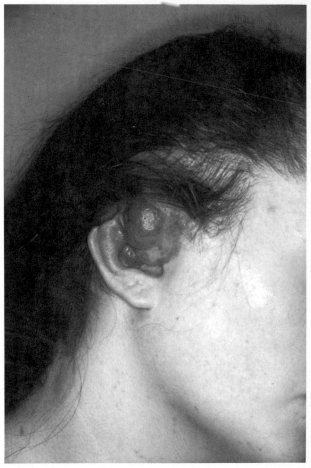

Figure 4   14-year-old girl with an arteriovenous malformation of the ear.

present with antenatal hydrops fetalis and may be fatal. AVM typically worsens over time and may lead to local ischemia, pain, bleeding, shunting, and heart failure.

- The most common combined vascular anomaly is Klippel-Trenaunay syndrome. This eponym denotes capillary-lymphatic-venous-malformation and overgrowth of an extremity. Typically, this syndrome involves the lower extremity and hemipelvis with overgrowth of the leg in both circumference and length. The foot may be massive. Neonatal therapy is not required, although the disfigured foot may require amputation. A shoe lift or epiphysiodesis may be required in childhood. The extremity hemihypertrophy is a local effect of the vascular anomaly, and these patients are not at risk for Wilms tumor and thus do not require serial ultrasonography.

Postnatal Diagnosis

Correct diagnosis of a vascular anomaly can be made by history and physical examination in 90% of patients. When the diagnosis is unclear, radiographic imaging is usually diagnostic; biopsy is rarely necessary.

Tumors

While superficial infantile hemangioma is readily diagnosed by history and physical examination, deep or congenital hemangioma may be more difficult to determine. Ultrasonography or Doppler examination will show high flow and a well-circumcised mass. MRI characteristics include isointensity on T1, hyperintensity on T2 (with fat saturation), and enhancement with contrast. When imaging is not characteristic for hemangioma, then biopsy to rule out malignancy may be indicated. Hemangioendothelioma, tufted angioma, hemangiopericytoma, fibrosarcoma, and lymphoma are proliferating lesions in childhood that can look similar to hemangioma. In the liver, hemangioma may be confused with hepatoblastoma or metastatic neuroblastoma.

Malformations

Like vascular tumors, 90% of vascular malformations may be diagnosed by history or physical examination. Capillary malformation is a superficial lesion and is diagnosed by physical examination. Lymphatic malformation has low flow on ultrasonography and Doppler examination. MRI will show isointensity on T1, hyperintensity on T2, and no enhancement with contrast. Like lymphatic malformation, venous malformation is a low-flow lesion. However, VM will enhance with contrast on MRI study. AVM is a high-flow lesion on ultrasonography with shunting. MRI will show flow voids due to the rapid blood flow through the lesion.

Management

TUMORS

Infantile Hemangioma

- In all, 90% of infantile hemangiomas do not require pharmacological treatment. Parents should be reassured that the lesion will regress. Typically, infantile hemangioma proliferates for approximately 10 months, and then involutes over the following 7 years. After involution, 50% of children have residual fibrofatty tissue or redundant skin that may necessitate resection.
- Approximately 10% of hemangiomas cause significant destruction of tissues, interfere with vital structures, or are life threatening. For example, facial lesions can have serious psychological morbidity. Periorbital tumors can cause amblyopia, astigmatism, or blindness. Subglottic lesions can rapidly asphyxiate the infant, and liver hemangiomas may lead to high-output cardiac failure.
- First-line treatment of problematic hemangioma is corticosteroid, which has an 85% response rate (accelerated involution or stabilization of growth), regardless of the location of the lesion. For small, well-localized lesions, intralesional corticosteroid may be administered. For larger hemangiomas, oral corticosteroid 2 to 3 mg/kg/d of the prednisone equivalent is used for 1 month and then tapered slowly over the next 6 to 8 months. A response should be evident within 7 to 10 days. If there is no response, the steroid dose may be increased up to 5 mg/kg/d.
- Many practitioners are hesitant to give steroids to preterm infants with hemangioma because of data suggesting that corticosteroids

may increase the child's risk of cerebral palsy. Although the risks of giving steroid therapy to any preterm infant must be carefully weighed, there are important safety advantages in the use of corticosteroids to treat hemangioma compared with pulmonary immaturity/chronic lung disease (CLD). Corticosteroid's negative effect on neurodevelopment is dependent on the type of steroid, the infant's weight and gestational age, and the timing of administration. Hemangioma is treated with oral prednisone and not with intravenous dexamethasone. The treatment for hemangioma is initiated at a much older age than for CLD. Infants with CLD receive pharmacotherapy typically in the first few days to weeks of life, whereas the average age and weight of a child treated for problematic hemangioma is 3 months and 5.7 kg, respectively. This is because hemangioma is usually not diagnosed until after 2 weeks of age, and 1 to 2 months of postnatal growth is necessary before the tumor can be identified as problematic, requiring drug treatment. Thus, even in the event that a hemangioma is found to be troublesome in a premature child, several weeks will have passed since birth at the time therapy is initiated.

- Complications of systemic corticosteroid for the management of problematic hemangioma have been studied, and no adverse effects on neurodevelopment have been found. Short-term morbidity includes cushingoid face (71%), personality change (29%), gastric irritation (21%), fungal (oral or perineal) infection (6%), decreased gain in height (35%), and decreased gain in weight (43%). These findings resolve after the completion of therapy. For example, more than 90% of children return to their pretreatment growth curve for height by 24 months of age. The risk of a temporary decrease in height gain falls to 12% for patients given prednisone after 3 months of age and for a course of less than 6 months.

- If steroids fail, interferon-α-2b (2 to 3 million units/m2/d) may be administered. Of note, this therapy is associated with an increased risk for developing spastic diplegia; therefore, the risks and benefits must be very carefully weighed, and the child must be followed by a neurologist. Vincristine also may be considered for children who fail corticosteroid therapy. Subglottic hemangioma may be controlled using endoscopic laser therapy while the lesion is responding to drug treatment.

- A diffuse hemangioma replacing hepatic parenchyma necessitates thyroid stimulating hormone monitoring to prevent irreversible mental retardation. Hypothyroidism results from the expression of a deiodinase by the hemangioma, which cleaves iodine from thyroid hormone and inactivates it. Massive intravenous thyroid replacement may be necessary until the hemangioma regresses. In contrast to diffuse hepatic hemangioma, a large single hemangioma in the liver is often a RICH and does not require intervention. Similarly, multiple small hepatic hemangiomas do not cause morbidity unless significant shunting is present.

Congenital Hemangioma

- RICH is managed by observation because it rapidly involutes postnatally. Most lesions are completely resolved by 12 months of age. Rarely, a large lesion may cause high-output cardiac failure and thus require excision or embolization.
- NICH does not undergo postnatal involution or respond to antiangiogenic therapy. Thus, excision is the mainstay of treatment.

Kaposiform Hemangioendothelioma

- Kaposiform hemangioendothelioma (KHE) with Kasabach-Merritt phenomenon can be fatal. Profound thrombocytopenia will not respond to platelet transfusion because the platelets are trapped in the lesion worsening the swelling. KHE only has a 10% response rate to corticosteroid and a 50% response rate to interferon. As a result, first-line therapy for KHE is often vincristine, which offers an 87% response rate.

MANAGEMENT: MALFORMATIONS

- The cutaneous stain of CM may be lightened with pulsedye laser (585 nm) therapy. Laser treatment also can retard the development of soft tissue overgrowth. Patients with bony overgrowth may require skeletal procedures, including orthognathic treatment.
- Macrocystic LM with channels greater than 5 mm are treated with sclerotherapy. Common sclerosing agents include

doxycycline, 100% ethanol, sodium tetradecyl sulfate, and OK-432 (killed group A *Streptococcus pyogenes*). Excision of macrocystic LM also is possible and may follow sclerotherapy. The only treatment for microcystic LM is resection. Patients with repeated infections may require prophylactic antibiotic treatment. Compression is helpful for extremity lesions.

• First-line treatment for symptomatic VM is compression and aspirin for the prevention and treatment of painful phlebothromboses. Like macrocystic LM, sclerotherapy may effectively shrink VM and can be performed prior to excision to facilitate the resection.

• Treatment of AVM is reserved for symptomatic lesions because intervention can exacerbate its growth. Thus, when excising an AVM, complete extirpation should be the goal, although it is rarely possible. Management of AVM includes embolization, sclerotherapy, excision, or a combination of techniques. Large neonatal high-flow AVMs may require embolization or amputation to control high-output cardiac failure. Typically, embolization is performed 24 to 36 hours prior to resection to reduce bleeding and to facilitate the removal of the AVM.

Recommended Readings

Amir J, Metzker A, Krikler R, Reisner SH. Strawberry hemangioma in preterm infants. Pediatr Dermatol 1986;3:331–2.

Barlow CF, Priebe C, Mulliken JB, et al. Spastic diplegia as a complication of interferon α-2a treatment of hemangiomas of infancy. J Pediatr 1998;132:527–30.

Barnes CM, Huang S, Kaipainen A, et al. Evidence by molecular profiling for a placental origin of infantile hemangioma. Proc Natl Acad Sci U S A 2005;102:19097–102.

Boon LM, Fishman SJ, Lund DP, Mulliken JB. Congenital fibrosarcoma masquerading as congenital hemangioma: report of two cases. J Pediatr Surg 1995;30:1378–81.

Boon LM, MacDonald DM, Mulliken JB. Complications of systemic corticosteroid therapy for problematic hemangioma. Plast Reconstr Surg 1999;104:1616–23.

Christison-Lagay ER, Burrows PE, Alomari A, et al. Hepatic hemangiomas: subtype classification and development of a clinical practice algorithm and registry. J Pediatr Surg 2007;42:62–7.

Finn MC, Glowacki J, Mulliken JB. Congenital vascular lesions: clinical application of a new classification. J Pediatr Surg 1983;18:894–900.

Greene AK, Kieran M, Burrows PE, et al. Wilms tumor screening for Klippel-Trenaunay syndrome is unnecessary. Pediatrics 2004;113:E326–9.

Greene AK, Fishman SJ. Complications of vascular anomalies. In: Caty MG, Levitt MA, Haynes JH, editors. Complications in pediatric surgery: An Individual and Systems Approach. New York, Taylor and Francis (in press).

Huang SA, Tu HM, Harney JW, et al. Severe hypothyroidism caused by type 3 iodothyronine deiodinase in infantile hemangiomas. N Engl J Med 2000;343:185–9.

Marler JM, Fishman SJ, Upton J, et al. Prenatal diagnosis of vascular anomalies. J Pediatr Surg 2002;37:318–26.

Marler JJ, Mulliken JB. Current management of hemangiomas and vascular malformations. Clin Plast Surg 2005;32:99–116.

Mulliken JB, Glowacki J. Hemangiomas and vascular malformations in infants and children: a classification based on endothelial characteristics. Plast Reconstr Surg 1982;69:412–22.

Mulliken JB, Young AE. Vascular birthmarks: hemangiomas and malformations. Philadelphia (PA): WB Saunders; 1988.

Mulliken JB, Fishman SJ, Burrows PE. Vascular anomalies. Curr Prob Surg 2000;37:517–84.

Mulliken JB, Anupindi S, Ezekowitz RA, et al. Case records of the Massachusetts General Hospital. Weekly clinicopathological exercises. Case 13-2004. A newborn girl with a large cutaneous lesion, thrombocytopenia, and anemia. N Engl J Med 2004;350:1764–75.

SIX

Respiratory Disorders

Part 1: Esophageal Atresia and Tracheoesophageal Fistula

Anne R. Hansen, MD, MPH, and
Craig Lillehei, MD

Embryology

- The respiratory system, including the trachea, develops as a ventral outpouching of the primitive foregut when the embryo is 4 weeks old. The esophagotracheal septum forms to separate the esophagus from the trachea. Esophageal atresia (EA), with or without tracheoesophageal fistula (TEF), occurs if this septum fails to completely separate the trachea from the esophagus.
- Types of fistula
  1. EA, distal TEF, 86%
  2. Pure EA, no TEF, 7% (see below)
  3. TEF, no EA, "H type," 4% (see below)
  4. EA, proximal TEF, 3%
  5. EA, with double (distal and proximal) TEF, <1%

Incidence

- The incidence of EA is 1 in 3,000 to 5,000 live births.

Prenatal Diagnosis

- The mother may present with polyhydramnios owing to inability of the fetus to swallow amniotic fluid. A prenatal fetal sonogram is most often normal, although it may show a dilated

pharynx and proximal esophageal pouch and/or small stomach
bubble.
- Polyhydramnios can precipitate preterm labor/delivery.
- Chromosomal analysis should be offered, given the association
between EA/TEF and genetic abnormalities such as trisomies,
especially 18.

Postnatal Clinical Presentation

- Inability to pass a nasogastric suction catheter in delivery
room
- Excessive salivation/drooling/vomiting
- Respiratory distress secondary to aspiration of oral secre-
tions/milk or reflux of gastric secretions through the fistula
- Abdominal distention secondary to air-trapping within the
gastrointestinal tract, especially if bag mask ventilation was
required in the delivery room

Diagnosis

- The first stage of diagnosis is the inability to pass a nasogastric
tube (generally 8 to 10 cm of the tube will pass before encoun-
tering atresia).
- Plain radiography: The tip of the nasogastric tube is seen in an
often-dilated proximal esophageal pouch. The presence of gas
within the gastrointestinal tract helps to distinguish TEF from
isolated EA and may show an associated duodenal atresia.
- Contrast swallow fluoroscopy: Generally, this procedure is
not necessary because air will adequately outline the EA
pouch. It may be helpful for diagnosis of an H-type fistula
but is unreliable.
- Bronchoscopy may be useful for detecting fistulae, particularly
H type and proximal fistulae.

Differential Diagnosis

- Dyscoordinated suck/swallow: The infant spits feedings and
may have associated cyanosis. Diagnostic tests are normal, and
symptoms improve daily.

- Pharyngeal/esophageal perforation (pharyngeal pseudodiverticulum): This is usually caused by attempted passage of an endotracheal or nasogastric tube. If the nasogastric tube is left in place, the falsely tracked tube on plain film can be seen, usually coiled in the right chest. If the tube has been pulled out, the site of perforation can be identified by contrast fluoroscopy.

Preoperative Management

- Gently pass a suction tube (Replogle) into the proximal esophageal pouch. Keep the infant's head elevated 30° to minimize risk of aspiration of oral secretions.
- Discontinue any further enteral intake. Start intravenous fluid. Send blood for pH, PCO_2, PO_2, complete blood count, culture, electrolytes, type, and cross-match.
- Start broad-spectrum antibiotics (generally ampicillin and gentamicin).
- Avoid positive pressure ventilation (ie, CPAP or endotracheal intubation with mechanical ventilation) if possible. If intubation is necessary and there is a distal TEF, the case should be considered a surgical emergency and every effort should be made to transfer the patient to a surgical center as safely and expeditiously as possible.
  1. If the infant must be intubated, position the endotracheal tube just above the level of the carina in the hope of bypassing the fistula.
  2. Rotate the endotracheal tube to position with the bevel facing ventrally, giving the best chance that the (posterior) fistula is sealed off by the endotracheal tube.
  3. If the patient has adequate respiratory effort, provide a trial of spontaneous breathing without additional positive pressure ventilation to avoid preferential passage of air through the fistula into the esophagus instead of the trachea.
  4. If unable to ventilate because of progressive abdominal distention and pulmonary atelectasis owing to the above-described preferential flow through the fistula into the distal esophagus, high-frequency ventilation, purposeful right mainstem intubation, and/or bronchoscopic

placement of a Fogarty catheter into the fistula can be life saving.

- Monitor for abdominal distention owing to flow of air into the gastrointestinal tract from the trachea into the esophagus.[1] Can cause respiratory compromise and decreased venous return secondary to diaphragmatic rise. Treatment is emergency gastrostomy. Failure to treat can lead to gastric perforation, progressive respiratory distress, diminishing cardiac output, and cardiac arrest.

- Avoid heavy sedation and muscle relaxants because spontaneous respiratory effort generates tidal volume with negative rather than positive pressure.

- Assess for associated anomalies, usually other midline defects (seen in more than half of cases).

  1. Cardiac malformations in 20 to 37%: ventricular septal defect, atrial septal defect, patent ductus arteriosus, tetralogy of Fallot, transposition of great arteries, endocardial cushion defects with trisomy 21, and right aortic arch or other aortic arch anomalies[2]

  2. Gastrointestinal anomalies (imperforate anus, duodenal atresia, malrotation) in 21%

  3. Anomalies of the tracheobronchial tree

  4. Musculoskeletal abnormalities (vertebral, rib, or extremity defects)

  5. Chromosomes should be analyzed; approximately 7% of patients with EA/TEF have trisomies, especially 18, but also 13 and 21

  6. Vertebral, anal, cardiac, tracheal, esophageal, renal, and limb (VACTERL) association seen in 5 to 10%:

     a. Vertebral: When the patient is stable postoperatively obtain spine film to assess for vertebral anomalies, and spinal sonogram to assess for tethered cord.

     b. Anus, imperforate: Physical examination is adequate for diagnosis.

     c. Cardiac: See 1. above. In addition, the suspicion of coronary heart disease should be raised by an abnormal position of the umbilical arterial catheter, if present. It is important to have an echocardiogram before surgery or anesthesia to determine presence of congenital heart disease and sidedness of aortic arch.

     d. TEF

   e. Renal: Obtain renal sonogram when the patient is stable postoperatively.

   f. Limb: Physical examination with palpation of radial bone and examination of the thumb is likely adequate; however, plain films are the most thorough way to evaluate for minor anomalies, and radiographic evaluation should certainly be pursued for those with abnormalities detected by physical examination.

   Hydrocephalus (VACTERL-H) has most recently been added to the growing list of associated VATER-type syndromes. Diagnosis is made by head ultrasound if clinically indicated (eg, macrocephaly or a full anterior fontanel).

7. Also seen in association with other multiple anomalies, including CHARGE association (Coloboma, Heart defect, Atresia choanae, Retarded growth, Genital hypoplasia, and Ear anomalies); Potter's syndrome (renal dysfunction with pulmonary hypoplasia); SCHISIS syndrome (cleft lip and palate, omphalocele, and hypogenitalism); and Feingold syndrome (microcephaly, hand and foot abnormalities, esophageal/duodenal atresia)

Anesthesia

- There is a risk of positive pressure breaths preferentially entering the esophagus via the fistula rather than entering the lung. Until the fistula is controlled or a gastrostomy tube is inserted to decompress the stomach, the patient must be carefully monitored to avoid hypoventilation, gastric distention, and decreased venous return.

Surgical Management

A primary repair can usually be accomplished shortly after birth, even in very small infants. Risk factors include severe prematurity, associated congenital anomalies, and pneumonia. With the exception of an H-type fistula (discussed below), repair is performed via a thoracotomy, usually on the infant's right side. The TEF is controlled within the chest to prevent further insufflation of the stomach or gastric reflux into the tracheobronchial tree. After sufficient mobilization of the proximal and distal esophageal pouches, an end-to-end anastomosis is typically performed. There may be considerable size disparity between the bulbous proximal pouch and narrow distal esophagus. If the gap is excessive, the anastomosis may be under considerable tension, which increases the risk of anastomosis leak and/or subsequent esophageal stricture. A chest tube is positioned intraoperatively to drain potential esophageal leakage. If an extrapleural approach is used, this chest tube does not communicate with the free pleural space.

Long gap EA is often defined as a 2.5 to 3 cm distance between the proximal and distal esophageal pouch and is suspected when the proximal pouch does not enter the thoracic inlet as seen on plain chest films. If a gastrostomy tube is placed for feeding and/or gastric decompression, a contrast study through the gastrostomy tube will determine the gap between the proximal pouch and the distal stump. Long gap EA usually occurs in patients without a TEF or if a fistula is present, it is usually more proximal.

There are several approaches to long gap EA. One is to maintain decompression of the proximal pouch and allow growth of the esophagus over an approximately 3-month period and subsequent thoracotomy and repair. Other surgical options include a thoracotomy and a lengthening procedure using myotomies and a primary anastomosis at the same time. In a more recent approach described by Foker, sutures are placed into the proximal and distal pouch and tension is progressively applied to stretch the two ends until they approximate each other. This requires a second thoracotomy and anastomosis between the two esophageal stumps and may be performed entirely thoracoscopically.

The native esophagus is the best conduit. With the above approaches, esophageal replacement surgery with colon, a stomach tube interposition or jejunum is rare. Indications for esophageal replacement include a previously removed or absent esophagus, failure of the above techniques, poor function of the esophagus after primary closure, and long strictures.

ISOLATED EA (WITHOUT TEF)

Embryology, pre and postnatal presentation, diagnosis and management are as above for TEF, except that if the gap between the proximal and distal esophagus is excessively long, the patient may require delayed treatment until the two ends can be approximated. Colonic interposition is increasingly rare.

TEF (WITHOUT EA): H-TYPE FISTULA

Embryology is as above for other TEFs, but lack of EA changes pre and postnatal presentation, diagnosis, and management. The condition is generally not suspected until the infant presents with episodic feeding intolerance, and/or respiratory distress, pneumonia, or abdominal distention. An esophagram with careful lateral views may yield diagnosis. If not, bronchoscopy may be required to visualize the fistula. Surgical repair is performed via a cervical approach.

Postoperative Management

- Continue broad-spectrum antibiotics during the perioperative period.
- Decompress the stomach via continuous drainage of the nasogastric or gastrostomy tube. Because of the risk of injuring the fresh esophageal anastomosis, if the surgeon elects to place a nasogastric tube rather than a gastrostomy tube, it should be placed intraoperatively by the surgeon and should never be passed blindly postoperatively.
- Minimize the volume of swallowed saliva by frequent oral suctioning, with care taken not to insert the suction catheter into the esophagus to the depth of the anastomotic site.
- Maintain pulmonary toilet, again with careful attention to the depth of insertion of the suction catheter to avoid contact with the site of fistula repair.
- Maintain intubation until the risk of extubation failure is low given the risk of reintubation of a freshly postoperative trachea. Infants have an increased risk of tracheomalacia, often responsive to prone positioning, sometimes requiring reintubation, and very occasionally requiring aortopexy.
- If a nasogastric tube is placed in the operating room, it may be left in place until a dye study documents the integrity of the surgical repair (generally obtained 1-week postoperatively). Suck reflex is not consistent or adequate until approximately 34 to 36 weeks' gestation; therefore, the nasogastric tube should be left in place even after dye study until oral feedings are established in infants with a postmenstrual age of < 36 weeks. An oral or naso-gastric tube should never be inserted blindly past a fresh esophageal anastamosis. If a baby is unable to PO feed and does

not have an indwelling gavage tube, the surgeon should be called to discuss the risks and benefits of passing an oral or naso-gastric tube.

- Maintain the chest tube until a dye study shows the integrity of the anastomosis. Extrapleural effusion (looks like pleural effusion by chest radiograph) may be associated with anastomotic leakage.
- All babies s/p EA repair should be treated with antigastro-esophageal reflux (GER) medications including acid blockade +/– a promotility agent. The EA repair itself increases the risk of GER because of tension on the lower esophagus. Furthermore acidic gastric contents will irritate the anastomotic site and increase the risk of stricture.

Complications/Outcome

- The overall survival rate is about 95%. Infants with severe associated anomalies are at the highest morbidity or mortality risk, with survival rates falling to 30 to 50%.
- Common complications include the following[3]:
  1. Esophageal leak owing to development of a postoperative fistula. It generally spontaneously closes in 1 to 2 weeks. The site of the fistula remains at increased risk for later stricture development.
  2. Gastroesophageal reflux. Approximately 40% of patients suffer from gastroesophageal reflux, likely multifactorial, including primary abnormality of esophageal motility, possibly exacerbated by surgical repair, and further exacerbated by a short component of the intra-abdominal esophagus, with resultant effect on the competency of the lower esophageal sphincter. It can usually be treated with thickened, small-volume feedings, prokinetic agents, and H2 blockers but occasionally requires antireflux surgery.
  3. Anastomotic stricture (exacerbated by reflux), which can be monitored with serial esophagrams and treated with dilation.[4] The cause of these strictures is generally multifactorial including tension, GER, and anastomotic leak.
  4. Tracheomalacia may be caused by compression of the proximal trachea by the distended esophagus during fetal development. It may require prolonged positive pressure ventilation. Tracheomalacia usually improves spontaneously

as the tracheal rings harden; however, it sometimes requires treatment with aortopexy.

5. Recurrent aspiration. The source can be a missed fistula, recurrent TEF, pooling of esophageal secretions proximal to a stricture, GER or injured recurrent laryngeal nerve. Treatment is determined by etiology.

6. Injured recurrent laryngeal nerve (particularly with repair of an H-type TEF). It may present as hoarse cry/voice +/– recurrent aspiration. Especially if the injury is unilateral, it generally improves over time and can be managed conservatively with observation and evaluation for aspiration (see chapter 3).

• The long-term effects of original surgery as well as the above-described complications can result in poor growth, recurrent respiratory infections and wheezing, chest wall deformities, and scoliosis.

References

1. Seibens AA. Mechanisms of gastric distention in esophageal atresia with distal tracheoesophageal fistula. Dysphagia 1996;11:90–2.

2. Canty TG Jr, Boyle EM Jr, Linden B, et al. Aortic arch anomalies associated with long gap esophageal atresia and tracheoesophageal fistula. J Pediatr Surg 1997;32:1587–91.

3. Tsai JY, Berkery L, Wesson DE, et al. Esophageal atresia and tracheoesophageal fistula: surgical experience of two decades. Ann Thorac Surg 1997;64:778–83 [Discussion 783–4].

4. Allmendinger N, Hallisey MJ, Markowitz SK, et al. Balloon dilation of esophageal strictures in children. J Pediatr Surg 1996; 31:334–6.

Recommended Readings

Dillon PW, Krummel TM. Chest. In: Levine BA, Copeland EM III, Howard RJ, et al, editors. Current practice of pediatric surgery. Vol XVIII. New York: Churchill Livingstone; 1994. p. 9–12.

Foker JE, Linden BC, Boyle EM, et al. Development of a true primary repair for the full spectrum of esophageal atresia. Ann Surg 1997; 226:533–43.

Georgeson KD, Robertson DJ. Minimally invasive surgery in the neonate: review of current evidence. Semin Perinatol 2004;28:212–20.

Manning PB, Morgan RA, Coran AG, et al. Fifty years' experience with esophageal atresia and tracheoesophageal fistula. Ann Surg 1986;204:446–53.

Nakayama DK. Esophageal atresia and tracheoesophageal fistula. In: Nakayama DK, Bose CL, Chescheir NC, Valley RD, editors. Critical care of surgical newborn. Armonk (NY): Futura; 1997. p. 227–47.

Orford J, Cass DT, Glasson MJ. Advances in the treatment of oesophageal atresia over three decades: the 1970's and the 1990's. Pediatr Surg Int 2004;20:402–7 [Epub 2004 May 18].

Spitz L. Esophageal atresia: past, present, and future. J Pediatr Surg 1996;31:19–25.

Van der Zee, DC, Vieirra-ravassos, Kramer, WLM, Tytgat S. Thoracoscopic elongation of the esophagus in long gap esophageal atresia. J Pediatr Surg 2007;42:1785–8.

Part 2: Congenital Diaphragmatic Hernia and Diaphragmatic Eventration

Monica E. Kleinman, MD, and
Jay M. Wilson, MD

Embryology

- 8 to 10 weeks gestation: A diaphragmatic defect occurs because of failure of closure of the pleuro-peritoneal canal, most commonly in the posterolateral aspect of the diaphragm (Bochdalek hernia). The abdominal viscera may herniate into the thoracic cavity on the ipsilateral side at any time after return of the midgut structures to the abdomen at 9 to 10 weeks of gestation.
- The presence of abdominal viscera in the thoracic cavity prohibits lung growth and development, resulting in pulmonary hypoplasia with reduction in the total number of bronchial and arterial branches and medial muscular hypertrophy of the preacinar and intra-acinar arterioles. While the ipsilateral lung is most severely affected, the contralateral lung may also have abnormal architecture and decreased mass because of mediastinal shift or, potentially, intrinsic pulmonary developmental abnormalities.

Classification

- Left-sided hernia: ~ 80%
- Right-sided hernia: ~ 20%
- Bilateral hernias: < 1%

Incidence

- ~ 1 in 4,000 live births
- Male:female ratio = 1:1
- Associated anomalies (occur in 50%):
  1. Chromosomal disorders and syndromes
     a. Trisomy 18
     b. Turner syndrome (45XO)
     c. Fryns syndrome

      d. Chromosome 27 deletion (small arm)
      e. Goldenhar syndrome
      f. Beckwith-Wiedemann syndrome
      g. Pierre-Robin sequence
      h. Goultz-Goulen syndrome
      i. Congenital rubella syndrome
      j. Pallister-Killian syndrome (tetrasomy 12p)
      k. Wolf-Hirschhorn syndrome (4p deletion)
2. Structural malformations
      a. Congenital heart disease
      b. Neural tube defects
      c. Skeletal anomalies
      d. Intestinal atresias
      e. Renal anomalies

Prenatal Diagnosis

- Pregnancy may be notable for polyhydramnios.
- Prenatal ultrasound can detect the presence of intestinal contents in the thorax as early as ~12 weeks of gestation. However, the lesion may still not be detectable at the routine 16-week ultrasound. This will be falsely reassuring if there are no other complications (eg, polyhydramnios) prompting a follow-up ultrasound.
- The importance of prenatal diagnosis is related to the following:
  1. Evaluation for associated anomalies or genetic syndromes
  2. Maternal counseling regarding delivery in a center with expertise in the management of congenital diaphragmatic hernia (CDH)
  3. Consideration of prenatal surgical intervention in clinical trials
  4. Anticipation of high-risk delivery by neonatology and surgical teams, including the option for ex-utero intrapartum therapy (EXIT)

Postnatal Clinical Presentation

- Most infants with CDH have onset of respiratory distress and cyanosis in the delivery room.

- Approximately 5% will be minimally symptomatic or asymptomatic at birth and will be diagnosed later in infancy or childhood.
- Physical examination may also show:
  1. a scaphoid abdomen,
  2. absence of breath sounds (and, perhaps, presence of bowel sounds) on the ipsilateral side, and
  3. displacement of heart sounds to the contralateral side.

Differential Diagnosis

- Intrathoracic masses
  1. Congenital cystic adenomatoid malformation
  2. Bronchogenic cyst
- Diaphragmatic eventration

Preoperative Management

DELIVERY ROOM RESUSCITATION

- For those infants with an antenatal diagnosis of CDH, avoid positive pressure ventilation via bag and face mask. Tracheal intubation should be performed rapidly by a skilled member of the resuscitation team.
- Immediately after the airway is secured, a large-bore multiple hole sump naso- or orogastric tube should be placed and attached to continuous suction.

Interfacility Transport

TEAM COMPOSITION

- A specialized neonatal transport team should respond to provide pretransport stabilization and ongoing critical care.

PRETRANSPORT STABILIZATION

- Any infant with a suspected CDH should undergo tracheal intubation before transport. Nasal continuous positive airway pressure (CPAP) is contraindicated.
- If not already performed, place a large-bore multiple hole sump naso- or orogastric tube and attach to continuous suction.

MODE OF TRANSPORT

- The decision to transport by air or ground should take into consideration the potential risks and benefits of each mode.
- If air transport is planned, rotor wing aircraft should fly at the lowest possible safe altitude. For fixed-wing air transport, the cabin should be pressurized to as close to sea level as possible, to avoid worsening of hypoxemia and/or expansion of air in the intrathoracic intestinal tract, which may further compromise cardiopulmonary function.

Preoperative Intensive Care Unit Management

MONITORING

- All infants admitted to the ICU with a diagnosis of congenital diaphragmatic hernia should be monitored with standard cardiorespiratory, NIBP, and temperature monitors. Pulse oximetry probes placed preductally (right arm or earlobe) and postductally (lower extremities) will indicate the presence of right-to-left ductal shunting, which, in turn, reflects the degree of pulmonary hypertension.
- An indwelling arterial catheter should be placed to provide continuous monitoring of blood pressure and frequent analyses of blood gases. Ideally, a right radial arterial catheter is placed to measure preductal PaO_2. The use of an umbilical arterial catheter may be less useful because it reflects postductal oxygen levels. In addition, umbilical arterial catheters may need to be removed in the process of surgical repair using a transabdominal approach.
- Central venous pressure monitoring may be useful to titrate intravascular volume administration. However, it may be technically difficult to pass an umbilical venous catheter into a central location because of displacement of the ductus venosus and right atrium. Percutaneous central venous access may be considered to provide vascular access for vasoactive infusions. Cannulation of the internal and external jugular veins should be avoided in the event that extracorporeal support is required.

RESPIRATORY CARE

- In the presence of significant pulmonary hypoplasia, the newborn will attempt to compensate with tachypnea. Preferably, intubated newborns with congenital diaphragmatic hernia should be permitted to breathe spontaneously using a synchronized ventilator mode. One option is neonatal pressure support, a mode that provides an assist-control, time-cycled, pressure-limited ventilatory pattern that is flow-triggered and provides a back-up control rate. This mode permits the newborn to determine its own tidal volume and respiratory rate, and can support even the most tachypneic infants because of the short inspiratory time. If SIMV is used, the rate is adjusted to provide adequate ventilatory support while maintaining patient-ventilator synchrony, usually 25 to 35 breaths/min.

- Goals for gas exchange should include a strategy of permissive hypercarbia so as to avoid ventilator-induced lung injury:

  1. Respiratory acidosis should be tolerated as long as arterial pH $\geq$ 7.25. Peak inspiratory pressure should be adjusted to achieve a tidal volume of 3 to 5 mL/kg and, ideally, should not exceed 25 cm H_2O. Low levels of PEEP (3 to 4 cm H_2O) are preferred.

  2. Preductal oxygen saturations are used to monitor oxygenation. The FiO_2 is adjusted to maintain preductal $SpO_2 \geq 90\%$ and the patient is monitored for metabolic acidosis and elevated lactate as an indicator of inadequate tissue oxygen delivery. $NaHCO_3$ 1 to 2 meq/kg or THAM 1 to 2 mL/kg may be administered as buffers if needed. However, continued metabolic acidosis and increasing lactate are indications for extracorporeal membrane oxygenation (ECMO).

  3. Significant respiratory or metabolic acidosis despite a pressure limit (PIP) $\geq$ 30 cm H_2O, or persistent hypoxemia while using an FiO_2 of 1, should prompt consideration of alternative modes of respiratory support:

     a. High frequency oscillatory ventilation may be used as a rescue therapy if adequate gas exchange cannot be achieved with conventional ventilation, but may not be successful. It has shown promise when used as a primary mode of ventilation.

b. Inhaled nitric oxide has been shown to reduce the need for ECMO for all causes of hypoxemic respiratory failure in term and near-term infants *with the exception of congenital diaphragmatic hernia*. However, its use to decrease right ventricular hypertension and dysfunction may be beneficial.

c. Surfactant replacement therapy has been advocated because the lungs of both human and animal subjects with CDH have been shown to be surfactant deficient. However, there have been no clinical trials to support the recommendation for exogenous surfactant administration on a routine basis. If exogenous surfactant is used it should be administered slowly, as bolus therapy has been reported to cause acute deterioration.

d. ECMO has been used as a rescue therapy for those infants who fail aggressive yet less invasive treatment.

Criteria for initiation of ECMO support in the neonate with CDH include persistent hypoxemia (preductal PaO_2 < 50 mm Hg) or hypotension (MAP < 35 mm Hg) with inadequate oxygen delivery despite optimal ventilatory and/or hemodynamic support. The decision to use venovenous versus veno-arterial ECMO is based on the evaluation of right heart function. For patients with insufficient gas exchange but good ventricular function, veno-venous ECMO may be adequate. Infants with right ventricular failure are candidates for veno-arterial ECMO to decompress the right heart and support cardiac output.

CARDIOVASCULAR SUPPORT

- Hypotension is a common finding during the initial stabilization of the infant with CDH. The presence of a mass-occupying lesion in one hemithorax and subsequent midline shift distort the relation of the great veins to the right atrium, reducing venous return and cardiac output. Positive-pressure ventilation further reduces venous return. Elevated pulmonary vascular resistance results in right ventricular hypertension with subsequent bowing of the interventricular septum into the left ventricle, reducing end-diastolic volume, and stroke volume.

- For term newborns, the systolic blood pressure should be maintained ≥ 45 to 50 mm Hg. The initial approach to hypotension is the judicious use of IV fluids. Small (5 to 10 mL/kg) boluses of normal saline or 5% albumin may be used to improve cardiac filling. However, the pulmonary function of infants with CDH is exquisitely sensitive to intravascular volume. The use of vasopressors such as dopamine should be considered early during initial stabilization if the infant remains hypotensive despite approximately 20 mL/kg of IV fluids.

- All infants with a diagnosis of CDH should undergo a cardiac ECHO to evaluate for the presence of congenital heart defects, to assess left ventricular size and volume, and to estimate right ventricular pressure. Even if the prenatal ECHO shows normal anatomy, abnormalities such as coarctation of the aorta may be difficult to diagnose in utero. The left ventricle often appears small because of decreased preload in the setting of high pulmonary vascular resistance as well as septal deviation and compression by the hypertensive right ventricle. In the absence of mitral or aortic valve abnormalities, this is not considered true "hypoplasia."

- Right ventricular dysfunction may occur because of suprasystemic pulmonary artery pressures, and is an indication for inotropic support with an infusion of dopamine or dobutamine. Reduction of right ventricular afterload can be achieved with medications such as milrinone, a phosphodiesterase inhibitor that also increases contractility. Because systemic vasodilation may necessitate the need for additional volume therapy, the use of inhaled nitric oxide as a selective pulmonary vasodilator may be preferable. Although nitric oxide has not been shown to alter outcome in a large population of infants with CDH, it may be useful to reduce right ventricular afterload in those patients with severe pulmonary hypertension and evidence of significant right ventricular dysfunction. If the ductus arteriosus is restrictive, some centers have advocated for the use of a PGE_1 infusion to improve ductal patency so that right-to-left shunting can help to decompress the hypertensive pulmonary artery.

- Persistent hypotension, including the need for an epinephrine infusion to maintain minimal systolic blood pressures, is indicative of right ventricular failure and should lead to strong consideration for use of ECMO.

FLUIDS, ELECTROLYTES, AND NUTRITION

- During the preoperative phase, intubated infants with CDH have approximately the same insensible water losses as those with a comparable gestational age being cared for on a radiant warmer.
- An infusion of 10% dextrose in water should be provided, with electrolyte supplementation when indicated by routine monitoring of serum electrolytes. Significant losses via the nasogastric tube should be replaced if the volume exceeds 10 mL/kg every 12 hours. A urine output of 0.5 to 1 mL/kg is indicative of adequate renal perfusion, although may not be reliable in the first 24 hours of life. A screening renal ultrasound is recommended after birth because of the association of CDH with renal anomalies.
- Because a prolonged period of non-enteral nutrition can be anticipated, total parenteral nutrition should be initiated on the second or third day of life. Central venous access via a percutaneous catheter should be considered early in the ICU course to provide adequate caloric intake.
- As with other newborn infants, a minimum glucose infusion of 5 to 7 mg/kg/min is required to meet metabolic demands. Calcium supplementation is frequently required in the stressed newborn.

PAIN MANAGEMENT AND SEDATION/NEUROLOGIC CONSIDERATIONS

- Intubated newborns with CDH may benefit from intermittent sedation to tolerate mechanical ventilation. However, sedatives should be administered judiciously because of the risk of respiratory depression, which could necessitate conversion to a controlled mode of ventilation.
  1. Fentanyl, 1 to 2 mcg/kg and midazolam, 0.05 to 0.1 mg/kg are usually effective. Midazolam should be avoided in infants less than 35 weeks gestation because of possible neurologic side effects.
  2. Neuromuscular blockade should be avoided if possible because the conversion to a control mode of mechanical

ventilation usually results in worsening gas exchange and hemodynamics.

- A baseline head ultrasound should be obtained on all infants admitted to the ICU with a diagnosis of CDH to assess for the presence of intracranial hemorrhage, in anticipation of the potential need for ECMO therapy. If the infant requires ECMO, head ultrasounds should be performed at least every other day or more frequently if there are changes in the infant's neurologic exam.

INFECTIOUS DISEASE

- All infants with CDH should receive empiric antibiotic therapy with ampicillin and gentamicin to protect against perinatally acquired infections. If the infant requires ECMO, oxacillin should be added to cover nosocomially-acquired gram-positive organisms.
- Other antimicrobial therapy should be considered based on maternal history and clinical assessment.

HEMATOLOGY

- Routine admission laboratory work should include a complete blood count and differential.
- A type and screen will facilitate the availability of blood products should they be needed for preoperative stabilization and/or priming of an ECMO circuit.
- If dysmorphic features or other anomalies are present, a sample of blood for chromosomal analysis should be obtained before red blood cell transfusion.

Surgical Management

TIMING OF OPERATION

- Operative repair of the defect should be delayed until such time as the infant has achieved an acceptable state of cardiorespiratory stability in the setting of a transitional circulation.
  1. In patients without evidence of significant pulmonary hypertension or hemodynamic lability, surgery can usually be performed safely at 24 to 36 hours of age. Newborns

with evidence of significant pulmonary hypertension or right ventricular dysfunction are best served by delaying surgery until hemodynamic stability is achieved.

2. For patients on ECMO, repair can be successfully performed at any point unless there are complicating factors such as infection or other co-morbidities. Earlier repair is easier because there is less edema but carries with it the risk of bleeding. Repair can also be performed after decannulation from ECMO if desired.

SURGICAL TECHNIQUES

- The abdominal approach is preferable to the thoracic approach in all situations.
- A subcostal incision on the side of the defect is performed and the intestinal contents are removed from the chest.
- If the patient is not on ECMO, the posterior diaphragmatic lip can be mobilized in an attempt to achieve a primary repair. If this is not possible, a patch of artificial material such as Gore-Tex can be fashioned and used. It is sutured in place with non-absorbable sutures.
- If the baby is on ECMO, no attempt should be made to dissect the posterior flap because that is frequently the site of postoperative bleeding. A generous patch should be fashioned and sutured with interrupted absorbable sutures to the diaphragmatic remnants. Laterally where the diaphragmatic remnant disappears, sutures should be placed around the ribs.
- The abdominal closure should be without significant tension if a generous enough patch has been fashioned.

TUBES AND LINES

- In patients not on ECMO, it is not necessary to place an ipsilateral chest tube as the resulting pneumothorax is because of the absence of lung tissue. Some surgeons believe that placement of a chest tube may facilitate expansion of the hypoplastic lung by draining some of the fluid which ultimately fills the void in the pleural space.
- Patients on ECMO may benefit from a chest tube in the ipsilateral chest to monitor postoperative blood loss. It can be removed shortly after decannulation.

- Central venous lines are generally placed at the conclusion of the operative repair to facilitate postoperative management including parenteral nutrition.

INTRAOPERATIVE AND POSTOPERATIVE ANALGESIA

- In patients not on ECMO, it is desirable to place an epidural catheter before the operation to minimize the intraoperative stress response. This epidural catheter can be maintained for several days postoperatively which allows more effective use of spontaneous ventilator modes by avoiding the respiratory depressant effects of parenteral narcotics.
- Because the standard anesthesia machines have a high dead space, patients may benefit from intraoperative ventilation with the same ventilator used in the intensive care unit using SIMV mode because of neuromuscular blockade. For this reason, a narcotic technique is typically favored over use of inhalation anesthetics.

Postoperative Management

RESPIRATORY CARE

- In the immediate postoperative period, the newborn will require controlled ventilation while still under the effects of anesthesia and neuromuscular blockade. As soon as there is adequate recovery of spontaneous respiratory effort, the patient should be converted back to a synchronized, assisted ventilatory pattern. Tidal volume monitoring should be performed to establish trends in lung volume over time.
- The initial postoperative chest radiograph is likely to show a large pneumothorax on the side of the repaired diaphragmatic hernia. The air collection may appear to be under tension because the mediastinal structures do not immediately return to the midline after reduction of the intrathoracic intestines.
- If a chest tube has been placed at the time of surgery, it is placed to water seal or to a very low level of suction (ie, −5 cm H_2O) because its purpose is to drain air or fluid under pressure. Placing the chest tube to suction produces a negative pressure in the hemithorax and may cause undesirable

hemodynamic effects by prematurely reducing the midline shift and placing tension on the great vessels.
- Over time, the pneumothorax is gradually replaced with fluid and there is progressive expansion of the hypoplastic lung. Chylothorax occurs in up to 20% of newborns following repair of a diaphragmatic hernia and may be an indication for continued chest drainage and/or placement of a thoracostomy tube if one was not placed intraoperatively.
- Weaning from mechanical ventilation may occur over days to weeks, depending upon the degree of pulmonary hypoplasia and perinatal and/or perioperative complications. The pressure limit (PIP) is reduced by 1 to 2 cm H_2O per day while monitoring respiratory rate, pH and P_{CO_2}, and exhaled tidal volume. Criteria for extubation include:
  1. Minimal ventilator settings, usually a pressure support level of 12 over a PEEP of 3 to 4 cm H_2O (PIP 16 over PEEP 3 – 4), with an exhaled tidal volume of 4 to 5 mL/kg, and low FiO_2 (< 0.04).
  2. low FiO_2 ($\leq$ 0.4).
  3. Adequate gas exchange without excessive work or rate of breathing, although the respiratory rate is expected to be elevated. $PaCO_2$s are typically elevated as with other forms of chronic lung disease and are tolerated as long as they are not excessive. A partially compensated metabolic alkalosis commonly develops in the setting of hypercarbia and may be exacerbated but the use of diuretics.

CARDIOVASCULAR SUPPORT

- Blood loss with congenital diaphragmatic hernia repair is usually minimal.
- Fluid and pressor requirements are not typically increased in the postoperative period. As with the preoperative phase, fluids should be administered judiciously to prevent significant changes in lung compliance.
- Significant hypotension or oliguria in the immediate postoperative period should prompt a search for sources of bleeding and/or reduced venous return, such as tension pneumothorax or abdominal compartment syndrome (see below).

FLUIDS, ELECTROLYTES, AND NUTRITION

- Parenteral nutrition should be continued or initiated in the post-operative period. Routine monitoring of electrolytes, glucose, and calcium is indicated, with supplementation as required.
- Urine output must be closely monitored. Intestinal reduction is usually well tolerated, but, in some infants, there is an acute increase in intra-abdominal pressure with development of abdominal compartment syndrome, manifested as a tense abdomen with plethora and edema of the lower extremities from venous congestion. Ultimately, renal perfusion will be compromised, as manifested by oliguria and rising serum creatinine. In severe cases, the abdominal fascia may need to be opened to relieve pressure.
- Diuretic therapy is almost always indicated after any perioperative capillary leak has resolved. If renal function is normal or only mildly impaired, lasix can be administered up to four times per day or by continuous infusion if intermittent diuresis is not tolerated hemodynamically. Hypokalemia and hypochloremia are common with use of lasix, and supplemental potassium chloride should be administered as needed to maintain a serum potassium > 3 meq/L. Excessive use of diuretics, coupled with chronic respiratory acidosis, may lead to a state of metabolic alkalosis that may benefit from a single dose of acetazolamide, to transiently promote excretion of bicarbonate and to avoid severe hypochloremia.
- Enteral feedings are delayed until bowel function has clearly been established, as evidenced by minimal nasogastric drainage, presence of bowel sounds, and passage of stool. The majority of infants will not tolerate gastric feeds because of delayed gastric emptying and gastro-esophageal reflux. A transpyloric tube is frequently difficult to place at the bedside because of malposition of the intestines, and may require use of fluoroscopy. Continuous feeds are initiated at 1 mL/kg/h and gradually advanced as tolerated.
- Following extubation, caloric needs may be significantly increased by tachypnea and increased work of breathing. Weight must be monitored closely and caloric intake adjusted

as needed; up to 180 kcal/kg/d has been required to achieve growth in some patients with chronic lung disease.

PAIN MANAGEMENT AND SEDATION/NEUROLOGIC CONSIDERATIONS

- The use of epidural analgesia has been a major advantage for neonates undergoing thoraco-abdominal surgery, including CDH repair. An infusion of bupivicane and fentanyl is commonly used, and the catheter left in place for 3 to 4 days, whereas the infant is permitted to recover from surgery and to breathe in a spontaneous, assisted mode with adequate analgesia.
- Following removal of the epidural catheter, intermittent doses of morphine and acetaminophen should be administered based on regular assessments of the infant's level of discomfort.
- Newborns who require cannulation for ECMO before surgical repair of the diaphragmatic hernia cannot receive epidural analgesia because of the risks of catheter placement associated with systemic heparinization. Those infants are commonly treated with continuous infusions of morphine for analgesia before surgery, and narcotic needs are expected to increase postoperatively. Although fentanyl may have a superior hemodynamic profile, it binds to the membrane oxygenator, making dosing needs unpredictable during ECMO. Morphine is the preferred agent for analgesia while the infant is receiving extracorporeal support.
- Sedation is usually required postoperatively to ensure tolerance of mechanical ventilation. Lorazepam or midazolam are acceptable choices and may be administered intermittently or by continuous infusion, depending on assessment of the infant's comfort. High doses of lorazepam should be avoided because of the potential toxicity of its medium, propylene glycol, which can cause hyperosmolarity and metabolic acidosis. Midazolam should be avoided in infants less than 35 weeks' gestation because of potential neurologic side effects.

INFECTIOUS DISEASE

- Postoperatively, empiric antibiotic therapy should be continued with ampicillin and gentamicin, as well as oxacillin if the infant is receiving ECMO. In general, antibiotics are continued until removal of invasive lines and chest tubes.

- Late deterioration of the infant treated with a long course of antibiotic therapy should prompt evaluation for resistant nosocomially acquired organisms or fungal infection.
- Infants whose postoperative course is complicated by a chylothorax may be at risk for lymphocyte depletion and hypogammaglobulinemia if there is a significant volume of drainage daily. These patients should have immunoglobulin levels monitored and replacement therapy with IVIG once IgG levels are below normal. Prolonged lymphopenia places the infant at risk for viral, fungal, and atypical infections.

HEMATOLOGY

- Many newborns with CDH will require transfusion with red blood cells during the course of hospitalization.
- Those infants treated with ECMO invariably receive multiple transfusions of blood products. To minimize postoperative bleeding complications, infants on ECMO receive aminocaproic acid (Amicar™) for at least 72 hours following surgery.

Complications/Outcome

MORTALITY

- Survival rates vary greatly among tertiary care centers. With the adoption of a strategy of permissive hypercapnea to minimize ventilator-induced lung injury, survival rates of 80 to 90% have been reported. The volume–outcome relationship is another consideration, with increased survival reported in centers that have developed a standardized approach to management with an adequate number of patients per year.
- Good prognostic factors include absence of liver herniation into the thorax, late (> 25 weeks) herniation into the hemithorax, and absence of co-existing congenital anomalies. The co-existence of CDH and congenital cardiac malformations significantly decreases survival. Defect size, as reflected by the necessity of patch repair, is also associated with survival.
- Recently the use of lung-to-head ratio (LHR) has been used to identify high-risk infants who may be appropriate candidates for fetal surgery. Calculated by ultrasound between 24 and 26 weeks

gestation, no fetuses with an LHR of < 1 survived, and all with an LHR of > 1.4 survived. LHR values between 1 and 1.4 correlated with a survival rate of 38% and a high rate of ECMO use (75%).

MORBIDITY

Chronic Lung Disease

Chronic pulmonary conditions can include reactive airway disease, chronic lung disease with oxygen and/or diuretic dependence, or bronchiectasis.

Cardiac Sequelae

In the absence of structural heart disease, most infants born with congenital diaphragmatic hernia will have normal cardiac function after recovery from surgery. A subset of patients will continue to manifest clinically significant pulmonary hypertension that may require prolonged treatment. Recently, the use of sildenafil has shown promise for those infants with persistent ECHO-documented pulmonary hypertension. Systemic hypertension may co-exist, necessitating the use of antihypertensive medications such as hydralazine or captopril.

Fluids, Electrolytes, and Nutrition

Persistent problems with gastro-esophageal reflux and oral aversion frequently necessitate placement of a gastrostomy tube with Nissen fundoplication for long-term nutritional management.

Neurologic Sequelae

All infants with CDH, including those who do not require treatment with ECMO, should receive close developmental and neurologic follow-up because of the risks of neurologic sequelae such as hearing loss, developmental delay, and motor deficits.

Infectious Disease

Infants with CDH who survive with chronic lung disease should receive routine childhood vaccinations. Immunization to attenuate infection from respiratory syncytial virus is indicated for the first 2 years of life. Palizumab (Synagis) may be administered as a monthly IM injection during RSV season, usually November through April. Once the infant reaches 6 months of age, annual immunization against influenza is recommended.

Diaphragmatic Eventration

DEFINITION

Eventration occurs when there is substantial thinning of the diaphragmatic leaflets, permitting abdominal contents to enter into the chest cavity. Eventration and sac-like diaphragmatic hernia represent a continuum of diaphragmaric developmental abnormalities.

ETIOLOGY

- Eventration of the diaphragm may be either congenital or acquired. The acquired lesion is often because of the paralysis of the phrenic nerve.
- The congenital form is frequently indistinguishable from a diaphragmatic hernia with a sac.

SYMPTOMS

- Even large eventrations may be completely asymptomatic.
- Frequent symptoms include wheezing, respiratory infections, exercise intolerance. Severe eventrations are associated with pulmonary hypoplasia.

DIAGNOSIS

- Diagnosis is best made with fluoroscopy of the chest where the diaphragm will move paradoxically with the respiratory motion.
- CT or MRI scan are now used frequently used to make the diagnosis as well.

TREATMENT

- Small everntrations may be left untreated.
- Large eventrations should be repaired even when asymptomatic to allow ipsilateral lung growth.

- Repair may be performed through either the abdomen or chest but usually the thoracotomy is best.
- Repair is achieved through pleating of the diaphragm with a non-absorbable suture.

References/Recommended Readings

Congenital Diaphragmatic Study Group. Defect size determines survival in infants with congenital diaphragmatic hernia. Pediatrics 2007;120:e651–7.

Glick PL, Leach CL, Besner GE, et al. Pathophysiology of congenital diaphragmatic hernia . III. Exogenous surfactant therapy for the high-risk infant with CDH. J Pediatr Surg 1992;27:866–9.

Harrison MR, Mychaliska GB, Albanese CT, et al. Correction of congenital diaphragmatic hernia in utero IX: Fetuses with poor prognosis (liver herniation and low lung-to-head ratio) can be saved by fetoscopic temporary tracheal occlusion. J Pediatr Surg 1998;33:1017–23.

Javid PJ, Jaksic T, Skarsgard ED. Survival rate in congenital diaphragmatic hernia: the experience of the Canadian neonatal network. J Pediatr Surg 2004;39:657–60.

Kaiser JR, Rosenfeld CR. A population-based study of congenital diaphragmatic hernia: Impact of associated anomalies and preoperative blood gases on survival. J Pediatr Surg 1999;34:1196–202.

Kays DW, Langham MR, Ledbetter DJ, Talbert JL. Detrimental effects of standard medical therapy in congenital diaphragmatic hernia. Ann Surg 1999;3:340–51.

Lin AE, Pober BR, Adatia I. Congenital diaphragmatic hernia and associated cardiovascular malformations: Type, frequency, and impact on management. Am J Med Genet Part C Semin Med Genet 2007;145:201–16.

Logan JW, Rice HE, Goldberg RN, Cotten CM. Congenital diaphragmatic hernia: A systematic review and summary of best-evidence practice strategies. J Perinat 2007;27:535–49.

Muratore, DS, Wilson, JM. Congenital diaphragmatic hernia: where are we and where do we go from here? Semin Perinatol 2000;24:418–28.

Nio M, Haase G, Kennaugh J, et al. A prospective, randomized trial of delayed vs. immediate repair of congenital diaphragmatic hernia. J Pediatr Surg 1994;29:618–21.

The Congenital Diaphragmatic Hernia Study Group. Does extracorporeal membrane oxygenation improve survival in neonates with congenital diaphragmatic hernia? J Pediatr Surg 1999;34:720–5.

The Neonatal Inhaled Nitric Oxide Study Group (NINOS). Inhaled nitric oxide and hypoxic respiratory failure in infants with congenital diaphragmatic hernia. Pediatrics 1997;99:838–45.

Wilson JM, Lund DP, Lillehei CW, Vacanti JP. Congenital diaphragmatic hernia—a tale of two cities: the Boston experience. J Pediatr Surg 1997;32:401–5.

Wung JT, Sahni R, Moffitt ST, et al. Congenital diaphragmatic hernia: survival treated with very delayed surgery, spontaneous respiration, and no chest tube. J Pediatr Surg 1995;30:406–9.

Part 3: Pneumothorax and Air Leak

Steven A. Ringer, MD, PhD, FAAP

Most pulmonary disease in the neonate is attributable to those processes that affect the air spaces, such as respiratory distress syndrome (RDS) and pneumonia. With appropriate medical treatment, these disorders are usually acute and time limited and neither require nor are amenable to surgical intervention. As such, those disorders are not included in this review, with the exception of air leaks, which can occur as a complication of these disorders. The focus will be on those congenital and developmental abnormalities that require intervention at birth or in the neonatal period.

Definitions and Incidence

Air leak (not including pneumoperitoneum) refers to an abnormal collection of gas outside the alveoli of the lung that originates from the alveoli. These collections may occur in the pleural space (pneumothorax), the lung parenchyma (interstitial emphysema), the mediastinum (pneumomediastinum), the pericardial space (pneumopericardium), or the vascular space (systemic air embolus).

Air leak is more common in the neonate than in any other age group, with the vast majority being pneumothoraces. The incidence of pneumothorax in otherwise healthy infants is approximately 0.1%, the majority of which are spontaneously occurring and asymptomatic. Most of these are never detected or are discovered only as an incidental finding during evaluation for another problem. Only about 1 in 10,000 healthy infants will have a symptomatic air leak.

The incidence is much higher in infants with underlying lung disease, particularly those who require mechanical ventilation including continuous positive airway pressure. The peak times of occurrence are in the immediate period after birth when higher distending pressures may be used to ventilate the baby, and in the resolution phase of RDS, when lung compliance may be rapidly increasing. Even in these cases, the incidence has dramatically decreased with the advent of surfactant therapy and antenatal treatment with corticosteroids.

Pneumothoraces are usually unilateral, of which about two-thirds are right sided. Bilateral pneumothoraces are present in about 20% of cases. In either instance, the air collection may vary in size and position, although it is usually found proximate to the uppermost area of the lung. Tension pneumothorax refers to a pneumothorax of sufficient size to cause deviation of the position of the heart, which may result in compression of major vessels, diminished cardiac return, and subsequent cardiovascular compromise and hypotension. Some authors consider the presence of cardiovascular symptoms to be necessary for diagnosis of significant tension pneumothorax.

Etiology

Air leak syndromes are not congenital anomalies or defects in the structure of the lung, although hypoplasia of the lung will predispose to the occurrence of these disorders. They result instead from a rise in the pressure of gas within an alveolus to a level sufficient to disrupt the integrity of the alveolar wall, allowing gas to escape into the interstitial tissues of the lung. The gas can either remain in the interstitium as interstitial emphysema or track along a path of lowest resistance until it enters and collects in another tissue space. The identity of this space determines the type of air leak. Most commonly, the gas will enter the pleural space, resulting in pneumothorax.

Predisposing factors include decreased or nonhomogeneous lung compliance, excess gas pressure in the alveolus, or a rapid change in lung compliance, resulting in alveolar overdistention. Decreased compliance is most often the result of lung immaturity and surfactant deficiency, but it may also result from pneumonia, maldevelopment, or lung hypoplasia. In these latter settings, efforts to effectively ventilate the baby may require the use of pressures high enough to rupture a normally noncompliant alveolus. Most typically, air leak owing to low compliance occurs early in the clinical course. The risk of air leak also increases when lung compliance changes rapidly, such as following surfactant administration or during the resolution phase of untreated hyaline membrane disease. If they are not adjusted as the infant's clinical condition changes, elevated ventilating pressures can cause overdistention and rupture of alveoli that have become normally compliant. In these circumstances, the occurrence of air leak may also be a result of alveolar compliance that is not homogeneous throughout the lung. The pressures or volumes required to ventilate or maintain the patency of low-compliance alveoli may be high enough to cause overdistention and rupture of the alveoli with normal compliance.

This is also the likely mechanism for spontaneous pneumothoraces or pneumomediastina that may occur during a baby's own first breaths. As infants begin to breathe, they may generate very high negative inspiratory pressures to open alveoli for the first time. These pressures may be required to open many alveoli but may, at the same time, be high enough to overdistend others, resulting in rupture and the development of air leak.

In babies with pneumonia or an aspiration syndrome, especially meconium aspiration syndrome, plugs of debris can produce a ball valve mechanism of air trapping that can result in the overdistention of distal alveoli, subsequent rupture, and an air leak. In a similar manner, airway compression or obstruction by intrathoracic masses can result in air trapping and subsequent pneumothoraces.

Presentation

- Small spontaneous pneumothoraces are typically asymptomatic and thus usually escape detection. They may be found incidentally on radiographs obtained for another purpose but should cause no alarm or a search for additional underlying diagnoses. Recurrent spontaneous pneumothoraces are abnormal and suggest an underlying problem in the lung.
- Symptomatic pneumothorax present with tachypnea, grunting, flaring, and retractions. The infant may be cyanotic or have episodes of apnea and bradycardia.
- Clinical signs include asymmetry of the chest, with expansion on the side of the pneumothorax. The cardiac impulse may be shifted if the air collection is large enough, and the breath sounds are often diminished on the affected side. If there are bilateral pneumothoraces, these signs may be less obvious or absent.

- In addition to tachypnea, there may be an alteration in other vital signs. Initially, tachycardia may occur, but larger air collections ultimately lead to a diminution in cardiac output, with resultant hypotension, hypoxemia, and bradycardia.
- The presentation may be relatively subtle and worsen over time but often includes a sudden change in vital signs and the onset of clinical symptoms. An acute change in oxygenation and blood pressure, often with associated bradycardia, should first prompt evaluation of the patency of the airway. If the airway is secure, immediate attention should be directed toward determining whether a pneumothorax is present.

Diagnosis

- The diagnosis should be suspected in the presence of the signs and symptoms described above.
- Transillumination of the infant chest with a focused high-intensity light is a very useful way to quickly show the presence of a pneumothorax, indicated by the presence of a wider area of chest illumination over an extrapulmonary air collection, especially when compared with the contralateral chest. The reliability of a positive transillumination is high, but falsely negative results are common, especially in edematous infants or in extremely small infants, in whom clinically significant air collections may be of low enough volume to be unapparent.
- The chest radiograph is the mainstay of diagnosis. An anteroposterior view of the chest is most useful and may show air collected between the visceral and parietal pleura, most common laterally over the apices or at the lung bases. It may be possible to discern an abrupt lateral truncation of lung markings next to relative lateral hyperlucency. The rib cage will appear larger as the loss of negative intrathoracic pressure allows it to expand. Anterior collections of air may result in a hyperlucent hemithorax, and medial collections may appear as hyperlucent "bubbles" along the cardiac border, with sharpening of that border. If the anteroposterior view is equivocal, a decubitus view, with the side of suspected air leak placed superiorly, is a more sensitive way to show the presence of a pneumothorax. A cross table view is less likely to be helpful.

- Needle thoracentesis may be used as both a diagnostic and a therapeutic tool in a rapidly deteriorating situation in the presence of signs and symptoms of a pneumothorax. If the infant's condition deteriorates in the delivery room or during transport, this may be the only diagnostic tool available for use.

Treatment

- Small pneumothoraces with minimal or no associated symptoms require no intervention other than observation. If the infant has no symptoms, a repeat chest radiograph is not necessary. If the infant has mild symptoms such as tachypnea alone, without an increased oxygen requirement, again, observation is appropriate. Many pneumothoraces will resolve both clinically and radiographically over 12 to 24 hours.
- Larger pneumothoraces with mild associated symptoms may be treated with observation and additional oxygen as needed. In some instances, treatment with 100% oxygen may shorten the duration of the clinical symptoms by hastening the resolution of the air collection. This "nitrogen washout" technique is postulated to work by washing out nitrogen from the baby's bloodstream, creating a concentration gradient that favors absorption of nitrogen within the air pocket. Whether this technique has any value or role in care of the newborn remains a matter of controversy.
- In the presence of underlying lung disease or significant symptoms, a pneumothorax should be drained. The most rapid method is thoracentesis with a butterfly needle. This method is used for rapid decompression of a pneumothorax in infants with hemodynamic compromise, as an adjunct to delivery room resuscitation, and for drainage of air collections in spontaneously breathing infants without evidence of continuing air leak, in whom re-collection of the air is unlikely.
  1. A 23-gauge butterfly needle is attached to a 20 mL syringe through a three-way stopcock.
  2. The infant is placed in a supine position, and the area overlying the air pocket is cleaned with an antibacterial solution. Almost always, because air rises above the lung, the air pocket will be located under the second or third intercostal

space in the midclavicular line, and entry at this location is likely to drain the air pocket. The Neonatal Resuscitation Program of the American Academy of Pediatrics recommends using an approach in the anterior axilllary line, similar to that used for chest tube placement (see below).

3. The needle wings are gripped with the operator's thumb and third finger, and the index finger is placed over the needle to limit the depth of entry. The needle is placed in the intercostal space, just over and perpendicular to the top of the lower rib, and advanced into the pleural space. As the needle is advanced, suction is applied to the syringe. As soon as airflow is established, the advance of the needle is stopped, and the needle is stabilized while the air is withdrawn. In this way, the risk of injury to the underlying lung is minimized. Once drainage is complete, the needle is withdrawn, and a radiograph is taken to assess success.

4. If it is necessary to repeat this procedure more than a second time, strong consideration should be given to placing an indwelling chest tube.

- A chest tube should be placed to evacuate pneumothoraces in patients receiving mechanical ventilation or in those with recurrent collections of air after needle thoracentesis. These are the situations in which the air leak is likely to be continuous and result in significant compromise if untreated.

1. The smallest effective chest tube should be used to minimize trauma and mechanical compromise from the intrathoracic volume occupied by the tube. For extremely low-birth-weight infants, an 8 French catheter should be used; a 10 or 12 French catheter should be used in larger babies.

2. In newborns, chest tubes are placed in the anterior axillary line to avoid injury to the nipple, the muscles of the chest wall, and the axillary artery. The area is widely cleaned from the third to the sixth intercostal space. The patient is given narcotic analgesia, and the area over the fifth rib is infiltrated with lidocaine.

3. An incision of about 5 mm is made in the skin, parallel to and overlying the fifth rib. The subcutaneous tissue is then gently dissected over the rib with a small curved hemostat,

and a track is made to the fourth intercostal space. The hemostat is then stabilized with the operator's index finger, and the tip is used to enter the pleural space just over the third rib. The index finger will limit the depth of entry. The pleural opening is enlarged with the hemostat tip.

4. Two methods are acceptable for inserting the chest tube. The preferred method is to grip the end of the tube within the curved tip of the hemostat. The infant is rolled slightly onto the side contralateral to the insertion site, and the tube is introduced into the incision, with the operator's hands moving from posterior toward anterior. The tube (with the trocar removed) is guided into the pleural space using the hemostat tip, and the curve of the tip is used to ensure that it is angled anteriorly. The tube direction is dictated by the identified location of the air pocket, either superior, midthoracic, or inferiorly, but the most common position is anterior and superior. The hemostat is then released and removed, and the tube is gently advanced 2 to 4 cm into the pleural space. Care should be taken not to advance the tube too far but to ensure that both the end and side holes are within the pleural space.

5. The other insertion method is to remove the chest tube trocar and break off the sharp tip using a large hemostat. The trocar is then bent into the shape of a hockey stick, with the "blade" about 1.5 cm in length, and the blunt trocar is reinserted into the tube. The tube is then inserted into the incision and subcutaneous track and then through the opening into the pleural space. The curved end is used to direct the tube into the pleural space and then to ensure that it is aimed anteriorly. The back end of the trocar is then held, and the tube is slipped off into the chest as the trocar is removed.

6. Once positioned, the tube is attached to an underwater drainage system, and 15 and 20 cm H_2O negative pressure is applied to the system. Water vapor in the tube and bubbling drainage confirm that the placement is in the air pocket. The position should be confirmed by radiography.

7. The tube is sutured in place using circumferential knots and secured to the chest wall with tape or a transparent

semipermeable dressing. The tube should be positioned and secured in a posterior to anterior direction, with the superior or inferior direction dictated by the site of the air collection.

8. Chest tubes are painful, and the patient should always be given adequate analgesia, both during placement and for the duration that the chest tube remains indwelling.

- Unusual air collections may be difficult to drain with an anterosuperiorly placed chest tube. Most air collections are anterosuperior when the infant is placed in a supine position. Air collections below the base of the lung are usually loculated and less likely to produce clinical compromise, but if the collection is large, the tube should be intentionally angled inferiorly to attempt drainage. Larger collections or those that cannot be completely drained by one tube may respond to an additional chest tube placed through the fifth intercostal space, but this situation is rare. Medial air collections usually communicate with anterior collections and are drained by anterosuperior tube position. On occasion, it may be necessary to reposition the infant to move the air toward the tube position. For example, the infant can be placed in a head-up incline, and air should rise toward the apex of the lung, where it can be drained. It may also be desirable to use needle thoracentesis to drain loculated air collections after a chest tube has been placed to drain the main collection.

- The chest tube is left in place, with suction drainage, until all bubbling drainage has ceased. Once drainage has stopped for 24 hours or longer, suction is discontinued, the tube is placed to water seal, and the baby is monitored for reaccumulation of air. Tubes should not be cross-clamped before removal because this procedure will permit air to reaccumulate in the pleural space and produce symptoms. The use of water seal avoids reaccumulation but permits assessment of any persistent air leak. If none has occurred within 12 to 24 hours and a radiograph confirms lack of air collection, the tube is removed, and a small occlusive dressing is placed over the wound. Ideally, the chest tube should be pulled during the portion of the respiratory cycle least likely to introduce air into the pleural space.

This is during expiration for a spontaneously breathing infant and during inspiration for an infant receiving positive pressure ventilation. A single suture may be needed to close the wound before dressing.

Complications

Pneumothoraces may be complicated by additional air leaks of the types described above. Sudden changes in blood pressure and perfusion that may accompany a pneumothorax can result in intraventricular hemorrhage in the premature infant. The syndrome of inappropriate secretion of antidiuretic hormone may result from a pneumothorax.

Chest tube placement may be complicated by laceration of the lung or airways or potential injury to other mediastinal structures, including the heart and major vessels. If the entry wound is made too large, it may not seal around the tube, and air may be drawn into the infant's chest, mimicking a persistent air leak.

The nipple area in small premature infants is often indistinct. Great effort must be made to identify this area, and to avoid it during the placement of a chest tube. This will avoid damage or obliteration of breast tissue.

Pneumomediastinum

Pneumomediastinum should be suspected when heart sounds are distant and the infant is tachypneic. The chest may have an increased anteroposterior diameter. Diagnosis is made by chest radiography.

Other than discomfort and tachypnea, few symptoms result from pneumomediastinum. Drainage is not indicated, and treatment should consist of observation. If the infant is receiving mechanical ventilation, efforts should be made to reduce mean airway pressure as much as possible.

Pneumopericardium

Pneumopericardium should be suspected when heart sounds are distant or muffled; pulse pressure is narrowed and mean arterial pressure is decreased, often to a very low level. The cardiac impulse will generally not be palpable, and electrocardiographic voltages may be diminished. Often the presentation occurs acutely in a patient requiring mechanical ventilation.

Diagnosis

The diagnosis is made by chest radiograph, on which a ring of air density is seen around the heart, sharply outlining it within the pericardial sac. The diagnosis may be made on clinical criteria during an emergent situation in which waiting for a radiograph will unnecessarily delay treatment of hypotension.

Treatment

In the presence of significant hypotension and cardiac compromise, emergent drainage is indicated.

The infant is placed in a supine position, and the area below the sternum is cleaned with an antibacterial solution.

A 22 g intravascular catheter is introduced below the sternum and advanced superiorly and slightly posteriorly, towards the left shoulder of the patient. Some operators will connect an ECG lead to the trochar to permit identification of contact with the myocardium, but usually the entry into the air pocket is obvious as pressure is released and blood pressure increases.

The trochar is withdrawn as the catheter is advanced slightly, and a 10 ml syringe is attached. Any remaining air is drained, and the catheter is removed.

Rarely, continuous airleak into the pericardial space requires that a small catheter be left in the space and attached to low suction.

Recommended Readings

Allen RW, Jung AL, Lester PD. Effectiveness of chest tube evacuation of pneumothorax in neonates. J Pediatr 1981;99:629–34.

Banagle RC, Outerbridge EW, Aranda JV. Lung perforation: a complication of chest tube insertion in neonatal pneumothorax. J Pediatr 1979;4:973–5.

Brann BS, Mayfield SR, Goldstein M, et al. Cardiovascular effects of hypoxia/hypercarbia and tension pneumothorax in newborn piglets. Crit Care Med 1994;22:1453–60.

Chernick V, Reed MH. Pneumothorax and chylothorax in the neonatal period. J Pediatr 1970;76:624.

Greenough A, Wood S, Morley CJ, Davis JA. Pancuronium prevents pneumothoraces in ventilated premature babies who actively expire against positive pressure inflation. Lancet 1984;i:1–4.

McIntosh N, Becher JC, Cunnningham S, et al. Clinical diagnosis of pneumothorax is late: use of trend data and decision support might allow preclinical detection. Pediatr Res 2000;48:408–15.

Rainer C, Gardetto A, Fruhwirth M, et al. Breast deformity in adolescence as a result of pneumothorax drainage during neonatal intensive care. Pediatrics 2003;111:80–6.

Watkinson M, Tiron I. Events before the diagnosis of a pneumothorax in ventilated neonates. Arch Dis Child 2001;85: F201–3.

Part 4: Chylothorax

Mark Puder, MD, PhD, and
Arin K. Greene, MD

Chyle is a lymphatic fluid that contains fat secreted by intestinal cells. The fluid is transported to the thoracic duct into the left subclavian vein and into the circulation. A chylothorax is a collection of this fluid in the pleural space and is the most common cause of pleural effusion in the newborn.

Development of the Lymphatic System

The lymphatic system develops at 6 weeks gestation, 2 weeks after the primordial of the cardiovascular system. Lymphatic capillaries develop with blood vessels and connect to the venous system. At the end of the embryonic stage, six primary lymph sacs are present.

Two jugular lymphatic sacs at the junction of the subclavian and internal jugular veins drain the head, neck, and upper limbs. Two iliac sacs at the junction of the iliac veins and the posterior cardinal veins drain the lower trunk and lower limbs. The retroperitoneal sac on the posterior abdominal wall at the base of the mesentery and the cisterna chyli dorsal to the retroperitoneal sac drain the primitive gut.

Lymphatic capillaries then join the lymph sacs and travel along with the veins. The jugular and cisterna chyli lymph sacs are then connected by the right and left thoracic ducts. The main thoracic duct forms from the caudal part of the right thoracic duct, the anastomosis between the thoracic ducts, and the cranial part of the left thoracic duct. In the adult, the right lymphatic duct is derived from the cranial portion of the right thoracic duct. The right lymphatic duct and thoracic duct drain into the venous system at the junction of the internal jugular and subclavian veins.

Because the main thoracic duct is formed from the right and left thoracic ducts, many variations of the thoracic duct in the adult are present. In the newborn, the duct begins in the abdomen at the cisterna chyli and then travels in the posterior mediastinum through the aortic hiatus. The duct then courses left at the fifth thoracic vertebra behind the aortic arch, above the clavicle, and then downward into the junction of the subclavian and jugular veins.

When the right and left thoracic ducts do not develop properly into the main thoracic duct, chylothorax occurs in the newborn period. A malformation of the lower duct causes an effusion into the right chest, whereas a malformation of the upper portion of the duct usually causes an effusion into the left chest.

Etiology

- The majority of cases are idiopathic.
- Trauma includes hyperextension of the cervical spine.
- Malformations include thoracic duct atresia, congenital fistulae caused by failure of lymphatic channels to connect with main lymphatic network, congenital heart disease, lobar sequestration, or pulmonary lymphangectasia, and an abnormal prominence of subpleural and interlobular lymphatics
- Genetic syndromes: Turner's, Noonan's, and Down syndromes
- Post operative or "iatrogenic" chylothorax includes thoracic duct injury during placement of left subclavian central venous lines, congenital diaphragmatic hernia repair, thoracic surgery cases such as tracheoesophageal fistula repair, excision of tumors, and especially cardiac surgery (which accounts for up to 2.5% of cases). Any thoracic operation in which lymphatics are injured may produce chylothorax. Postoperative chylothorax occurs within 25 days with an average of 7 days.
- Vascular thrombosis (superior vena cava, subclavian vein)
- Malignancy: Neuroblastoma or any mass producing obstruction, rupture, or invasion of lymphatics

Prenatal Diagnosis and Management

In-utero diagnosis of chylothorax by ultrasonography offers the potential for prenatal treatment. In general, conservative antenatal management is recommended because many chylothoraces resolve spontaneously. A fetal thoracentesis can be used for diagnosis but is of limited therapeutic value owing to the rapid reaccumulation of fluid. Pleuroamniotic shunts have been placed to help lung development, decrease polyhydramnios, or minimize hydrops fetalis. Gestational age at the time of diagnosis, duration, and severity of chylothorax are major factors predicting the degree of pulmonary hypoplasia.

Postnatal Presentation

- Fifty percent of congenital chlyothoraces present within the first week of life.
- It is often associated with systemic lymphatic malformations.
- It usually presents as respiratory distress with diminished breath sounds.

Postnatal Diagnosis

- Chest radiography shows pleural effusion(s).
- Pleural tap shows lymphocytosis. Chyle appears clear to light yellow in the absence of feeds. It turns milky after feedings have been initiated because of the presence of chylomicrons and elevated triglycerides.

Medical Management

CARDIOPULMONARY

- Respiratory failure can occur because of a combination of atelectasis (secondary to compression of lungs by effusions), chest wall edema, and pneumonia. If the infant is preterm, surfactant deficiency can further complicate the respiratory status. Cardiovascular collapse can result from compression of mediastinal structures and inhibition of venous return. If the effusions have been present for a prolonged period antenatally, the infant may have significant pulmonary hypoplasia and/or hydrops.
- Respiratory failure will often require support with endotracheal intubation and mechanical ventilation. Relatively high positive end-expiratory pressure and diuretic therapy can be helpful if pulmonary edema is present.
- Treatment of cardiovascular failure includes support of circulating intravascular volume and treatment of myocardial dysfunction with pressors as indicated.

- The pleural effusions may be treated with pleural taps. If repeated taps are necessary, a chest tube should be placed.

Chest Tube Placement

Site: For fluid drainage, our preferred site is the midaxillary line at the level of the nipple lateral to the pectoralis major muscle. Direct the chest tube posteriorly to allow for dependent drainage. This contrasts with the desired anterior chest tube tip position for the drainage of pneumothoraces. Another option is to locate the chylous fluid by ultrasound and place the chest tube directly into the fluid. The second intercostal space in the mid-clavicular line lateral to the sternal boarder is not safe in infants owing to the large thymus. Chest tubes should not be placed with a trocar.

Chest Tube Sizes: A 12 French tube (eg, Argyle) is usually used in term infants. Smaller tubes are needed for preterm infants. Larger tubes are also available in increments of 4 French.

Insertion Technique: Prepare and drape the site using sterile technique and anesthetize with 1% lidocaine. Locate the site of insertion and estimate the length of the intrathoracic chest tube. Make a small skin incision approximately 1 cm below the selected intercostals space to allow for tunneling the chest tube under the skin.

Use a curved hemostat to tunnel a tract superiorly and subcutaneously over the next higher rib and into the pleural cavity. To prevent bleeding, avoid the neurovascular bundle located on the inferior edge of each rib. Spread the hemostat to enlarge the opening. Tunnel the tube to avoid introducing a pneumothorax on removal of the chest tube because infants have minimal subcutaneous fat to occlude the hole in the chest. Then introduce the chest tube into the chest cavity. All side holes of the chest tube must be within the chest. Secure the tube with sutures and cover with a sterile occlusive dressing. Place the Pleurovac to approximately 10 cm of H_2O suction. Obtain a chest radiograph immediately to determine the placement of the chest tube, and the effectiveness of reducing the chylothorax volume as well as to ensure that the procedure was not complicated by a pneumothorax.

Chest Tube Removal

When fluid has stopped draining from the chest tube for at least 24 hours, place the chest tube to water seal and obtain a chest radiograph to assess for reaccumulation of effusions. Because chylous fluid is produced at an increased rate when being fed, it is important for the infant to be challenged with enteral feedings before confidently removing a chest tube (see section on Fluids, Electrolytes, and Nutrition below).

If evaluation of the patient and radiograph are consistent with resolution of the effusion, the chest tube is clamped and the sutures are removed. A vaseline occlusive dressing is applied over the tube. The chest tube is pulled during the portion of the respiratory cycle when the risk of introducing a pneumothorax is lowest. If the baby is not intubated, the tube is pulled during expiration (Valsalva's maneuver in older children). If the baby is intubated, the tube is pulled during inspiration. Once pulled, the incision site is immediately sealed with the gauze and occlusive tape. Another chest radiograph is taken. The tube site usually seals in a matter of hours, but the dressing is left in place for at least 24 hours.

Fluids, Electrolytes, and Nutrition

Chyle is rich in phospholipids, cholesterol, triglycerides, and albumin. Loss of these components when chylous fluid is drained makes the management of fluid, electrolytes, and nutrition quite challenging. The nutritional goal is to balance adequate caloric intake with minimal chyle production. The rate of chyle production is monitored with the chest tube. Enteral feedings with long chain fatty acids increase chyle flow and worsen the chylothorax. Medium chain triglycerides (MCTs) enter directly into the portal circulation and not the lymphatics. Therefore, a diet with MCTs as the only source of fat will reduce chyle production. If a diet with only MCTs does not diminish the output, the patient should be placed on total parenteral nutrition (TPN). Exclusive parenteral nutrition is often successful in decreasing chyle production and frequently shortens time until resolution of the chyle leak. Somatostatin infusion may be helpful in decreasing the duration of chylothorax.

Immunologic/Hematologic

Chyle also contains immunoglobulins, T lymphocytes, and fibrinogen. Patients draining substantial volumes of chyle must be monitored for evidence of immunologic or hematologic compromise and treated accordingly.

Surgical Management

Patients are often given 2 to 4 weeks of the above nonoperative therapy before surgical therapy is considered. Earlier surgical intervention may be indicated if the pulmonary or nutritional complications are unmanageable. Options include thoracic duct ligation either through a thoracotomy or thorascopically, pleurodesis, sclerosis, pleuroperitoneal shunts, and pleurectomy. These must be tailored to the specific cause of the chylothorax.

- Thoracic duct ligation is preferred when thoracic duct injury is suspected and there are no contraindications to surgery. The duct is ligated at the aortic hiatus. It may be possible to identify the chyle leak by open thoracotomy or thoracoscopy and ligation of the leaking area.
- Pleurodesis and sclerosis may be combined with the thoracic duct ligation. This procedure creates adhesions in an attempt to obliterate chylous leaks. Some have used fibrin glue and sclerosing agents such as talc, OK-432, or the antimalarial agent quinacrine.
- Pleuroperitoneal shunts can be used if the above interventions fail. Some surgeons proceed directly to shunt after expectant management. One advantage of shunt over drainage is that the chyle is reabsorbed by the peritoneum and therefore limits fluid, electrolyte, and nutritional losses. It is also a relatively conservative intervention that allows time for the possible development of new lymphatic channels. This therapy is ineffective in the presence of either inferior vena cava obstruction or high right atrial pressures.

Complications

- Risks of repeated pleural taps include lung injury with pneumothorax, bleeding, and infection.
- Complications of a pleuroperitoneal shunt include shunt failure and infection.

Prognosis

Resolution of chylothorax is reported in up to 80% of cases treated with MCT, TPN, and chest tube drainage. Most patients with refractory chylothorax are those who present with superior vena cava obstruction or congenital lymphatic malformations.

Reported mortality rates range from 0 to 50%. Increased mortality risk is associated with prematurity, associated congenital anomalies, and hydrops fetalis, low apgar scores, and early high ventilator settings.

References

1. Al-Tawil K, Ahmed G, Al-Hathal M, et al. Congenital chylothorax. Am J Perinatol 2000;3:121–420.
2. Beghetti M, La Scala G, Belli D, et al. Etiology and management of chylothorax. J Pediatr 2000;136:653–7.
3. Dubin P, King IN, Gallagher PG. Congenital chylothorax. Curr Opin Pediatr 2000;12:505–9.
4. Moore KL, Persaud TVN. The developing human. 6th ed. Philadelphia: WB Saunders; 1998.
5. O'Neill JA, Rowe MI, Grosfeld JL, et al. Pediatric surgery. 5th ed. St. Louis: Mosby; 1998.
6. Rocha G. Pleural effusions in the neonate. Curr Opin Pulm Med 2007;13:305–11.
7. Abrams ME, Meredith KS, Kinnard P, Clark RH. Hydrops fetalis: a retrospective review of cases reported to a large national database and identification of risk factors associated with death. Pediatrics 2007;120:84–9.

  8. Chan GM, Lechtenberg E. The use of fat-free human milk in infants with chylous pleural effusion. J Perinatol 2007; 27:434–6.

  9. Chan SY, Lau W, Wong WH, Cheng LC, Chau AK, Cheung YF. Chylothorax in children after congenital heart surgery. Ann Thorac Surg 2006;82:1650–6.

 10. Stajich GV, Ashworth L. Octreotide. Neonatal Netw 2006;25:365–9.

Part 5: Thoracic Mass Lesions

Steven A. Ringer, MD, PhD, FAAP, and
Jay M. Wilson, MD

Congenital Cystic Adenomatoid Malformation

Congenital cystic adenomatoid malformation (CCAM) of the lung is a rare pulmonary anomaly. Although there are reports of cystic disease of the lung dating back to the seventeenth century, CCAM was first reported in the English literature in 1949. CCAMs communicate with large conducting airways via tiny pores of Kohn, and the vascular supply is from the pulmonary circulation.

Embryology

- The conducting airways arise from an outpouching of the foregut (endoderm) at about the fourth week of gestation, whereas the respiratory component of the lungs arises from mesenchyma that are concentrated around the tips of the developing bronchi. CCAM is thought to develop when there is a disruption of the connection between the two tissues before the fifth week of gestation, with subsequent overgrowth of the terminal bronchioles.
- The cystic mass is of variable size and may be large enough to deform the lung, shift the mediastinum, or even compress the contralateral lung. A classification system was proposed by Stocker in 1977, based on the gross and pathologic findings:
  1. Type 1: 50% of postnatal cases, characterized by a small number of large cysts up to 7 cm in diameter. These are lined with pseudostratified epithelium.
  2. Type 2: 40% of postnatal cases, characterized by many small cysts of variable size, usually less than 2 cm in diameter, and lined with tall columnar epithelium. These are more likely to be associated with other anomalies and thus have a worse prognosis.

3. Type 3: 10% of cases, characterized by a homogeneous microcystic mass lined with cuboidal epithelium, interspersed with irregular small structures lined by nonciliated cuboidal epithelium. These lesions have the worst prognosis because of their tendency to grow and cause compression, as well as their association with other anomalies.

This classification scheme has been reviewed primarily because specimens obtained from fetal sections suggest that the histopathology of antenatally detected lesions may differ from that suggested by ultrasound. Adzick proposed classifying lesions as either macrocystic or microcystic, based on ultrasonographic and pathologic findings. Macrocystic lesions have single or multiple large cysts, greater than 5 cm in diameter, that are echolucent on ultrasonography. The less common microcystic lesions are generally solid echogenic masses with multiple small cysts and carry a worse prognosis. Cha and coworkers identified two histologic patterns, which they proposed to represent the different stages at which the arrest in development occurred. Others have identified hybrid lesions that sonographically appear to be CCAMs, but have a systemic blood supply.

Incidence

CCAM is a rare lesion that has been reported in small series or as individual cases. It is, therefore, impossible to estimate a true incidence, but improved imaging techniques has led to increased identification during fetal life. At least 15 to 20% of CCAMS will either resolve or significantly shrink in size before birth; hence, postnatal reports almost certainly underestimate the true rate of occurrence. The peak growth of these lesions tends to occur by 28 weeks of gestation. They are almost always unilateral, and only one lobe of the lung is affected in 80 to 95% of cases. There is no side predilection, and both sexes are affected equally.

Prenatal Diagnosis

Prenatal diagnosis is made by ultrasonography, with type 1 and 2 lesions appearing as echolucent cystic masses of varying size and number, whereas type 3 lesions are more echogenic and solid. There may be a mediastinal shift, and hydrops may be present. In almost three-fourths of cases, there is polyhydramnios caused by esophageal compression, which may precipitate preterm labor. Doppler studies show the absence of a systemic vascular supply. There may be associated anomalies, including cardiac, gastrointestinal, or renal. Ultrafast magnetic resonance imaging (MRI) is also useful, especially for differentiating CCAM from other diagnoses such as sequestration. MRI can be used to obtain an accurate measurement of fetal lung volumes, which may allow a prediction of whether there is sufficient lung to sustain extrauterine life. This modality also permits a more accurate assessment of the relationship of the lesion to other structures in the thorax so that operative intervention can be planned more reliably.

The course of the lesions during fetal life is variable, depending on the size of the cysts. Larger masses may cause a shift of the mediastinum, with compression of venous return and compromise in cardiac function, with resultant hydrops fetalis. If the mass is large enough, it may compress the lung and result in pulmonary hypoplasia, or it may compress the esophagus and cause polyhydramnios. The presence of hydrops is a grave prognostic sign, with only isolated cases of survival reported.

Conversely, many large lesions will steadily decrease in size and may even appear to completely resolve during gestation. In the largest published series, 20% of the lesions diagnosed in the second trimester decreased in size and showed resolution of the mediastinal shift. There are no factors that allow prediction of which lesions will resolve and which will continue to progress during fetal life, although small lesions that change little over a 3-week period around 28 weeks usually have a benign course and only require expectant management and postnatal evaluation. Determining which lesions fall in this category can be difficult. Consequently, frequent imaging throughout pregnancy is essential.

If the CCAM does not resolve or regress, the severity of presentation relates to the volume of the mass and to the associated findings. The presence of hydrops and pleural effusion is the most important among these factors. When hydrops and pleural effusions are present and the mass remains large, the outcome has been reported as almost uniformly fatal, but intervention and in-utero decompression of pleural effusions have resulted in anecdotal survival. In cases in which antenatal diagnosis has been made but no hydrops is present, the outcome is much better, with 100% survival reported following close fetal surveillance and postnatal resection of the mass.

Postnatal Presentation

Postnatal presentation is as variable as the fetal presentation. Some patients will present with respiratory distress in the neonatal period, whereas others will develop recurrent pulmonary infections during later childhood. The majority of patients will have symptoms by 2 years of age. About half of patients with a type 1 lesion and most of those with types 2 and 3 are likely to be symptomatic on the first day of life, except those cases in which significant regression has occurred. Neonatal presentation also depends on the presence and severity of pulmonary hypoplasia. Although often accompanied by hydrops, pulmonary hypoplasia may occur independently because of the mass effect of CCAM. Infants with pulmonary hypoplasia may require support with high-frequency ventilation and are often more difficult to manage after surgery because of associated pulmonary hypertension. If the mass has significantly regressed during fetal life, the clinical presentation after birth may be normal. These infants should have imaging studies performed to assess the status of the mass. If plain radiographs do not show the lesion, computed tomography (CT) or MRI should be employed. In all patients, postnatal CT scans have reported persistent abnormalities, even when the chest radiograph is normal and the infant is free of symptoms.

Differential Diagnosis

Differential diagnosis of cystic thoracic masses generally includes CDH, bronchogenic cyst, or bronchopulmonary sequestration (BPS), although rare tumors such as pleuro-pulmonary blastoma may mimic these cystic lesions. Mediastinal lesions, such as neuroblastoma, may present with a similar appearance on chest radiography, although ultrasonography or CT will permit differentiation of these lesions. The differentiation of CCAM from BPS is made by the demonstration of a systemic vascular supply in sequestration.

Surgical Management

Surgical management begins during fetal life, when a decision must be made as to whether intervention should be done at that time or safely delayed until after birth. The presence of hydrops before 32 weeks of gestation generally makes the fetus a potential candidate for prenatal intervention because of the poor outcome without intervention. Little is generally gained by simple aspiration of a cyst, as the fluid tends to reaccumulate. Percutaneous laser ablation of the blood supply has been described in case reports, but these attempts are currently in the early experimental stage. Those cases presenting with hydrops later than 32 weeks are usually managed by treating the mother with betamethasone and then delivering the baby, with subsequent resection of the lesion. There have also been reports of resolution of the hydrops after the maternal betamethasone treatment, although the mechanism for this remains unknown. The fetus with a large CCAM, with or without hydrops and pleural effusions, should be delivered at a facility with the capacity for neonatal intensive care and emergent pediatric surgery, including the availability of high-frequency ventilation and ECMO. Initial management should be aimed at stabilization of the symptomatic infant, after which surgical resection of the mass should be undertaken. When hydrops is present, it will be the cause of the most severe symptoms in the immediate neonatal period, and immediate therapy must be directed toward managing fluid collections, supporting ventilation, and correcting hypotension. Pleural effusions should be drained by either intermittent needle thoracocentesis or insertion of a thoracostomy tube for continuous drainage. Once stabilized, immediate resection of the mass is indicated in all infants with clinical symptoms. Even for children with no symptoms, postnatal resection of all CCAMs is commonly recommended because multiple reports have shown an association between CCAM and the later development of pulmonary rhabdomyosarcoma, arising from within the cystic lesion.

Complications and Associated Anomalies

Although most cases are not associated with other anomalies, some reports have found them in about 25% of cases. The reported anomalies include bilateral renal agenesis or dysplasia, truncus arteriosus, tetralogy of Fallot, hydrocephalus, jejunal atresia, and diaphragmatic hernia. Deformities of the clavicles and spine, including sirenomelia, have also been reported.

BPS

BPSs are segments of nonfunctioning lung with an anomalous blood supply from the systemic circulation and no connection to the tracheobronchial tree.

Embryology

The tracheobronchial tree derives from an outpouching of the foregut, and sequestrations arise either from a separate outpouching or as a lung segment that has lost its connection with the rest of the tracheobronchial tree. If this separation occurs before the pleura are formed, then the sequestration will be adjacent to the normal lung and surrounded by the same pleura (intralobar sequestration). If the separation occurs later, then the sequestered lung will have its own pleura (extralobar sequestration). Extralobar sequestrations are by far the most common. The sequestered lung may also rarely connect to the gastrointestinal tract. A distinguishing feature of sequestrations is that the blood supply arises from the aorta, frequently below the diaphragm, and not from the pulmonary artery. This indicates that the disruption in development occurs before the separation of the pulmonary and aortic circulations. In extralobar sequestration, venous drainage is also systemic, but in intralobar sequestration, it is via the pulmonary veins. Because of its foregut origin, BPS may be associated with bronchogenic or esophageal duplication cysts or CCAMs on either side of the chest or within the BPS itself.

Incidence

Owing to the rarity of the lesion, the true incidence has not been determined exactly, but sequestrations represent between 0.15 and 6.4% of all pulmonary anomalies. Essentially all the lesions are unilateral and located in the lower lobe, and about two-thirds of them are left sided. There is a distinct male predominance, especially among the extralobar form.

Prenatal Diagnosis

Prenatal diagnosis is generally made based on the ultrasonographic finding of a homogeneous, hyperechoic mass in the lung, usually in the lower lobe. Doppler ultrasonography will often be helpful if it shows blood supply arising from a systemic artery, which is most commonly from the aorta, but may also arise from any of the major thoracic arteries. The presence of a systemic vascular connection (frequently from below the diaphragm) distinguishes BPS from CCAM, but this information may be difficult to obtain. As a result, the diagnosis is often difficult to confirm, and in one series, only 29% of BPS cases were correctly identified. It is especially difficult to diagnose BPS late in gestation because, characteristically, the echogenicity of the lesion decreases, and it becomes less possible to distinguish it from the lung that surrounds it. Increasingly, MRI has become more useful in the diagnosis and definition of this lesion.

Postnatal Presentation

Postnatal presentation is variable. Intralobar sequestrations usually present after the age of 2 years as recurrent pneumonia and abscess formation within the sequestration and surrounding normal lung. Because of the systemic blood supply, a significant arteriovenous shunt may occur through the sequestration, and result in high-output heart failure or massive hemoptysis later in life.

Postnatal Diagnosis

In the absence of prenatal evaluation, the diagnosis of BPS should be considered in an infant with respiratory distress or hydrops and an intrathoracic mass. Sonographic diagnosis may be complicated by the presence of an air-filled lung surrounding the mass, but Doppler studies may be important in showing the anomalous systemic vascular supply of the lesion. MRI and angiography can greatly aid in both diagnosis and determining the extent of the lesion, and these are increasingly becoming imaging studies of choice. Extralobar sequestrations may be found below the diaphragm in the region of the adrenal gland. Chest wall deformities, CDH, and congenital heart disease are all associated with extralobar sequestrations.

Differential Diagnosis

As noted above, the differentiation of BPS from other mass lesions may be difficult. Most commonly, it is confused with CDH, bronchogenic cyst, cystic adenomatoid malformation (type III), or a mediastinal tumor such as neuroblastoma or teratoma. The identification of anomalous systemic vascular supply is an important feature of this lesion.

Surgical Management

Extralobar sequestration rarely requires resection unless a symptomatic shunt exists. Most recent studies support the practice of serial monitoring of the mass during childhood, with intervention reserved for those patients who develop symptoms. Sequestrations in association with CDH are the most likely to be symptomatic because of the associated pulmonary hypoplasia. Intralobar sequestrations are electively resected because of the infections that invariably occur.

Complications

The outcome for an asymptomatic patient is usually good. Complications are rare in unresected extralobar sequestrations and are usually limited to recurrent infections in intralobar sequestrations. Complications of surgery are usually a result of failure to identify one or more systemic arteries, which retract below the diaphragm during thoracotomy leading to silent exsanguination into the abdominal cavity.

Bronchogenic Cyst

EMBRYOLOGY

Bronchogenic cysts are cystic structures filled with mucoid material and lined with bronchial (ciliated columnar) epithelium. They, like BPS and CCAM, result from abnormal budding of the foregut during early embryogenesis between 4 and 6 weeks. Bronchogenic cysts occur earlier than the other lesions, in the period before the bronchi are formed, and therefore may occur within the wall of the bronchus or other airway. They most typically remain attached to the primitive tracheobronchial tree and are most commonly located within the mediastinum, along the trachea, or within the pulmonary parenchyma itself. In some cases, the foregut out-pouching separates from its original site and subsequently migrates into the mediastinum, neck, or more distant locations, including within the pericardium or below the diaphragm. The blood supply of these cysts arises from the pulmonary circulation, as distinguished from BPS, for which the arterial supply arises from an anomalous systemic artery.

The histology of these cysts includes a lining of columnar cylindrical epithelium, and many also have components of smooth muscle, cartilage, and bronchial glands. These features permit straightforward distinction from other cystic structures that occur in the mediastinum, such as cystic malformations of the esophagus.

INCIDENCE

These lesions are extremely rare in neonates and are often asymptomatic. Therefore, an exact incidence cannot be determined, although they may represent as many as 50% of congenital malformations of the lung. They may present clinically at any time from the prenatal period through adulthood, or they may escape detection entirely. Many are discovered as they become symptomatic later in life or are incidental findings on radiographs in adults. Sometimes the diagnosis is made in adult-hood during the removal of a suspicious thoracic tumor. The prenatal diagnoses of bronchogenic cysts will likely increase as prenatal evaluation becomes more universal, as well as increasingly sensitive and specific, although many of these diagnosed lesions will not be clinically significant.

PRENATAL DIAGNOSIS

Prenatal detection is more sensitive than postnatal detection because in the fetus the cyst is filled with fluid, making it easily detectable by ultrasonography. Following birth, a fluid-filled cyst is very likely to be missed on plain radiographs and even air-filled cysts of moderate size can be difficult to appreciate. In one report of intrathoracic anomalies diagnosed during fetal life, 5 of 22 cases were bronchogenic cysts. It is unusual for bronchogenic cysts to result in clinical compromise of the fetus, but rare cases have been reported in which progressive growth of the cyst has led to compromise of fetal cardiac function, which has, in some cases, progressed to hydrops fetalis. Sometimes intrabronchial location of a small cyst can create significant obstruction, leading to a fluid-filled lung easily identifiable on MRI.

POSTNATAL PRESENTATION AND MANAGEMENT

In most patients, both fetal and neonatal, there is no need for immediate intervention because compromise is unusual. Indeed, bronchogenic cysts are commonly asymptomatic in the newborn period, and clinical symptoms may not present until at least 6 months of age or as late as adulthood. The diagnosis may be suspected when a cystic lesion is seen on a chest radiograph obtained for another indication, but most often the air-filled cysts will be difficult or impossible to discern on plain radiographs. Conservative management of the asymptomatic patient has been advocated, although the risks of late complications, including recurrent pneumonia, or possible malignant transformation, have prompted other authors to advocate for surgical removal early in life. It is likely that with increasing sensitivity of prenatal diagnosis, there will be an opportunity to more accurately define true incidence and progression so that it will be possible to better determine the correct management of the asymptomatic patient.

DIFFERENTIAL DIAGNOSIS

The differential diagnosis includes CCAM, BPS, and Congenital lobar emphysema (CLE), as well as cysts derived from non-pulmonary origin. Location and delineation of arterial supply, as well as the solitary nature of bronchogenic cyst compared with the cysts in CCAM, are often helpful in increasing diagnostic accuracy.

PREOPERATIVE MANAGEMENT

Preoperative management is dictated by the location of the cyst and the presenting symptom. Infections should be treated before operation. Respiratory or cardiovascular symptoms are rare, but, occasionally, a cyst arising within a bronchus can cause life-threatening respiratory distress that requires more urgent resection.

SURGICAL MANAGEMENT

Surgical management depends on the location of the cyst. All bronchogenic cysts diagnosed in childhood should be excised because of the high incidence of infectious complications and a definite association with malignancy later in life. Mediastinal cysts are easily excised by enucleation. Cysts within the lung itself require segmentectomy or lobectomy.

POSTOPERATIVE MANAGEMENT

Postoperative management is usually straightforward and rarely complicated by the pulmonary hypoplasia or hypertension seen with CCAM or CDH.

COMPLICATIONS

Complications such as pneumonia or abscess are common in unresected cysts. Malignancies such as rhabdosarcoma and adenocarcinoma have also been reported in long-standing cysts. Complications following resection are rare.

CLE

EMBRYOLOGY

CLE occurs almost always within a single pulmonary lobe as a result of air-trapping within the affected lobe. This in turn may be caused by a large variety of quite different underlying lesions or developmental events; thus, there is no single definable embryologic etiology. Even when an underlying lesion is found, its presence does not always fully explain the development of the emphysematous changes.

INCIDENCE

As with the other cystic lesions of the lung, the rarity of these conditions makes incidence difficult to determine. Even those that have been suggested are subject to later revision as reported experience accumulates and large case reviews are completed. With this caveat, the reported experience does indicate that not all lobes are equally affected. In one review, 43% of the cases involved the left upper lobe, 32% involved the right middle lobe, and 20% involved the right upper lobe. In one-fifth of the cases, there was bilateral involvement. There is a male predominance in reported cases, although this may be related to a gender difference in the incidence of underlying causes.

PRENATAL DIAGNOSIS

The development of emphysema requires air trapping, obviously a postnatal event. Although the potential underlying cause for this development may be present during fetal life, without the lung expansion, the condition cannot be diagnosed prenatally. If an underlying cause is identified by ultrasonography, MRI will sometimes show CLE lobes that are expanded and fluid filled in the fetus, which may become a useful marker.

POSTNATAL PRESENTATION

The underlying etiology leading to CLE appears to be air trapping, owing to some type of bronchial compression. This mechanism may explain the predominance of upper lobe involvement. Intrinsic bronchial abnormalities have been identified as the root cause. In some cases, a deficiency of bronchial cartilage predisposes the airway to collapse, with subsequent ball-valve trapping of air in the distal portion of the affected lobe. Similar situations have been reported to occur when the bronchial mucosa is abnormally ridged or invaginated or if a plug of inspissated mucus obstructs a branching bronchus.

Obstruction may also be caused by extrinsic compression resulting from a bronchogenic cyst, enteric duplications, BPS, mediastinal tumors or lymphadenopathy, or vascular rings. Although it is extraordinarily unlikely in the neonate, aspiration of a foreign body could theoretically lead to the development of an emphysematous lobe by the same mechanism. In at least 50% of reported cases, however, no apparent obstruction could be found. This suggests that an additional mechanism or contributing factor may be present in the development of some CLE, such as an underlying defect in the lung parenchyma that results in tissue that is easily overdistended in a particular setting. There is an association with congenital cardiac or vascular abnormalities in about 13% of cases.

POSTNATAL DIAGNOSIS

Diagnosis is made during the early postnatal period in an infant with worsening respiratory distress and an increasing oxygen requirement. The chest radiograph shows the presence of an overdistended, emphysematous lobe in one lung, which is usually one of the upper lobes. The unilobar appearance and marked overdistention in a neonate are nearly pathognomonic for this condition.

DIFFERENTIAL DIAGNOSIS

The presentation of CLE is unique and rarely confused with another cystic lesion. There are several aspects of CLE that are not seen with other lesions: the absence of prenatal findings, the involvement of a single lobe, and the progressive nature of the clinical presentation beginning with an infant who is initially well.

With incomplete information, CLE could be confused with CCAM or a large bronchogenic cyst, but these diagnoses can usually be quickly ruled out. The rare possibility of an aspirated foreign body with subsequent air trapping should also be considered if the history is suggestive.

PREOPERATIVE MANAGEMENT

Preoperative management depends on the severity of symptoms and can vary from oxygen therapy and semielective resection to emergent intubation and urgent resection. The indication for surgical intervention is life-threatening progressive pulmonary insufficiency from compression of adjacent normal lung. Treatment of the asymptomatic hyperlucent lobe is controversial. There is no evidence that leaving it impairs development of the remaining lung. But infectious complications such as pneumonia are more common, and their incidence should be used to help guide decisions about resection.

SURGICAL MANAGEMENT

Surgical management is straightforward and requires resection of the involved segment or lobe. Occasionally, it is possible to spare the lung by resecting a mass that has caused an extrinsic compression. In the most symptomatic cases, emergent thoracotomy without delay is mandatory. Once the hyperinflated lung is released from the thoracic cavity, ventilation of the remaining normal units becomes much easier.

POSTOPERATIVE MANAGEMENT

Postoperative management is straightforward as symptoms of respiratory distress rapidly subside once the involved lobe has been resected.

COMPLICATIONS

Complications of untreated CLE can be fatal in the most symptomatic cases. Long-term follow-up of treated infants shows no evidence of impairment of pulmonary function.

References/Recommended Readings

Adzick NS. The fetus with cystic adenomatoid malformation. In: Harrison MR, Golbus MS, Filly RA, (eds). The unborn patient. 2nd ed. Philadelphia: WB Saunders; 1991. p. 320.

Adzick NS, Harrison MR, Cromblehome TM, Flake AW, Howell LJ. Fetal lung lesions: management and outcome. Am J Obstet Gynecol 1998;179:884.

Adzick NS, Harrison MR, Flake AW, et al. Fetal surgery for cystic adenomatoid malformation of the lung. J Pediatr Surg 1993;28:806.

Al-Salem AH, Gyamfi YA, Grant CS. Congenital lobar emphysema. Can J Anaesth 1990;37:377.

Case records of the Massachusetts General Hospital (case 32-1990). N Engl J Med 1990;323:398.

Cass DL, Cromebleholme TM, Howell LJ, et al. Cystic lung lesions with systemic arterial blood supply: a hybrid of congenital cyctic adenomatoid malformation and bronchopulmonary sequestration. J Pediatr Surg 1997:32;986–90.

Cha I, Adzick NS, Harrison MR, Finkbeiner WE. Fetal congenital cystic adenomatoid amlformations of the lung: a clinicopathologic study of eleven cases. Am J Surg Pathol 1997;21:537–44.

Ch'in KY, Tang MY. Congenital adenomatoid malformation of one lobe of a lung with anasarca. Arch Pathol 1949;48:155.

Clark SL, Vitale DJ, Minton SC, Stoddard RA, Sabey PL. Successful fetal therapy for cystic adenomatoid malformation associated with second trimester hydrops. Am J Obstet Gynecol 1987;157:294.

d'Agostino H, Bonoldi E, Dante S, et al. Embryonal rhabdomyosarcoma of the lung arising in cystic adenomatoid malformation: case report and review of the literature. J Pediatr Surg 1997;32:1381.

Dale PJ, Shaw NJ. Bronchogenic cyst presenting in the neonatal period. Acta Paediatr 1994;83:1102.

Dolkart L, Reimer F, Helmuth W, et al. Antenatal diagnosis of pulmonary sequestration. A review. Obstet Gynecol Surv 1992;47:515.

Donovan CB, Edelman RR, Vrachliotis TG, Frank HA, Kim D. Bronchopulmonary sequestration with MR angiographic evaluation. J Vasc Dis 1994;45:239.

Engle WA, Lemons JA, Weber TR, Cohen MD. Congenital lobar emphysema due to a bronchogenic cyst. Am J Perinatol 1984;1:196.

Haddon MJ, Bowen A. Bronchogenic and neurenteric forms of foregut anomalies: imaging for diagnosis and management. Radiol Clin North Am 1991;29:241.

Krieger PA, Ruchetti Ed, Mahboubi S, et al. Fetal pulmonary malformations: defining histopathology Am J Surg Pathol 2006:30;643–9.

Kwittken J, Reiner L. Congenital cystic adenomatoid malformation of the lung. Pediatrics 1962;30:759.

Laisaar T. Intralobar pulmonary sequestration of the upper lobe combined with congenital lobar emphysema. Chest 1999;116:401S.

Langer JC, Donato L, Riethmuller C, et al. Spontaneous regression of fetal pulmonary sequestration. Ultrasound Obstet Gynecol 1995;6:33.

Lopoo JB, Goldstein RB, Lipshutz GS, et al. Fetal pulmonary sequestration: a favorable congenital lung lesion. Obstet Gynecol 1999;94:567.

Meizner I, Levy A. A survey of non-cardiac fetal intrathoracic malformation diagnosed by ultrasound. Arch Gynecol Obstet 1994;255:31.

Monin P, Didler F, Vert P, Prevot J, Plenat F. Giant lobar emphysema: neonatal diagnosis. Pediatr Radiol 1979;8:259.

Morris E, Constatine G, McHugo J. Cystic adenomatoid malformation of the lung: an obstetric and ultrasound perspective. Eur J Obstet Gynecol 1991;40:11.

Murphy JJ, Blair GK, Fraser GC, et al. Rhabdomyosarcoma arising within congenital pulmonary cysts: report of three cases. J Pediatr Surg 1992;27:1364.

Murray GF, Talbert JL, Haller Jr JA. Obstructive lobar emphysema of the newborn infant: documentation of the "mucous plug syndrome" with successful treatment by bronchotomy. J Thorac Cardiovasc Surg 1967;53:886.

Ong SS, Chan SY, Ewer AK, et al. Laser ablation of Foetal microcystic lung lesion: successful outcome and rationale for its use. Fetal Daign Ther 2006:21:471–4.

Rahmani MR, Filler RM, Shuckett B. Bronchogenic cyst occurring in the antenatal period. J Ultrasound Med 1995;14:971.

Sade RM, Clouse M, Ellis Jr FH. The spectrum of pulmonary sequestration. Ann Thorac Surg 1974;18:644.

Sakala EP, Perott WS, Grube GL. Sonographic characteristics of antenatally diagnosed extralobar pulmonary sequestration and congenital cystic adenomatoid malformation. Obstet Gynecol Surv 1994;49:647.

Sauerbrei E. Lung sequestration: duplex Doppler diagnosis at 19 weeks gestation. J Ultrasound Med 1991;10:101.

Savic B, Birtel FJ, Tholen W. Lung sequestration: report of seven cases and review of 540 published cases. Thorax 1979;34:96.

Schoenenberger AW, Weder W, Meyenberger C. Check-up at 40 years of age. Schweiz Rundsch Med Prax 1996;85:798.

Scully RE, Mark EJ, McNeely WF, et al. Weekly clinicopathological exercises. N Engl J Med 1997;337:916–24.

Slotnick RN, McGahan J, Milio L, et al. Antenatal diagnosis and treatment of fetal bronchopulmonary sequestration. Fetal Diagn 1990;5:33.

Smith RP, Illanes S, Denvow ML, Soothill PW. Outcome of fetal pleural effusions treated by thoracoabdominal shunting. Ultrasound Obstet Gynecol 2005:26;63–6.

Stocker JT, Madewell JER, Drake RM. Congenital cystic adenomatoid malformation of the lung: classification and morphologic spectrum. Hum Pathol 1977;8:155.

Warner JO, Rubin S, Heard BE. Congenital lobar emphysema: a case with bronchial atresia and abnormal bronchial cartilages. Br J Dis Chest 1982;76:177.

SEVEN

Gastrointestinal Disorders

Part 1: Gastroschisis

Camilia R. Martin, MD, MS, and
Steven J. Fishman, MD, FACS, FAAP

Embryology

NORMAL GASTROINTESTINAL FORMATION AND ROTATION

At 4 Weeks' Gestation

The primordial gut is formed from the yolk sac and is comprised of three different sections: the foregut, the midgut, and the hindgut.

- The foregut gives rise to the pharynx, lower respiratory system, esophagus, stomach, duodenum proximal to the bile duct, liver, pancreas, and biliary apparatus.
- The midgut gives rise to the duodenum distal to the bile duct, jejunum, ileum, cecum, appendix, ascending colon, and right portion of the transverse colon.
- The hindgut gives rise to the left portion of the transverse colon, descending and sigmoid colon, rectum, and the superior portion of the anal canal.

At 6 Weeks' Gestation

The midgut forms a U-shaped intestinal loop that protrudes from the abdominal cavity into the proximal portion of the umbilical cord (yolk sac). While in the umbilical cord, this midgut loop rotates counterclockwise 90°.

At 10 and 11 Weeks' Gestation

The midgut loop starts to return to the abdominal cavity while rotating another 90°. In the 11th week, after returning to the abdominal cavity, the intestines rotate a final 90°, for a total rotation of 270°.

Etiology

The etiology of gastroschisis remains controversial. Several mechanisms have been proposed.

- Early embryology of the umbilicus includes two umbilical veins. The left umbilical vein persists and later migrates toward the central ventral position. The right umbilical vein normally regresses. It has been postulated that this involution creates a potential weak spot at the junction of the right aspect of the umbilical ring and the abdominal wall that may allow for rupture and bowel herniation.[1] This event most likely occurs sometime after the sixth week of gestation but before the return of the intestines into the abdominal cavity, which normally occurs around the tenth week of gestation.
- Exposure to teratogenic agents, such as solvents, colorants, aspirin, ibuprofen, pseudoephedrine, and cocaine, have been associated with an increased risk of gastroschisis. Many of these substances are vasoconstrictive agents, which supports a vascular contribution to the pathogenesis of gastroschisis.[2]
- Genetic influences have been implicated, with several reports of familial occurrences, including multiple affected siblings and vertical transmission from mother to son.[3,4]

Incidence

- The incidence of gastroschisis is 1 in 4,000 to 20,000 live births.
- Maternal risk factors include very young age, primigravidity, lower socioeconomic status, and lower body mass index.[5]

Prenatal Diagnosis and Treatment

- Elevated alpha fetoprotein levels are associated with abdominal wall defects.
- Antenatal ultrasonography can accurately diagnose gastroschisis in the second trimester of pregnancy.
- An amniocentesis is not necessary for simple or isolated cases; the incidence of associated chromosomal abnormalities in infants with isolated gastroschisis is very low.[6]
- There is a higher incidence of oligohydramnios, fetal growth restriction, and meconium-stained amniotic fluid.[7,8] If intestinal atresia is present, there may be polyhydramnios.
- Regular fetal monitoring and antenatal testing have been shown to reduce perinatal mortality.[7]
- Although, delivery at an earlier gestational age has been previously suggested, current data does not support this practice.[9–11]
- The presence of dilated bowel is not an absolute indication for delivery.[12,13]
- Delivery at a regional center has been associated with improved outcomes, including earlier enteral feedings and shorter lengths of stay.[14]
- When the diagnosis is known prenatally, surgical and neonatal consultations should be obtained to adequately prepare the family as well as the specialty services.

PREFERRED ROUTE OF DELIVERY

The preferred route for delivery remains controversial. Elective cesarean section has been advocated to reduce additional bowel injury that may occur during the passage through the birth canal.[15] Conversely, delivery by elective cesarean section has not been shown to be advantageous in multiple recent studies.[14,16,17] However, some of these studies do not distinguish cesarean sections performed before the onset of labor from those performed after the onset of labor, which may be an important distinguishing feature.[15,18,19]

- Currently, there is not enough strong evidence to recommend or mandate a specific route of delivery for an uncomplicated gastroschisis.

- A cesarean section is recommended for rare large lesions with the liver exposed to avoid damage to the liver and bleeding.

Postnatal Presentation

- Gastroschisis presents as eviscerated intestinal loops, without a covering sac, protruding through an abdominal wall defect located just right of the umbilical cord.
- The umbilical cord is intact.
- The intestinal loops may be thickened, foreshortened, and covered with a fibrous peel.

Postnatal Diagnosis

Gastroschisis should be readily identifiable by the lack of a covering sac and the placement of the abdominal wall defect to the right of an intact umbilical cord.

ASSOCIATED DEFECTS

- All of these infants will have abnormal rotation and fixation of the intestines (malrotation).
- Of infants with gastroschisis, 8 to 16% will have other gastrointestinal (GI) anomalies, including midgut volvulus, intestinal atresia, intestinal stenosis, and/or intestinal perforation.[1,20]
- Chromosomal or non-GI structural anomalies are rare (in contrast to an omphalocele). In a recent, large international study, 86% of cases were isolated while 12% were associated with multiple congenital anomalies, and 2% were associated with a recognizable syndrome.[21]

Differential Diagnosis

- Omphalocele. See Table 1-1 for a comparison of these two abdominal wall defects. If omphalocele sac is ruptured, it confuses distinction from gastroschisis.
- Rule out ruptured omphalocele and umbilical cord hernia.

Continued

TABLE 1   Clinical Distinction between Gastroschisis and Omphalocele

Characteristic	Gastroschisis	Omphalocele
Incidence	1 in 4,000 to 20,000	1 in 3,000 to 10,000
Maternal age	Younger	Older
Male: female ratio	1:1	3:1
Location of defect	Right of the umbilical cord	Within umbilical ring
Umbilical cord	Intact, normal insertion	Insertion onto covering sac
Size of defect	Usually < 4 cm	Usually > 4 cm
Organs extruded, other than bowel	Stomach	Liver, spleen, bladder, uterus, ovaries
Cover sac	Absent	Present, may be ruptured
Appearance of bowel	Matted, foreshortened, edematous	Usually normal
Additional anomalies	10 to 20%	45 to 80%
Gastrointestinal, other than malrotation	16%, intestinal atresia, midgut volvulus, intestinal stenosis	Rare

TABLE 1 Continued

Characteristic	Gastroschisis	Omphalocele
Nongastrointestinal	Rare	Common [Cardiac (28%), genitourinary (20%), craniofacial (20%), diaphragmatic hernia (12%), musculoskeletal]
Chromosomal	Rare	50%, trisomies common
Syndromes	None	Pentalogy of Cantrell [Beckwith-Wiedemann syndrome OEIS complex]
Surgery	Primary closure in 80%	Often primary closure for lesions < 5 cm, multi staged for larger lesions
Bowel function after surgery	Usually slow	Normal to slow
Survival	> 90	90% in absence of associated anomalies, 60 to 70% in presence of multiple associated anomalies

Adapted from Torfs et al. Gastroschisis. J Pediatr 1990;116:1–6.
OEIS = omphalocele, extrophy of the bladder, imperforate anus, and spinal deformity.

Preoperative Management

- The exposed intestinal loops must be handled carefully to avoid additional injury to the bowel wall.
- Use latex-free gloves and other latex-free products.
- Avoid contamination when handling the bowel.
- The dressing options are as follows:
  1. It is preferred to encase the intestinal contents in a bowel bag (eg, Vi-Drape Isolation Bag®) as this will be less directly abrasive to the bowel serosa. Place the lower two-thirds of the infant into a sterile bowel bag containing 20 mL of warmed sterile saline. Tie it at the nipple line.
  2. If a bowel bag is not available, saline-soaked dressings may be used. Make sure that the externalized bowel is not twisted or kinked before wrapping. Moisten gauze with warmed sterile saline. Wrap wide cotton gauze roll around the infant to hold the dressing in place. Place an 8 French (F) feeding tube into the gauze wrap to provide sterile access for subsequent hydration if surgical correction cannot be performed immediately, and then cover with plastic wrap. Moisten the dressing every 4 hours by drawing 20 to 30 mL of warmed sterile saline into a syringe and slowly injecting it into the 8 F feeding tube inserted under the plastic wrap.
- For small defects, the infant may be placed supine. For larger defects, the infant may be placed on his side, to avoid kinking of the mesenteric vessels over the abdominal fascial opening. Alternately, if supine, the wrapped bowel must be supported directly over the abdomen.
- For abdominal decompression, place a nasogastric tube to low continuous suction at 20 to 40 mm Hg.
- Give nothing by mouth (NPO). Insert an intravenous line (IV) in the upper extremity and provide IV fluids two to four times maintenance because of the increased insensible losses through the exposed bowel.
- Send blood for complete blood count (CBC), blood culture, electrolytes, hydrogen ion concentration (pH), and type and cross match.
- Start broad-spectrum IV antibiotics (generally ampicillin and gentamicin).

- Monitor temperature, blood pressure (BP), fluid balance, and acid-base status closely.
- Transfer to an appropriate facility for surgical correction and postoperative neonatal care.
- An extensive preoperative evaluation is not necessary, as associated major congenital anomalies are rare.[6]

Surgical Management

- Because of the lack of a covering sac, gastroschisis repair is conducted as soon as possible.
- Surgical correction can be made either by primary closure or delayed, staged closure using a prosthetic silo. The amount and condition of the exposed intestinal bowel loops, as well as the ratio of exposed abdominal contents to abdominal cavity development, will determine the type of closure that will be necessary.
  1. A primary closure is preferred unless there is a concern for cardiovascular, renal (compartment syndrome), or respiratory compromise. This can be achieved in approximately 80% of cases.[22–24]
  2. A staged repair with a prosthetic silo usually occurs over a period of 5 to 7 days.[22,23]
- Historically, surgical reduction was recommended with the infant intubated and under general anesthesia. However, several recent case series have reported successful bedside reduction without general anesthesia with similar or improved infant outcomes compared to cohorts managed with general anesthesia. Although these studies are small, their results warrant additional investigation with larger clinical trials.[25–27]
- For reduction under general anesthesia:
  1. Anesthesia preparations should include gastric decompression as well as induction, and intubation with the infant in a semiupright position.[28,29]
  2. High peak inspiratory pressures may be needed for adequate respiratory support, because of the impaired diaphragmatic mobility secondary to elevated intra-abdominal pressure. An increase in required peak inspiratory pressures during

the surgical correction is an indicator that a primary closure may not be tolerated well by the infant.

3. Anesthesia may include an inhalational agent with oxygen and an opioid. Nitrous oxide should be avoided as it will exacerbate bowel distention. Spinal anesthesia also has been reported to be an effective anesthetic for gastroschisis repair.

- The management of coexisting intestinal atresia is controversial. The atretic segment can be addressed at the time of the repair with a resection and primary anastomosis or by creation of a stoma. If the bowel integrity is concerning, repair can be deferred until the inflammation has resolved. The overall condition of the bowel at the time of surgery will dictate the preferred option. Although some proximal atresias may be safely managed with a delayed procedure, distal atresias are sometimes complicated by infarction and necrosis; therefore, early repair at the time of the initial surgery should be considered.[30]

- If intestinal perforation or necrosis is present, an enterostomy may be necessary at the time of the initial repair.

- At the time of surgery, placement of a central venous catheter (CVC) should be considered to provide long-term parenteral nutrition (PN). Umbilical arterial and venous catheters and lower extremity peripheral intravenous central catheters (PICCs) are generally not desirable.

Postoperative Management

- Monitor for complications of increased intra-abdominal pressure, including escalation of respiratory support, hemodynamic compromise, and inferior vena cava compression as demonstrated by cyanotic lower extremities, decreased perfusion, decreased urine output, and metabolic acidosis. Surgical decompression may be necessary if complications of a primary closure are severe.

- Maintain normothermia, neutral fluid balance, hemodynamic stability, and gastric decompression.

- Give respiratory support. The return of the abdominal viscera into the abdominal cavity with primary closure temporarily worsens pulmonary compliance. Pulmonary mechanics progressively improve over the subsequent 24 to 72 hours, after which time, progressive weaning from the ventilator should be possible.

NUTRITIONAL SUPPORT

- Recovering patients may have decreased GI motility and/or prolonged ileus, resulting in significant delay in tolerating full enteral feedings. If severe, mechanical obstruction should be excluded using a contrast study.
- The average length of time to achieve full enteral feeds is 2 to 3 weeks.[22,24]
- Prokinetic agents have not been documented to be helpful.[31,32]
- Nutritional requirements should be provided by PN until full enteral feedings are achieved.
- Potential GI complications include gastroesophageal (GE) reflux and necrotizing enterocolitis (NEC).

CONTROL OF PAIN

Adequate pain control can be achieved using IV narcotics (eg, morphine or fentanyl). High doses of narcotics will exacerbate issues of GI motility. For those infants who had an epidural catheter placed prior to the surgical repair, postoperative analgesia can be continued through this device.

ANTIBIOTIC COVERAGE

No published data exist regarding the optimal length of postoperative antibiotic coverage. Our practice is to continue broad-spectrum antibiotics for 72 hours after final closure, whether it is a primary or staged repair.

SEPSIS

Sepsis is a significant contributor to overall morbidity and mortality with gram-negative organisms being the most common etiologic agents.[22] A high suspicion for sepsis should be maintained throughout the hospital course. A CBC and blood culture should be drawn if an infection is suspected. Antibiotic regimens can be tailored based on the blood culture results.

Complications and Outcome

- The survival rate is > 90%.[1,22,24]
- The finding of dilated loops of bowel on an antenatal sonogram has been shown to correlate with bowel edema, longer repair time, later initiation of enteral feedings, and a higher rate of postoperative complications.[16,33]
- Prematurity, low birth weight, staged silo repair, and the presence of associated GI lesions (intestinal atresia, perforation, necrosis, and volvulus) are associated with a longer time to full enteral feedings, prolonged hospital stays, and increased hospital costs.[20,22,34]
- A minority of patients have cholestasis.
- Most patients experience good long-term health and growth.[35] Reported long-term complications include nonspecific abdominal pain and the need for additional abdominal surgery for strictures and scar revisions.[35,36]

References

1. Dillon PW, Cilley RE. Newborn surgical emergencies. Gastrointestinal anomalies, abdominal wall defects. Pediatr Clin North Am 1993;40:1289–314.
2. Torfs CP, Katz EA, Bateson TF, et al. Maternal medications and environmental exposures as risk factors for gastroschisis. Teratology 1996;54:84–92.
3. Nelson TC, Toyama WM. Familial gastroschisis: a case of mother-and son occurrence. J Pediatr Surg 1995;30:1706–8.
4. Schmidt AI, Gluer S, Muhlhaus K, Ure BM. Family cases of gastroschisis. J Pediatr Surg 2005;40:740–1.
5. Feldkamp ML, Carey JC, Sadler TW. Development of gastroschisis: review of hypotheses, a novel hypothesis, and implications for research. Am J Med Genet A 2007;143:639–52.
6. Gaines BA, Holcomb GW, Neblet WW. Gastroschisis and omphalocele. In: Ashcraft KW, editor. Pediatric surgery. WB Saunders Company; 2000. p. 639–49.
7. Adair CD, Rosnes J, Frye AH, et al. The role of antepartum surveillance in the management of gastroschisis. Int J Gynaecol Obstet 1996;52:141–4.

8. Chen CP, Liu FF, Jan SW, et al. Prenatal diagnosis and perinatal aspects of abdominal wall defects. Am J Perinatol 1996;13:355–61.

9. Charlesworth P, Njere I, Allotey J, et al. Postnatal outcome in gastroschisis: effect of birth weight and gestational age. J Pediatr Surg 2007;42:815–8.

10. Ergun O, Barksdale E, Ergun FS, et al. The timing of delivery of infants with gastroschisis influences outcome. J Pediatr Surg 2005;40:424–8.

11. Puligandla PS, Janvier A, Flageole H, et al. The significance of intrauterine growth restriction is different from prematurity for the outcome of infants with gastroschisis. J Pediatr Surg 2004;39:1200–4.

12. Alsulyman OM, Monteiro H, Ouzounian JG, et al. Clinical significance of prenatal ultrasonographic intestinal dilatation in fetuses with gastroschisis. Am J Obstet Gynecol 1996;175(4 Pt 1):982–4.

13. Sipes SL, Weiner CP, Williamson RA, et al. Fetal gastroschisis complicated by bowel dilation: an indication for imminent delivery? Fetal Diagn Ther 1990;5:100–3.

14. Quirk JG Jr, Fortney J, Collins HB II, et al. Outcomes of newborns with gastroschisis: the effects of mode of delivery, site of delivery, and interval from birth to surgery. Am J Obstet Gynecol 1996;174:1134–8; discussion 1138–40.

15. Lenke RR, Hatch EI Jr. Fetal gastroschisis: a preliminary report advocating the use of cesarean section. Obstet Gynecol 1986;67:395–8.

16. Adra AM, Landy HJ, Nahmias J, Gomez-Marin O. The fetus with gastroschisis: impact of route of delivery and prenatal ultrasonography. Am J Obstet Gynecol 1996; 174:540–6.

17. Logghe HL, Mason GC, Thornton JG, Stringer MD. A randomized controlled trial of elective preterm delivery of fetuses with gastroschisis. J Pediatr Surg 2005;40:1726–31.

18. Vegunta RK, Wallace LJ, Leonardi MR, et al. Perinatal management of gastroschisis: analysis of a newly established clinical pathway. J Pediatr Surg 2005;40:528–34.

19. White JJ. Outcome analysis for gastroschisis [letter; comment]. J Pediatr Surg 2000;35:398–9

20. Abdullah F, Arnold MA, Nabaweesi R, et al. Gastroschisis in the United States 1988–2003: analysis and risk categorization of 4344 patients. J Perinatol 2007;27:50–5.

21. Mastroiacovo P, Lisi A, Castilla EE, et al. Gastroschisis and associated defects: an international study. Am J Med Genet A 2007;143:660–71.

22. Driver CP, Bruce J, Bianchi A, et al. The contemporary outcome of gastroschisis. J Pediatr Surg 2000;35:1719–23.

23. Meller JL, Reyes HM, Loeff DS. Gastroschisis and omphalocele. Clin Perinatol 1989;16:113–22.

24. Novotny DA, Klein RL, Boeckman CR. Gastroschisis: an 18-year review. J Pediatr Surg 1993;28:650–2.

25. Cauchi J, Parikh DH, Samuel M, et al. Does gastroschisis reduction require general anesthesia? A comparative analysis. J Pediatr Surg 2006;41:1294–7.

26. Davies MW, Kimble RM, Cartwright DW. Gastroschisis: ward reduction compared with traditional reduction under general anesthesia. J Pediatr Surg 2005;40:523–7.

27. Owen A, Marven S, Jackson L, et al. Experience of bedside preformed silo staged reduction and closure for gastroschisis. J Pediatr Surg 2006;41:1830–5.

28. Bikhazi GB, Davis PJ. Anesthesia for neonates and premature infants. In: Motoyama EK, Davis PJ, editors. Smith's anesthesia for infants and children. Mosby; 1996. p. 455–7.

29. Palmer T. Anesthesia considerations for pediatric general surgery and gastrointestinal and hepatobiliary disease. In: Zaglaniczny K, Aker J, editors. Clinical guide to pediatric anesthesia. W.B. Saunders Company; 1999. p. 133–5.

30. Fleet MS, de la Hunt MN. Intestinal atresia with gastroschisis: a selective approach to management. J Pediatr Surg 2000;35: 1323–5.

31. Curry JI, Lander AD, Stringer MD. A multicenter, randomized, double-blind, placebo-controlled trial of the prokinetic agent erythromycin in the postoperative recovery of infants with gastroschisis. J Pediatr Surg 2004;39:565–9.

32. Langer JC. Gastroschisis and omphalocele. Semin Pediatr Surg 1996;5:124–8.

33. Piper HG, Jaksic T. The impact of prenatal bowel dilation on clinical outcomes in neonates with gastroschisis. J Pediatr Surg 2006;41:897–900.

34. Eggink BH, Richardson CJ, Malloy MH, Angel CA. Outcome of gastroschisis: a 20-year case review of infants with gastroschisis born in Galveston, Texas. J Pediatr Surg 2006;41:1103–8.

35. Davies BW, Stringer MD. The survivors of gastroschisis. Arch Dis Child 1997;77:158–60.

36. Koivusalo A, Lindahl H, Rintala RJ. Morbidity and quality of life in adult patients with a congenital abdominal wall defect: a questionnaire survey. J Pediatr Surg 2002;37: 1594–601.

Part 2: Omphalocele

Camilia R. Martin, MD, MS, and
Steven J. Fishman, MD, FACS, FAAP

Embryology

- For normal gastrointestinal formation and rotation, refer to "Embryology" in "Part 1: Gastroschisis."
- The union of the four somatic folds (cephalic, two lateral, and caudal) lead to the normal formation of the abdominal wall. Early in gestation, these four folds migrate centrally to join with the umbilical ring. This migration is completed by 18 weeks' gestation.
- An omphalocele occurs if the intestinal loops fail to return to the abdominal cavity at 11 weeks' gestation and/or the somatic folds fail to complete the formation of the abdominal wall by 18 weeks' gestation.
- Omphalocele is due to abnormal embryologic development, and, therefore, it has a high rate of associated defects and chromosomal anomalies.

Incidence

- The incidence is 1 in 3,000 to 1 in 10,000 live births.
- Vertical transmission across several generations in one family has been described suggesting, in rare circumstances, autosomal dominant inheritance.[1]

Prenatal Diagnosis and Treatment

- Abdominal wall defects are associated with elevated alpha fetoprotein levels.
- Omphalocele can be accurately diagnosed by antenatal ultrasound in the second trimester.
- A careful examination of other organ systems, including a fetal echocardiogram, should be performed due to the high rates of additional anomalies.

- An amniocentesis is recommended to rule out chromosomal abnormalities, which are found in almost 50% of cases.
- There is a higher incidence of prematurity and fetal growth restriction.[2] The risk of preterm birth is greater in multiparous versus nulliparous mothers.[3]
- There is a 3:1 male-to-female predominance.[4]
- Infants with small lesions may be delivered vaginally. Cesarean sections are recommended for large lesions that contain the liver.[5]
- When the diagnosis is known prenatally, consultation with a neonatologist and a surgeon should be arranged antenatally to adequately prepare the family as well as the specialty services.

Postnatal Presentation

- The amniotic sac and peritoneum protect the intestinal loops; however, the covering sac may be ruptured.
- The umbilical cord inserts onto the amniotic sac.
- The abdominal wall musculature is normal.
- The defect can vary in size. Larger lesions ("giant" omphalocele, > 5 cm) may contain the liver as well as intestinal loops, whereas smaller lesions contain only bowel.

Postnatal Diagnosis

- A careful physical examination should be performed for dysmorphic features and radiographic evaluation obtained if additional anomalies are evident.
- Echocardiography should be performed to evaluate for associated cardiac anomalies.
- All infants will have malrotation of the intestines. However, in contrast with gastroschisis, it is rare to have other intestinal anomalies.

ASSOCIATED DEFECTS

- Associated defects are present in as many as 80% of cases.[6]
- Chromosomal defects (most commonly trisomy 13, 18, or 21) can be seen in 48%[6] of cases. It has been reported that small lesions, those only containing bowel, have a greater likelihood of being chromosomal abnormalities.[7–9]

- Cardiac anomalies can be seen in 28% of cases. These include atrial septal defect, ventricular septal defect, patent ductus arteriosus, dextrocardia, tetralogy of Fallot, and bicuspid aortic valve.
- Genitourinary defects can be seen in 20% of cases.
- Craniofacial defects can be seen in 20% of cases.
- Diaphragmatic hernia can be seen in 12% of cases.
- Musculoskeletal, vertebral and limb, deformities can also be seen.
- Pulmonary hypoplasia secondary to thoracic maldevelopment, such as narrow chest deformity, can also be seen.[10,11]

Associated Syndromes

- Pentalogy of Cantrell with midline abdominal wall defect, ectopia cordis, sternal cleft, diaphragmatic hernia, and cardiac anomalies
- Beckwith–Wiedemann syndrome with macroglossia, hemihypertophy, hypoglycemia (hyperinsulinism), and umbilical anomalies
- OEIS complex with omphalocele, extrophy of the bladder, imperforate anus, and spinal deformity

Differential Diagnosis

If the amniotic sac and peritoneum rupture in utero, the defect must be differentiated from a gastroschisis. Refer to "Table 7-1" in "Part 1: Gastroschisis" for a comparison of the two abdominal wall defects.

Preoperative Management

- Use latex-free products, including latex-free gloves.
- Avoid contamination when handling the defect.
- The dressing options are as follows:
  1. If the sac is ruptured, it is preferred to encase the intestinal contents in a bowel bag (eg, Vi-Drape Isolation Bag®) as this will be less directly abrasive to the bowel serosa. Place the lower two-thirds of the infant into a sterile bowel bag containing 20 mL of warmed sterile saline. Tie the nipple line.
  2. If a bowel bag is not available or if the sac is intact, saline-soaked dressings may be used. Moisten gauze with warmed

sterile saline and wrap wide cotton gauze roll around the infant to hold the dressing in place. Place an 8F feeding tube into the gauze wrap to provide sterile access for subsequent hydration if operative correction is not performed immediately and then cover with plastic wrap. Moisten dressing every 4 hours by drawing 20 to 30 mL of warmed sterile saline into a syringe and slowly injecting it into the 8F feeding tube inserted under the plastic wrap.

- For abdominal decompression place a nasogastric tube to low continuous suction at 20 to 40 mm Hg.
- Keep the infant NPO. Insert an IV in the upper extremity and provide adequate hydration to compensate for increased insensible losses through the exposed abdominal contents.
- Send blood for CBC, blood culture, electrolytes, pH, and type and cross match.
- Start broad-spectrum IV antibiotics (generally ampicillin and gentamicin).
- Monitor temperature, blood pressure, fluid balance, and acid-base status closely.
- Transfer to an appropriate facility for surgical correction and postoperative neonatal care.

Surgical Management

- Primary repair is usually possible for lesions that are 5 cm or less.[6]
- The infant may not tolerate the primary closure of a large lesion due to an increase in abdominal cavity pressure resulting in hemodynamic, cardiorespiratory, and renal compromise.
- If a primary closure is not possible, several options exist for continuing management of the defect.[6]
  1. Skin closure alone can be performed creating a ventral hernia that can be closed several months later.
  2. A prosthetic silo can be created allowing for gradual, progressive compression with final closure in 7 to 10 days.
  3. When the above two options are not feasible in an infant with multiple underlying medical conditions (eg, additional anomalies, respiratory failure, and extreme prematurity), drying agents (alcohol, Mercurochrome, povidone-iodine,

silver nitrate, silver sulfadiazine) can be used to create an eschar with the final repair at a later date. These drying agents should be used sparingly as toxicity may develop. Mercury levels should be monitored with Mercurochrome use and thyroid function tests with povidone-iodine use.[11]

- Closure of giant omphaloceles represents a surgical challenge often requiring a multi-staged approach. Recently, additional strategies have been reported to facilitate the closure of giant omphaloceles including:
  1. Use of tissue expanders to lengthen the abdominal wall and increase the abdominal compartment[12,13] and
  2. Use of vacuum-assisted closure (VAC) device.[14]
- Anesthesia considerations are similar to those for gastroschisis repair. Please refer to "Part 1: Gastroschisis."
- At the time of surgery, placement of a CVC should be considered to provide long-term parenteral nutrition. Umbilical arterial and venous catheters and lower extremity PICCs are generally not desirable.

Postoperative Management

Principles of postoperative management are similar to those for gastroschisis repair. Please refer to "Postoperative Management" in "Part 1: Gastroschisis."

Complications and Outcome

- The survival rate is > 90% in patients with isolated omphalocele.[15]
- Mortality can be as high as 30 to 40% in the presence of multiple underlying complications. Factors affecting survival include a large defect, ruptured sac, low birth weight, the presence of additional congenital anomalies, and early respiratory failure.[11]
- Potential complications include decreased gastrointestinal motility (although to a lesser extent than with gastroschisis), bowel obstruction, perforated viscus, gastroesophageal reflux, and sepsis.
- Long-term morbidity and quality of life is determined by the associated malformations or syndromes. Long-term outcomes

for an isolated omphalocele are favorable with no greater morbidity than in the general population.[16,17]

References

1. Kanagawa SL, Begleiter ML, Ostlie DJ, et al. Omphalocele in three generations with autosomal dominant transmission. J Med Genet 2002;39:184–5.

2. Meller JL, Reyes HM, Loeff DS. Gastroschisis and omphalocele. Clin Perinatol 1989;16:113–22.

3. Salihu HM, Emusu D, Sharma PP, et al. Parity effect on preterm birth and growth outcomes among infants with isolated omphalocele. Eur J Obstet Gynecol Reprod Biol 2006;128:91–6.

4. Gilbert WM, Nicolaides KH. Fetal omphalocele: associated malformations and chromosomal defects. Obstet Gynecol 1987;70:633–5.

5. Gaines BA, Holcomb GW, Neblet WW. Gastroschisis and omphalocele. In: Ashcraft KW, editor. Pediatric surgery. WB Saunders Company; 2000. p. 639–49.

6. Dillon PW, Cilley RE. Newborn surgical emergencies. Gastrointestinal anomalies, abdominal wall defects. Pediatr Clin North Am 1993;40:1289–314.

7. Benacerraf BR, Saltzman DH, Estroff JA, Frigoletto FD Jr. Abnormal karyotype of fetuses with omphalocele: prediction based on omphalocele contents. Obstet Gynecol 1990;75:317–9.

8. Nicolaides KH, Snijders RJ, Cheng HH, Gosden C. Fetal gastro-intestinal and abdominal wall defects: associated malformations and chromosomal abnormalities. Fetal Diagn Ther 1992;7:102–15.

9. St-Vil D, Shaw KS, Lallier M, et al. Chromosomal anomalies in newborns with omphalocele. J Pediatr Surg 1996;31:831–4.

10. Langer JC. Gastroschisis and omphalocele. Semin Pediatr Surg 1996;5:124–8.

11. Tsakayannis DE, Zurakowski D, Lillehei CW. Respiratory insufficiency at birth: a predictor of mortality for infants with omphalocele. J Pediatr Surg 1996;31:1088–90; discussion 90–1.

12. De Ugarte DA, Asch MJ, Hedrick MH, Atkinson JB. The use of tissue expanders in the closure of a giant omphalocele. J Pediatr Surg 2004;39:613–5.

13. Foglia R, Kane A, Becker D, et al. Management of giant omphalocele with rapid creation of abdominal domain. J Pediatr Surg 2006;41:704–9; discussion 704–9.

14. Kilbride KE, Cooney DR, Custer MD. Vacuum-assisted closure: a new method for treating patients with giant omphalocele. J Pediatr Surg 2006;41:212–5.

15. Heider AL, Strauss RA, Kuller JA. Omphalocele: clinical outcomes in cases with normal karyotypes. Am J Obstet Gynecol 2004;190:135–41.

16. Koivusalo A, Lindahl H, Rintala RJ. Morbidity and quality of life in adult patients with a congenital abdominal wall defect: a questionnaire survey. J Pediatr Surg 2002;37:1594–601.

17. Lunzer H, Menardi G, Brezinka C. Long-term follow-up of children with prenatally diagnosed omphalocele and gastroschisis. J Matern Fetal Med 2001;10:385–92.

Part 3: Necrotizing Enterocolitis

Anne R. Hansen, MD, MPH, Biren P. Modi, MD, Y. Avery Ching, MD, and Tom Jaksic, MD, PhD

Incidence

The overall incidence of necrotizing enterocolitis (NEC) is 1 to 7% of admissions to the neonatal intensive care unit. Of affected infants, 90% are preterm, with risk inversely related to gestational age.

Pathophysiology

PATHOLOGY

Necrotizing enterocolitis involves coagulation necrosis, bacterial overgrowth, and inflammation of the bowel wall. Although any segment can be affected, NEC most commonly involves the terminal ileum and ascending colon. In the most severe cases, the entire bowel is involved (necrotizing enterocolitis totalis).

MULTIFACTORIAL ETIOLOGY

The etiology of NEC is likely multifactorial, including mesenteric ischemia and tissue hypoxia caused by inadequate vascular supply to the premature gut, infectious agents in the setting of an immature immune system, and enteral alimentation providing a luminal substrate for bacterial pathogens and increasing the oxygen demand of the intestine. Numerous molecular intermediaries have been implicated, including the pro-inflammatory cytokines, nitric oxide, and the cyclooxygenase-2/NF-κB pathway.[1,2]

RISK FACTORS

- Extreme prematurity is the single greatest and most consistent risk factor.

- The occasionally endemic or even epidemic occurrence of NEC fits the epidemiology of an infectious process. There are no specific causative organisms associated specifically with NEC; rather, the organisms colonizing the gut appear to become invasive pathogens.

- Enteral feedings are associated with NEC, with only 10% of cases occurring in infants who have never been fed enterally. Since enteral feedings are an essentially universal part of any infant's care, it is difficult to distinguish between causation and association.

- Most risk factors are forms of inadequate mesenteric perfusion and/or oxygenation and include the following: intrauterine growth restriction, asphyxia, hypotension, polycythemia, and hypoxia. These "risk factors" may actually be only proxies for prematurity and severity of illness.

- There is inconsistent evidence that umbilical arterial lines, positioned in either the "low" or "high" position, increase the risk of NEC.[3,4] Again, an infant's need for an umbilical artery catheter is a marker for prematurity and severity of illness.

- Intrauterine exposure to cocaine increases the risk of NEC.[5]

- Miscellaneous other risk factors include poor gut motility and hypoglycemia.

- It is controversial whether prenatal exposure to indomethacin as a tocolytic agent or postnatal exposure for the treatment of PDA increases an infant's risk of NEC.[6–9] Because PDA is itself a risk factor for NEC, it is extremely difficult to distinguish whether it is the duct, the indomethacin, or both that yields an increased incidence of NEC in this patient population. Given the potential cardiorespiratory and neurologic[10] benefits of indomethacin, the benefits appear to outweigh the risks of aggressive medical treatment of PDA with indomethacin unless contraindicated.[11]

- The risk of NEC is increased with medical conditions that may compromise mesenteric perfusion and/or oxygenation, such as congenital heart disease (left ventricular outflow tract obstruction, left-to-right shunt, or cyanotic lesion), and gastroschisis. It is important to consider the possibility of such an underlying condition, especially when NEC occurs in term infants who are otherwise at low risk.

Prevention

- Efforts should be aimed at provision of adequate mesenteric perfusion and oxygenation: maintain normal BP and partial pressure of oxygen (PaO_2), avoid hyperviscosity, and treat hemodynamically significant PDA.
- Feeding with breast milk rather than formula may decrease the risk of NEC.[12,13]
- Early introduction of trophic feedings (10 mL/kg/d) may also be protective.[14]
- Slower rate of advancement of enteral feedings may decrease the incidence of NEC, but it is unclear if this intervention improves survival or other pertinent outcomes.[15]

POTENTIAL PREVENTIVE STRATEGIES

There are many other potential preventive strategies that are still in the experimental phases of development and require further study before being introduced into standard practice:

- Prenatal exposure to steroids may be protective against NEC. Current studies suggest that this may be mediated through a maturational resistance to inflammation in the premature intestine.[16]
- Prevention of bacterial overgrowth by acidification of oral feedings has been shown to decrease rates of NEC. This concept is further supported by the demonstration of an increased risk of NEC in infants treated with histamine receptor blockade.[17,18] Though enteral acidification is not yet warranted, judicious use of acid blockade is a reasonable implementation at this point.
- Bowel decontamination with enterally administered antibiotics has been shown to decrease the incidence of NEC, but concerns about development of resistant bacteria persist. The routine use of enteral antibiotics to prevent NEC does not seem to be clinically warranted at present.[19]
- Probiotic prophylaxis with enterally administered *Lactobacillus acidophilus* and *Bifidobacterium infantis* has been suggested[20] but is not used clinically because of concern regarding potential bacterial translocation.
- Augmentation of intestinal growth and development with erythropoietin (epo). Infants receiving epo for prevention of

anemia of prematurity were noted to have a decreased incidence of NEC.[21]
- Passive immunization with oral IgG and IgA has been attempted in several studies but has not demonstrated any benefit in prevention of NEC or survival.[22]

Clinical Presentation

The typical age at onset of symptoms is 2 or 3 weeks, with the range being from the first week to as late as 12 weeks of age. In general, the age at onset is inversely related to gestational age, with gestationally more mature infants presenting sooner after birth.

SYSTEMIC SYMPTOMS

The symptoms of NEC include the following: increased frequency and/or severity of apnea and/or bradycardia of prematurity, irritability, lethargy, unstable temperature, poor perfusion, bleeding, and, when in its most extreme form, shock.

ENTERIC SYMPTOMS

The following enteric symptoms may be present.

- Decreased motility: hypoactive bowel sounds, increased volume and/or bile staining of residual milk, abdominal distention
- Bowel injury and/or necrosis: abdominal tenderness and/or bluish discoloration, bloody stool, ascites.

Diagnosis

The diagnosis of NEC is based on laboratory tests and imaging and surgical findings.

SPECIFIC DIAGNOSIS

- Imaging: pneumatosis with or without free intraperitoneal air is revealed on imaging of the kidney(s), ureter(s), and bladder (KUB).
- A laparotomy will show bowel necrosis.

NONSPECIFIC DIAGNOSIS

Blood Testing

- Blood tests will reveal the following: thrombocytopenia, metabolic and/or respiratory acidosis, leukocytosis or leukopenia with left shift (ratio of immature: total neutrophils > 0.2), hyponatremia, hyperkalemia, hypoglycemia or hyperglycemia. A recent prospective analysis demonstrated a significant increase in acidosis and hyperglycemia in the 24-hour period preceding NEC.[23]
- The relative indications for surgical intervention include refractory metabolic acidosis, thrombocytopenia, and neutropenia suggestive of necrotic and/or perforated bowel.

Stool Testing

The stool is positive for guaiac. Carbohydrate in the stool (positive Clinitest®) suggests malabsorption, which can be an early sign of altered bowel function caused by NEC.

Paracentesis

Paracentesis showing positive for stool or bacteria in the peritoneal fluid can be helpful in equivocal situations.

Imaging

RADIOGRAPHY

- KUB and cross-table lateral or left lateral decubitus radiography may show pneumatosis, edema of the bowel wall and distended, featureless, and/or fixed loops of bowel.[24] Portal venous air represents a progression of pneumatosis, while free peritoneal air supports the diagnosis of intestinal perforation.
- Free air is most easily seen in the left lateral decubitus position tracking above the right lobe of the liver.
- In an anteroposterior (AP) film, free air can be seen
  - as a "football" sign when it accumulates anteriorly in a football-shaped distribution, outlining the falciform ligament

that tracks from the start of the left lateral segment of the liver
to the umbilicus and

- in Morrison's pouch as a triangle-shaped collection of air in
  the right upper quadrant; or as visualization of both sides
  of the bowel wall.
- On the cross-table lateral view, free air can be seen as triangles of
  gas between the bowel loops and the anterior abdominal wall.

GASTROINTESTINAL SERIES

- An upper gastrointestinal (UGI) series is indicated, in the setting of bilious vomiting or aspirates, when trying to distinguish NEC from an anatomic obstruction such as malrotation
  with midgut volvulus.
- A lower gastrointestinal (LGI) study (eg, using a contrast
  enema performed with water-soluble, nonionic, iodinated
  contrast material) permits visualization of the bowel wall for
  areas of edema and ulceration.
- The potential diagnostic benefit of these procedures must be
  carefully weighed against the considerable risk of destabilization
  during the procedure and transport, as well as of intestinal perforation, especially during the enema.

ULTRASONOGRAPHY

When faced with an extremely ill infant who cannot tolerate an UGI
series, ultrasonography[25] can be useful for distinguishing between
NEC and malrotation by detecting thickening of the bowel, which
is indicative of possible ischemia, and by delineating the relationship
between the superior mesenteric artery and the superior mesenteric
vein. Ultrasonography has been shown to be more sensitive than
radiography for visualizing gas in the portal venous system.[26] The
clinical significance of this finding is not yet clear.

Bell Staging

Bell staging can be useful for predicting the need for surgical treatment, the outcome and mortality, and for comparing severity
before and after an intervention. In brief, there are three stages.

STAGE I

Suspected NEC. Clinical signs and symptoms are present but mild. The radiograph is nondiagnostic (showing a normal, mild dilation, or ileus).

- Stage Ia: the stool is positive for guaiac.
- Stage Ib: there is gross blood in the stool.

STAGE II

Definite NEC. Clinical signs and symptoms as in stage I plus pneumatosis or portal venous air can be seen on the radiograph.

- Stage IIa: Mildly ill
- Stage IIb: Moderately ill, systemic toxicity

STAGE III

Advanced NEC. Signs and symptoms and radiologic findings as in stage II plus critically ill infant.

- Stage IIIa: bowel intact
- Stage IIIb: bowel perforated

Differential Diagnosis

The differential diagnosis depends on the presenting symptoms.

- Poor bowel motility secondary to prematurity, medications (maternal $MgSO_4$, maternal or neonatal narcotics), or septic ileus
- Feeding intolerance
- Milk allergy
- Infectious enterocolitis, although diarrhea is unusual with NEC
- Bowel obstruction (eg, malrotation with midgut volvulus, intussusception, congenital bowel atresia, and/or stenosis)
- Isolated, usually gastric or ileal, perforation resulting from indomethacin or steroid therapy
- Mesenteric vessel thrombosis
- Inborn error of metabolism with resultant metabolic acidosis, electrolyte disturbances, glucose abnormalities, increased risk for sepsis (eg, galactosemia with *Escherichia coli* sepsis)

Preoperative Medical Management

CARDIOVASCULAR MANAGEMENT

- Support cardiovascular status to avoid hypotension and metabolic acidosis with resultant decrease in myocardial function.
- Patient may need intravascular volume expansion.
- Dopamine at low doses (ie, 1.25 to 2.5 mcg/kg/min) can increase mesenteric flow without causing systemic hypertension. This is not a common practice. If instituted, systemic hypertension with possible constriction of the mesenteric artery must be avoided. An increase, rather than decrease, in urine output is one functional measure of achieving a "low-dose" effect.
- Discontinue umbilical arterial access in order to maximize mesenteric perfusion. The patient may need placement of a peripheral arterial line to monitor continuous BP and arterial blood gases and to provide access for frequent blood draws.
- Weigh the risks and benefits of umbilical venous access. Consider the theoretical possibility of decreased venous return and a source of infection vs. the need for central access for intravascular volume resuscitation, pressor therapy, and parenteral nutrition.
- Central venous access will eventually be needed for long-term, high osmolarity nutrition and antibiotics. Given the high rate of bacteremia in the initial presentation of NEC, placement of central access should be deferred if possible until blood culture results are negative for 48 hours.

RESPIRATORY MANAGEMENT

- Support respiratory needs to avoid hypoxemia and respiratory acidosis. The infant may need intubation and mechanical ventilation.
- Respiratory failure may be multifactorial, including atelectasis and compromised diaphragmatic excursion secondary to abdominal distention, pulmonary edema secondary to fluid resuscitation and capillary leak, and pneumonia as a pulmonary manifestation of systemic sepsis.

GASTROINTESTINAL MANAGEMENT

- Discontinue all enteral intake – milk and medications.
- Decompress abdomen with Replogle® to continuous wall suction.
- KUB and cross-table lateral and/or left lateral decubitus radiographs will have been obtained as part of the diagnostic process. Serial abdominal radiographs should then be obtained to track progression and/or regression of disease and assist in determining the need for surgical intervention. Generally, radiographs are obtained every 6 to 8 hours for the first 24 hours, then at increasing intervals if the patient's condition stabilizes.
- Any suspicion of free air should be followed up with left lateral decubitus radiography.

MANAGEMENT OF FLUIDS, ELECTROLYTES, AND NUTRITION

- Monitor and, as needed, correct fluid and electrolyte balance carefully. Monitor weight, total input and outputs hourly, urine output, electrolytes, blood urea nitrogen (BUN), creatinine, and glucose.
- Anticipate an increase in the need for total fluids due to bowel wall edema, generalized capillary leak, and in extreme circumstances, cardiovascular collapse.
- Start parenteral nutrition as soon as possible, advance to maximum glucose, protein, and fat as appropriate (see Chapter 1, "General Considerations").

MANAGEMENT OF INFECTIOUS DISEASE

- Obtain a white blood cell count with differential and a blood culture.
- Perform lumbar puncture for cerebrospinal fluid glucose, protein, cell count, and culture when infant is stable enough to tolerate this procedure.
- Start broad-spectrum antibiotics for NEC beyond Bell stage I. We generally treat with Piperacillin-Tazobactam (Zosyn), a single, broad-spectrum antibiotic with excellent gram-negative and anaerobic coverage. Of note, it has limited CNS penetration and

so should not be used in the setting of associated meningitis. A traditional alternative is triple antibiotics with ampicillin, gentamicin, and clindamycin. The disadvantage of this regimen is the increased number of total antibiotic doses, the need to follow gentamicin levels, and the possible association between clindamycin and eventual stricture formation.

- Ensure that any organism identified by culture is sensitive to antibiotic regimen chosen. Because NEC can involve infection from multiple organisms, even if a single organism is identified, broad-spectrum antibiotic coverage should continue to be provided.
- Generally, the bacteremia of nonperforated NEC is gram positive, while that of perforated NEC is gram-negative, but this tendency cannot be relied upon for antibiotic selection.
- Consider adding fungal coverage (eg, amphotericin B), in selected patients at risk who do not respond to antibacterial therapy.

HEMATOLOGIC MANAGEMENT

- Monitor hematocrit (Hct). Hematocrit may drop as a result of GI blood loss. This may be masked by hemoconcentration, because of depletion of intravascular volume.
- Once the hydration status has been corrected, the patient should be transfused to keep Hct above 30 to 35 mL/dL, depending on the severity of illness.
- Monitor platelets. The platelet count may fall because of consumption at the level of the intestinal mucosa, with or without disseminated intravascular coagulation, as well as destruction caused by the hypoxia with or without sepsis.
- Our practice is to transfuse platelets as needed to eliminate clinical bleeding and keep the platelet count > 50,000/mm³, especially in the preterm infant at risk for intraventricular hemorrhage.

Indications for Surgery

- Evidence of free intraperitoneal air on the radiograph is an absolute indication for surgical intervention.

- A constellation of signs and symptoms that supports severe involvement with likely perforation or full-thickness bowel necrosis is a relative indication for surgery: erythema of the abdominal wall, persistent fixed loop(s) of bowel, refractory metabolic acidosis, severe thrombocytopenia, neutropenia, and recurrent positive blood cultures.
- If there is no identifiable surgical intervention (eg, removal of a discrete portion of affected bowel), then exploratory laparotomy is unlikely to be of use to the patient.

Anesthesia

- Avoid nitrous oxide to prevent further distention of the bowel.
- Have crossmatched blood available, especially in the event of liver laceration.
- Monitor the baby's temperature closely; avoid hypothermia.

Surgical Management

- The usual approach is laparotomy, with resection of the affected segment and the formation of a stoma. If the contamination is limited and the perforation localized, primary closure may be considered.
- In critically ill extremely low-birth-weight infants (< 1 kg), peritoneal drainage may be considered for stabilization or even definitive management.[27–32]
- A prospective, randomized clinical trial was recently reported demonstrating equivalent survival with peritoneal drainage as compared to laparotomy in preterm, low-birth-weight infants with perforated NEC.[29] Our current practice is determined by the characteristics of the individual patient. If the patient who is either too unstable to tolerate transfer to a facility with a pediatric surgeon and/or to tolerate the operation itself peritoneal drain placement may be employed as primary therapy. Failure to respond to drain placement may subsequently mandate formal operative exploration.
- For extensive necrosis, bowel conservation techniques may be appropriate.

Postoperative Management

- Monitor for ongoing bowel necrosis, especially if the margins of the resected bowel were of questionable integrity. This may include a repeat laparotomy for a "second-look" to assess for extension of bowel necrosis requiring further resection.
- Persistent thrombocytopenia, metabolic acidosis, and/or bacteremia support ongoing necrosis.
- Observation of the stoma and bowel just inside the stoma can offer valuable information about the condition of the segments most at risk.

Ongoing Management

- Aggressive fluid resuscitation is necessary because of the loss of intravascular fluid from the injured bowel wall and capillary leak.
- Careful monitoring of the heart rate, BP, respiratory status, inputs and outputs, and weight is required to provide adequate intravascular volume while avoiding the complications of fluid overload.
- Antibiotic therapy, NPO status, and PN should be continued for typically for 2 weeks. This period will may be shorter for the occasionally very mild presentation (Bell stage I) and longer for the very severe presentation.
- Bowel recovery is heralded by resolution of bilious aspirates from the nasogastric tube and passage of stool through the stoma and/or anus.
- After completion of this medical management, with or without surgical therapy, the antibiotics should be discontinued, and the patient should be given a cautious trial of enteral feedings.

General Considerations

The more proximal the stoma, the higher the risk of malabsorption. See Chapter 7, "Part 6: Short Bowel Syndrome" of this chapter for details on the management of malabsorption in the setting of short bowel syndrome (SBS).

- Generally, retention of < 50% of the entire length of bowel or < 20 cm beyond the ligament of Treitz is worrisome for significant malabsorption.
- Signs of malabsorption include watery stool, the presence of carbohydrate in stool (positive Clinitest®), and lack of weight gain.
- If the disease process was severe with substantial loss of bowel length, the initial feedings should be with a continuous, low volume of an elemental formula. Because these formulas are intended for term infants, the risks and benefits of their long-term use in the preterm infant must be assessed carefully.
  1. Elecare® and Neocate® are the most elemental formulas available using amino acids as their protein source. Elecare contains more MCT (33%) than Neocate (5%). Babies with fat malabsorption SBS will be able to absorb the most nutrients from Elecare. Neocate® is an elemental formula with the peptide fraction made of amino acids. It is intended for infants with severe protein allergies including cow's milk protein allergy, but it is also often well tolerated by patients after NEC resection.
  2. Alimentum®, Pregestimil® and Nutramigen® are semi-elemental, hypoallergenic formulas using protein hydrolysate rather than amino acids.
- Supplementation with fat and water-soluble vitamins may be necessary.

Complications and Follow-up Procedures

COMPLICATIONS

Strictures

The risk of strictures correlates directly with the severity of illness, having an overall incidence of 15 to 30% of NEC cases.

- Strictures are most commonly found distal to the stoma, generally in the colon.
- Therefore, if attempts at enteral feedings yield signs and symptoms of obstruction, a contrast enema of the distal bowel should be obtained to evaluate for strictures.

- In general, upper and lower gastrointestinal contrast studies are obtained prior to stoma reversal to assess for strictures that may have developed.

Short-Bowel Syndrome, Dumping Syndrome, Malabsorption and Malnutrition

- If > 50% of the jejunum and ileum is lost, the patient is likely to have some symptoms of SBS; loss of > 75% is associated with severe symptoms.
- Although the exact length of jejuno-ileum needed for survival continues to change as advances are made in management as SBS and in PN, 10 cm is generally considered minimal.
- The ileocecal valve is important both to slow the rate of transit through the small bowel and to prevent bacterial overgrowth of the small bowel from the colon. Surgical resection of the ileocecal valve may predict a longer period of PN dependence, but it does not appear to predict growth, outcome, or mortality[33,34] (see Chapter 7, "Part 6: Short-Bowel Syndrome" of this chapter for more on SBS).

Long-term Dependence on Parenteral Nutrition

The complications with long-term PN include the following:

- Infection or sepsis at the central venous catheter site
- Progressive secondary hepatic dysfunction, including cholestasis. Once diagnosed, every effort should be made to minimize PN and maximize enteral nutrition, including placement of feeding tubes and reestablishment of bowel continuity, if possible. Early research regarding the substitution of omega-6 fatty acids (Intralipid) with omega-3 fatty acids (Omegaven) shows a potential reduction in PN/lipid emulsion associated liver disease.[35]

RECURRENCE

Approximately 4% of patients with NEC have recurrence of the disease. Generally, the recurrent condition is managed the same way, with careful attention paid to identifying and treating any possible underlying cause of the recurrence.

FOLLOW-UP SURGICAL PROCEDURES

In addition to reestablishment of bowel continuity, follow-up surgical procedures such as bowel lengthening and tapering [ie, serial transverse enteroplasty (STEP) or the Bianchi procedure] may be useful.[36–39]

TRANSPLANTATION

Intestinal transplantation, with or without transplantation of the liver, has been life saving in infants with SBS who have developed life-threatening complications secondary to long-term PN dependence.[40] Recently reported 1-year and 3-year patient survival is as high as 83% and 60%, respectively.[41]

Long-term Outcome

- The overall survival rate is 60 to 70%.
- Intestinal adaptation takes up to 2 years, but it can result in functional outcomes that are superior to what was predicted on the basis of the remaining intestine at the time of initial disease.
- Although 75% of infants who survive surgical NEC have an excellent quality of life, there is a significantly higher rate of developmental morbidity that requires careful neurodevelopmental follow-up. A large retrospective study demonstrated significantly delayed growth and adverse long-term neurodevelopmental outcomes for infants with NEC requiring surgical intervention.[42]

References

1. Ford HR. Mechanism of nitric oxide-mediated intestinal barrier failure: insight into the pathogenesis of necrotizing enterocolitis. J Pediatr Surg 2006;41:294–9.
2. Chung DH, Ethridge RT, Kim S, et al. Molecular mechanisms contributing to necrotizing enterocolitis. Ann Surg 2001;233:835–42.
3. Kemply ST, Bennett S, Loftus BG, et al. Randomized trial of umbilical arterial catheter position: clinical outcome. Acta Paediatr 1993;82:173–6.

4. Rand T, Weninger M, Kohlhauser C, et al. Effects of umbilical arterial catheterization on mesenteric hemodynamics. Pediatr Radiol 1996;26:435–8.

5. Lopez SL, Taeusch HW, Findlay RD, Walther FJ. Time of onset of necrotizing enterocolitis in newborn infants with known prenatal cocaine exposure. Clin Pediatr 1995;34:424–9.

6. Ojala R, Ikonen S, Tammela O. Perinatal indomethacin treatment and neonatal complications in preterm infants. Eur J Pediatr 2000;159:153–5.

7. Vermillion ST, Newman RB. Recent indomethacin tocolysis is not associated with neonatal complications in preterm infants. Am J Obstet Gynecol 1999;181:1083–6.

8. Fowlie PW. Intravenous indomethacin for preventing mortality and morbidity in very low birth weight infants. Cochrane Database Syst Rev 2000;2:CD000174.

9. Grosfeld JL, Chaet M, Molinari F, et al. Increased risk of necrotizing enterocolitis in premature infants with patent ductus arteriosus treated with indomethacin. Ann Surg 1996;224:350–5.

10. Ment LR, Oh W, Ehrenkranz RA, et al. Low dose indomethacin and prevention of intraventricular hemorrhage: a multicenter randomized trial. Pediatrics 1994;98:543–50.

11. Gersony WM, Peckham GJ, Ellison RC, et al. Effects of indomethacin in premature infants with patent ductus arteriosus: results of a national collaborative study. J Pediatr 1983;102:895–906.

12. Sisk PM, Lovelady CA, Dillard RG, et al. Early human milk feeding is associated with a lower risk of necrotizing enterocolitis in very low birth weight infants. J Perinatol 2007;27:428–33.

13. Lucas A, Cole TJ. Breast milk and neonatal necrotising enterocolitis. Lancet 1990;336:1519–23.

14. Tyson JE, Kennedy KA. Trophic feedings for parenterally fed infants. Cochrane Database Syst Rev 2005;3:CD000504.

15. Kennedy KA, Tyson JE. Rapid versus slow rate of advancement of feedings for promoting growth and preventing necrotizing enterocolitis in parenterally fed low-birth-weight infants. Cochrane Database Syst Rev 1998;4:CD001241.

16. Nanthakumar NN, Young sC, Ko JS, et al. Glucocorticoid responsiveness in developing human intestine: possible role in

prevention of necrotizing enterocolitis. Am J Physiol Gastrointest Liver Physiol 2005;288:G85–92.

17. Carrion V, Egan EA. Prevention of neonatal necrotizing enterocolitis. J Pediatr Gastroenterol Nutr 1990;11:317–23.

18. Guillet R, Stoll BJ, Cotton CM, et al. Association of H2-blocker therapy and higher incidence of necrotizing enterocolitis in very low birth weight infants. Pediatrics 2006;117:e137–42.

19. Bury RG, Tudehope D. Enteral antibiotics for preventing necrotizing enterocolitis in low birthweight or preterm infants. Cochrane Database Syst Rev 2001;1:CD000405.

20. Hoyos AB. Reduced incidence of necrotizing enterocolitis associated with enteral administration of *Lactobacillus acidophilus* and *Bifidobacterium infantis* to neonates in an intensive care unit. Int J Infect Dis 1999;3:197–202.

21. Ledbetter DJ, Juul SE. Erythropoietin and the incidence of necrotizing enterocolitis in infants with very low birth weight. J Pediatr Surg 2000;35:178–81.

22. Foster J, Cole M. Oral immunoglobulin for preventing necrotizing enterocolitis in preterm and low birth-weight neonates. Cochrane Database Syst Rev 2004;1:CD001816.

23. Hallstrom M, Koivisto AM, Janas M, Tammela O. Laboratory parameters predictive of developing necrotizing enterocolitis in infants born before 33 weeks of gestation. J Pediatr Surg 2006;41:792–8.

24. Buonomo C. The radiology of necrotizing enterocolitis. Radiol Clin North Am 1999;37:1187–98.

25. Morrison SC, Jacobson JM. The radiology of necrotizing enterocolitis. Clin Perinatol 1994;21:347–63.

26. Bomelburg T, von Lengerke HJ. Sonographic findings in infants with suspected necrotizing enterocolitis. Eur J Radiol 1992;15:149–53.

27. Ein SH, Shandling B, Wesson D, Filler RM. A 13-year experience with peritoneal drainage under local anesthesia for necrotizing enterocolitis perforation. J Pediatr Surg 1990;25:1034–6.

28. Lessin MS, Luks FI, Wesselhoeft CW Jr, et al. Peritoneal drainage as definitive treatment for intestinal perforation in infants with extremely low birth weight (< 750 g). J Pediatr Surg 1998;33:370–2.

29. Pierro A, Hall N. Surgical treatments of infants with necrotizing enterocolitis. Semin Neonatol 2003;8:223–32.

30. Tepas JJ III, Sharma R, Hudak M, et al. Coming full article: an evidence-based definition of the timing and type of surgical management of very low-birth-weight (< 1000 g) infants with signs of acute intestinal perforation. J Pediatr Surg 2006; 41:418–22.

31. Moss RL, Dimmitt RA, Barnhart DC, et al. Laparotomy versus peritoneal drainage for necrotizing enterocolitis and perforation. N Engl J Med 2006;354:2225–34.

32. Fasoli L, Turi RA, Spitz L, et al. Necrotizing enterocolitis: extent of disease and surgical treatment. J Pediatr Surg 1999; 34:1096–9.

33. Ladd AP, Rescorla FJ, West KW, et al. Long-term follow-up after bowel resection for necrotizing enterocolitis: factors affecting outcome. J Pediatr Surg 1998;33:967–72.

34. Georgeson KE, Breaux CW Jr. Outcome and intestinal adaptation in neonatal short-bowel syndrome. J Pediatr Surg 1992;27:344–8.

35. Gura KM, Duggan CP, Collier SB, Jennings RW, Folkman J, Bistrian BR, Puder M. Reversal of parenteral nutrition-associated liver disease in two infants with short bowel syndrome using parenteral fish oil: implications for future management. Pediatrics 2006;118:197–201.

36. Kim HB, Fauza D, Garza J, et al. Serial transverse enteroplasty (STEP): a novel bowel lengthening procedure. J Pediatr Surg 2003;38:425–9.

37. Weber TR. Isoperistaltic bowel lengthening for short bowel syndrome in children. Am J Surg 1999;178:600–4.

38. Figueroa-Colon R, Harris PR, Birdsong E, et al. Impact of intestinal lengthening on the nutritional outcome for children with short bowel syndrome. J Pediatr Surg 1996;31:912–6.

39. Chaet MS, Farrell MK, Ziegler MM, Warner BW. Intensive nutritional support and remedial surgical intervention for extreme short bowel syndrome. J Pediatr Gastroenterol Nutr 1994;19:295–8.

40. Vennarecci G, Kato T, Misiakos EP, et al. Intestinal transplantation for short gut syndrome attributable to necrotizing enterocolitis. Pediatrics 2000;105:E25.

41. Kato T, Tzakis AG, Selvaggi G, et al. Intestinal and multivisceral transplantation in children. Ann Surg 2006;243:756–66.

42. Hintz SR, Kendrick DE, Stoll BJ, et al. Neurodevelopmental and growth outcomes of extremely low birth weight infants after necrotizing enterocolitis. Pediatrics 2005;115:696–703.

Recommended Readings

Henry MC, Lawrence Moss R. Surgical therapy for necrotizing enterocolitis: bringing evidence to the bedside. Semin Pediatr Surg 2005;14:181–90.

Part 4: Obstruction

DeWayne Pursley, MD, MPH, Anne R. Hansen, MD, MPH, and Mark Puder, MD, PhD

Embryology

Because many of the causes of neonatal gastrointestinal (GI) obstruction originate from abnormal fetal development, a review of GI embryology is informative.

WEEK 4

During the fourth week of gestation, the flat endoderm sheet folds ventrally into a tube, the endoderm tube, that runs the length of the embryo. Diverticula of the endoderm tube later give rise to the associated digestive organs. Lateral plate mesoderm will form the connective tissue and smooth muscle components of the GI system. As the endoderm folds, three separate regions are formed: the foregut, midgut, and hindgut.

Foregut Derivatives

The foregut derivatives include the mouth and pharynx, esophagus, stomach, and first third of the duodenum. A diverticulum at the end of the pharynx forms the lining of the respiratory system, and the surrounding mesoderm helps to create a septum between the future trachea and esophagus. Abnormal septation may result in esophageal stenosis (esophageal narrowing), or esophageal atresia (a blind lumen).

Diverticula at the end of the foregut will later develop into the pancreas, liver, and gall bladder. The liver and part of the pancreas derive from a ventral outpouching, which must rotate dorsally and to the left, later meeting with the dorsal bud of the pancreas. An annular pancreas can result from a portion of the ventral pancreatic bud growing around the ventral side of the duodenum before meeting the pancreas.

Midgut Derivatives

The derivatives of the midgut include the second third of the duodenum, the small intestines, the ascending colon, and two-thirds of the transverse colon. The midgut also remains connected to the yolk sac via the vitelline duct, which becomes the core of the umbilical cord. During gestational weeks 5 through 7, the midgut elongates, and this causes it to leave the abdominal cavity and herniate into the yolk stalk.

The apex of the herniated loop is where the endoderm of the midgut is continuous with the yolk sac through the vitelline duct, which is connected to the ileum. The midgut, and the future stomach and proximal duodenum of the foregut, rotate around the axis of the herniated loop. By week 9, after the abdominal cavity increases in size to accommodate the retracting gut, rotation is complete. The result is that the colon is now an inverted U-shape – with the cecum rotating counterclockwise and fixed in the right lower abdomen – and lies ventral to the small intestines. The duodenum rotates to the right, forming a C shape, and is fixed to the left of the midline at the ligament of Treitz.

Incomplete intestinal rotation with consequent inadequate fixation of the intestinal mesentery and arrest of the cecum in the right upper abdomen is referred to as malrotation. Torsion of a loop (generally on the axis of the superior mesenteric artery) adequate to cause obstruction is a volvulus. If the gut remains partially herniated through the body wall, an omphalocele or umbilical hernia will develop.

Hindgut Derivatives

The hindgut derivatives will form the lining of the distal portion of the large intestines and will include the distal one-third of the transverse colon, the descending colon, the rectum, and the anus.

WEEKS 6 AND 7

Through the sixth and seventh weeks of gestation, the endodermal epithelium proliferates to form multiple layers. During this period, many portions of the GI tract temporarily lose patency until the lumen is recanalized by weeks 8 to 10. Patency is essential at this point, because amniotic fluid, which is continually produced and, therefore, must be continually removed, is swallowed by the fetus and returned to the maternal circulation through the placenta after it is absorbed through the epithelial lining of the GI tract into the splanchnic vessels.

Duodenal atresia can result from failure to recanalize during development. Autonomic innervation of the GI tract smooth muscle results in peristalsis by week 10. Defective parasympathetic innervation of the descending colon and rectum will result in failure of ganglion formation and result in obstruction due to lack of peristalsis. This condition is referred to as aganglionic megacolon or Hirschsprung's disease.

Incidence

PROXIMAL OBSTRUCTION

- Esophageal atresia occurs in 1 in 3,000 to 5,000 live births.
- Pyloric stenosis is present in 1 in 300 to 1,000 live births; 80% of cases are males, and they are often the firstborn.

SMALL BOWEL OBSTRUCTION

There are several kinds of small bowel obstruction (SBO). Their incidence is as follows:

- Duodenal atresia occurs in 1 in 10,000 live births.
- Other atresias and stenoses occur in 1 in 5,000 live births.
- Meconium ileus is present in 1 in 10,000 to 16,000 live births; 90% of babies have cystic fibrosis (CF).

LARGE BOWEL OBSTRUCTION

There are several kinds of large bowel obstruction (LBO). Their incidence is as follows:

- Atresia and/or stenosis occurs in 1 in 20,000 live births.
- Hirschsprung's disease is present in 1 in 5,000 to 8,000 live births, more often in males than in females.
- Imperforate anus occurs in 1 in 2,500 to 5,000 live births.

Prenatal Diagnosis and Management

ESOPHAGEAL ATRESIA

Polyhydramnios may be present. Failure to visualize the stomach in serial examinations may lead to prenatal ultrasonographic diagnosis. The diagnosis is only possible in approximately 10% of cases. Esophageal atresia may be associated with cardiac (mostly atrial and ventricular septal defects) and genitourinary (GU) anomalies or Trisomies 18 and 21.

- Fetal echocardiography and karyotyping should be performed.
- After viability is determined, obstetric management is unaffected except in cases where severe polyhydramnios may lead to preterm labor.

PYLORIC ATRESIA

In addition to esophageal dilation and (single bubble) gastric distention, polyhydramnios is seen in most cases. Pyloric atresia has been reported in association with severe epidermolysis bullosa (EB) and, rarely, with esophageal atresia.

- An evaluation for EB should be considered when a fetal diagnosis of gastric outlet obstruction is made.
- Polyhydramnios may precipitate preterm delivery.

DUODENAL ATRESIA AND STENOSIS

Polyhydramnios is almost always present. Diagnosis depends on the presence of the double-bubble sign, representing simultaneous distention of the stomach and the first part of the duodenum. This is an isolated condition in one-third to one-half of cases.

- One-third of affected fetuses have trisomy 21.
- It may also be associated with vertebral, GI, cardiac, and renal anomalies.

OTHER INTESTINAL OBSTRUCTIONS

Polyhydramnios is often seen with proximal, but rarely with distal obstruction. Using ultrasonography, it is difficult to distinguish small from LBO. Bowel obstruction may be demonstrated by multiple markedly distended bowel loops with increased peristalsis and floating particulate matter.

- Patients with intestinal atresia or stenosis commonly have additional anomalies, including malrotation, duplication, microcolon, and esophageal atresia.
- In most cases, there is no need for a change in obstetric management, although significant polyhydramnios may result in preterm delivery.

MECONIUM ILEUS

Diagnosis may be made by demonstrating an echogenic mass in the abdominal cavity. Of note, the finding of echogenic bowel is common and of no significance in most cases. Diagnosis of meconium peritonitis may be easier, especially if calcification or ascites is noted.

- Because 90% of babies with meconium ileus have CF, the baby should be evaluated for this condition.
- Preterm delivery may be indicated after antenatal steroid administration, if there is rapid development of ascites.

General Approach to the Infant with a Bowel Obstruction

HISTORY

Obtain a complete maternal history, including family history, complications during pregnancy, dates, and results of ultrasonograms with particular attention to oligohydramnios or polyhydramnios, intra-abdominal calcifications, or dilated viscera. Note gestational age and maternal medications before and during labor. Further history should include overall clinical condition, how long after delivery symptoms began, whether vomiting is protracted, bilious or nonbilious, whether or when meconium was first passed and its characteristics.

PHYSICAL EXAMINATION

Complete a full physical examination, including vital signs, severity of illness, cardiac examination specifically in regard to PDA or other congenital anomaly, and respiratory status (drooling, respiratory distress, need for ventilator support). Abdominal distention may be minimal with high obstruction or marked with lower obstruction. A palpable mass may be present, such as an "olive" in pyloric stenosis, or bowel in intussusception. Tenderness suggests peritonitis.

- The inguinal region must always be examined to rule out a hernia as the cause of obstruction.
- Perineal examination is important to assess for such pathology as cloacal malformations, imperforate anus, and anal atresia.

LABORATORY STUDIES

Important laboratory studies that should be sent in preparation for possible surgical repair include: CBC; blood culture; electrolytes; BUN and creatinine; coagulation studies, including prothrombin time, partial thromboblastin time; and type and screen. Blood gases may be indicated depending on the condition of the infant.

RADIOGRAPHIC STUDIES

Generally, KUB and lateral views of the abdomen are obtained, and further studies may be indicated based on the history and symptoms (see below).

MANAGEMENT

Most patients with suspected obstruction must have an nasogastric tube (NGT) placed to continuous suction. Intravenous lines and fluids are essential because the infant will be NPO, and in many cases fluid shifts out of the vasculature into the bowel lumen.

- Antibiotics should be given since the obstruction leaves the patient at risk for sepsis.
- It is important to obtain prompt surgical consultation in any case of suspected bowel obstruction.

Postnatal Presentation and Management

For the management of tracheoesophageal fistula and esophageal atresia, see Chapter 4, "Cleft Lip/Palate and Robin Sequence."

ANTRAL AND PYLORIC WEBS

Webs are circumferential membranes that may cause intermittent partial obstruction.

Symptoms

The symptoms may include epigastric pain, intermittent nonbilious vomiting, and failure to thrive.

Diagnosis

Diagnosis is usually made with a UGI series and confirmed with endoscopy.

Treatment

The treatment is generally surgical repair. Balloon or laser ablation has also been used.

PYLORIC OR ANTRAL ATRESIA

This is a very rare autosomal defect that is occasionally associated with EB.

Signs and Symptoms

Gastric distention and a gasless abdomen are seen on KUB imaging.

Diagnosis

Diagnosis is made using a UGI contrast study demonstrating a complete gastric outlet obstruction.

Treatment

The treatment is surgical, consisting of a gastroduodenostomy or, if a web is thin, excision of the web.

PYLORIC STENOSIS

Pyloric stenosis usually occurs in the first 3 to 6 weeks of life.

Symptoms

The symptoms are nonbilious progressively projectile vomiting, dehydration, and in cases of delayed diagnosis, cachexia.

Physical Examination

Physical examination is by palpation of the "olive". The examiner may see abdominal distention and gastric peristaltic waves. A pacifier dipped in formula or in a glucose solution is given to relax the infant. Palpation of the upper abdomen just to the right of the midline may reveal a palpable moveable 2 to 3 cm (olive) mass and is diagnostic of pyloric stenosis.

Diagnosis

Ultrasonography is the most sensitive test to determine the diagnosis. A muscle thickness of > 4 mm and a pyloric channel length of > 17 mm have a sensitivity of 97% and specificity of 100% in infants > 1 month of age. Muscle thickness of > 3 mm is diagnostic in infants < 1 month of age. A barium study may reveal a typical "string" or "double-track" sign.

Treatment

The treatment includes initial hydration with a normal saline bolus of 10 to 20 mL/kg followed by a maintenance fluid of 5% dextrose in water (D5W) half normal saline at an appropriate rate to replace fluid deficits. Potassium should be added once good urine output is established. Surgical repair is essential: a pyloromyotomy may be performed using either an open or laparoscopic technique.

Postoperative Management

- The infant is made NPO until fully awake. A diluted formula or sugar water is begun postoperatively. We use the following regimen: D5W or Pedialyte® 30 mL every 3 hours for the first two feedings.
- Advance to full strength formula or breast milk ad lib every 3 hours for next two feedings.

- Mother may breast-feed once the patient tolerates at least 30 mL of expressed breast milk. If there is emesis, we wait 3 hours and then refeed. The IV is heparin locked once the first bottlefeed is tolerated.

Never place an NGT postoperatively for vomiting – this can perforate the pylorus because there is only mucosa left at the site of the pyloromyotomy.

If the duodenum or pylorus was inadvertently entered during the pyloromyotomy, the infant should receive nasogastric suction via the NGT that was placed in the operating room (OR). IV antibiotics should be given postoperatively for a minimum of 2 days.

DUODENAL ATRESIA AND WEB

This is believed to occur as a result of failure of complete recanalization of the duodenum. It may be associated with biliary atresia, agenesis of the gallbladder, and stenosis of the common bile duct.

Symptoms

Duodenal atresia and web usually present with gastric distention and vomiting that may be bilious.

Diagnosis

The double-bubble sign on plain radiography of the abdomen is pathognomonic. One-third of children with duodenal atresia have trisomy 21. These children may also have complex cardiac anomalies. Therefore, all infants with duodenal atresia require a cardiology evaluation prior to surgery.

Treatment

The treatment includes IV hydration and the placement of an NGT for decompression. If medically cleared for surgery, a duodenostomy is performed. Web excision is curative for duodenal web. Postoperatively, provide hydration and nasogastric suction until bowel function returns.

ANNULAR PANCREAS

Symptoms

Annular pancreas produces similar signs and symptoms to duodenal atresia.

Diagnosis

A double-bubble sign may be seen on plain radiography.

Treatment

The treatment is surgical bypassing of the obstruction.

MALROTATION AND MIDGUT VOLVULUS

This is a very common cause of intestinal obstruction in infants and must be considered in every infant with bilious emesis.

Symptoms

Infants can range from asymptomatic to acutely ill. More than 50% of cases present in the first month of life, 30% in the first week. Ninety-five percent have vomiting that becomes bilious. Bloody vomitus suggests bowel necrosis. Twenty-eight percent have bloody stools. Abdominal distention is common but can be absent. Abdominal tenderness varies. Rectal examination is usually guaiac positive.

Diagnosis

Midgut volvulus is one of the most serious emergencies seen in the newborn period. Delay in diagnosis can result in loss of the entire midgut, which is uniformly fatal. Any studies should be obtained expeditiously, since a few hours may be the difference between a totally reversible and a lethal condition.

Plain radiographs are most commonly normal, but may show either a gasless abdomen, dilated intestine suggesting SBO, or duodenal obstruction with a double bubble. With shock or other clear indication for exploration, no studies are necessary, and the infant should be brought directly to surgery. If the infant is stable, diagnosis should be confirmed by a UGI series documenting the location of the duodenum and ligament of Treitz.

Treatment

The treatment is always surgery. An NGT is placed to continuous suction, IV hydration and antibiotics are started, and the infant is transported immediately to the OR. The surgeon decompresses the volvulus in a counterclockwise fashion. Adhesions are lysed, the small bowel is placed in the right lower quadrant, and the cecum and colon into the left lower quadrant. An appendectomy is performed. Recurrent volvulus occurs in up to 8% of cases.

Postoperative Management

If all of the bowel appeared normal intraoperatively, feedings are begun once the ileus resolves. If there was bowel of questionable viability, a "second-look" operation may be necessary to determine whether bowel resection is necessary. If bowel necrosis is found at that time, resection is performed.

GASTRIC VOLVULUS

Gastric volvulus is often associated with diaphragmatic abnormalities, hiatal hernia, and paraesophageal hernia.

Symptoms

In the newborn, it usually presents as an acute event with sudden onset of abdominal pain and persistent vomiting. There may be abdominal distention with difficulty passing an NGT because of the obstruction. Peritoneal signs suggest ischemia and/or perforation.

Diagnosis

The KUB imaging may show gastric distention and a solitary air-fluid level in the midline or left upper quadrant. Contrast studies may show esophageal dilation without passage of contrast into the stomach.

Treatment

Prompt management is essential. Surgical management is reduction of the volvulus with gastric fixation with either a gastrostomy tube placement or anterior gastropexy. The diaphragm is examined and abnormalities and repaired.

INTESTINAL ATRESIA

Intestinal atresia occurs in decreasing order of frequency as follows: ileum, duodenum, jejunum, colon, and pylorus. A careful antenatal and perinatal history may help to localize the site of atresia. Prenatal ultrasonographic diagnosis of a dilated stomach and or duodenum may be indicative of duodenal atresia. Though intestinal atresias (except duodenal) are generally thought to be due to intrauterine vascular accidents with ischemic necrosis and bowel resorption, it is underappreciated that 15 to 30% of babies with jejunal and ileal atresias have CF.

Symptoms

Atresias usually present with abdominal distention except in the most proximal lesions. Vomiting usually occurs within the first 48 hours of life. Emesis is usually bilious.

Diagnosis

The KUB imaging may show multiple loops of dilated bowel, suggesting a distal atresia, or a few loops, suggesting a more proximal atresia. A contrast enema is helpful to identify a microcolon, which is a very reliable finding in distal SBO. This study also evaluates the patency of the colon.

Classification

Intestinal atresias are classified into four types.

Type I This is a complete obstruction from a membrane containing the mucosa and submucosa. The mesentery is intact. The total bowel length is usually normal.

Type II   This is an obstruction that ends blindly and connects with the more distal segment of bowel by a fibrous cord. The mesentery is intact, and the total bowel length is usually normal.

Type III   There are two kinds of type III. Type III(a) is similar to type II in that the proximal portion ends blindly but does not contain a fibrous band between the two ends and contains a V-shaped defect in the mesentery. The total bowel length is usually shortened.

Type III(b) is also known as the "Christmas tree" or "apple peel" deformity. There is usually an atresia near the ligament of Treitz, absence of the superior mesenteric artery beyond the takeoff of the middle colic branch, and a large mesenteric defect. The length of the intestine is usually severely compromised. The blood supply is usually by a single vessel off of the ileocolic or right colic artery. This is the one type that has been found to occur in some families. Survival from this deformity is approximately 50%.

Type IV   This is a combination of multiple atresias that include types I and III and appears as a string of sausages. The bowel is foreshortened.

COLONIC ATRESIA

This is thought to be secondary to vascular impairment or intrauterine volvulus. This may be associated with other bowel atresias, Hirschsprung's disease, or gastroschisis. It is also associated with hindgut defects and major GU and abdominal wall defects.

- Surgical therapy is intended to preserve as much bowel as possible and to ensure that no atresias are missed. Ideally, a preoperative contrast enema is obtained to clarify the patency of the colon. Otherwise, patency must be assessed using intraoperative saline injection. All bowel is measured intraoperatively. Anastomosis is performed between loops of bowel. Frequently, the proximal ends are very dilated and are either removed or plicated to match the small distal segment to preserve maximal bowel length.
- Colonic atresias are usually treated with a temporary colostomy and later repair.

- Prognosis is largely based on the length of functioning bowel. Short Bowel Syndrome is the biggest complication with these bowel abnormalities.

HIRSCHSPRUNG'S DISEASE

Hirschsprung's disease is another name for congenital aganglionic megacolon, and it is a frequent cause of neonatal intestinal obstruction. In this disease, there is an absence of ganglion cells, which causes ineffective conduction of peristalsis and a functional obstruction. The aganglionic segment may be limited to the rectosigmoid colon or extend proximally to involve the entire colon or small intestine.

Symptoms

The symptoms are nonspecific and include episodic abdominal distention, constipation, obstipation, or diarrhea. Failure to pass meconium in the first 48 hours of life with abdominal distention and vomiting are symptoms specific to the newborn.

Physical Examination

A digital rectal examination or insertion of a thermometer often produces an explosive release of stool. The rectal tone is usually increased, and the rectum is usually empty.

Associated Anomalies

Urogenital, cardiovascular, and GI anomalies are associated. Approximately 3% have trisomy 21. Congenital atresias of the small and large intestine, meconium ileus, and imperforate anus are also associated with Hirschsprung's disease.

Diagnosis

- Abdominal radiographs may show air-fluid levels in the colon. A contrast enema should be obtained. This classically shows a transition zone at the narrowed rectum with a dilated colon proximally. However, this finding is often absent in infants. If the contrast enema is normal and there is a high suspicion for Hirschsprung's disease, one should obtain a plain radiograph of the abdomen on the following day. Retained contrast

in the colon on this follow-up film is highly suspicious for Hirschsprung's disease.
- The diagnosis is confirmed using suction mucosal rectal biopsy or full-thickness rectal biopsy showing an absence of ganglion cells and hypertrophied nerves in the myenteric plexus of the muscularis layer. There is increased acetylcholinesterase in the aganglionic rectum.

Management

- Initially, Hirschsprung's disease is managed with saline rectal irrigations every 6 hours. As long as the child passes stool with irrigations and the abdomen decompresses appropriately, the child may be fed ad lib.
- Neonatal primary perineal pull-through, with or without laparoscopic assistance, may be performed once an infant is stabilized. We currently avoid colostomy in most cases; however, a colostomy is standard at many institutions. Rectal dilations usually are continued for several months, as recommended by the surgeon.
- Colostomy is indicated for enterocolitis or the inability to obtain adequate decompression with irrigation. Long-segment Hirschsprung's disease may also require a stoma. Despite the removal of the aganglionic segment, the remaining bowel is not completely normal. The internal sphincter itself is also aganglionic and, therefore, continues to have high tone. Parents and caretakers must understand that this surgery, although very helpful, does not eliminate the need for follow-up. These children remain at risk for enterocolitis that may be life threatening.

Complications

Overall, excellent results are reported in 90% of cases.

Early
- Anastamotic leak will require diversion.
- Anastamotic stricture may require dilation or revision of anastomosis.
- Wound infection

Late

- Constipation may require bowel regimen, sphincter dilation, and sphincterotomy.
- Enterocolitis will require bowel decompression, NGT, antibiotics, and resuscitation.
- Encopresis

MECONIUM ILEUS

Meconium ileus accounts for almost one-third of all neonatal SBOs. 90% of babies with meconium ileuse have CF and 15% of babies with meconium ileus have CF. The incidence of CF in the United States is 1 in 3,000 live births. It is extremely rare in non-white populations. Male and females are equally affected.

Signs and Symptoms

Meconium ileus is suspected in the infant, who develops generalized abdominal distention, bilious vomiting, and failure to pass meconium in the first 24 to 48 hours. A family history of CF is common and there is a history of polyhydramnios in 20% of patients.

Physical Examination

On physical examination, the meconium may be palpable as a doughy substance in the dilated loops of distended bowel. The anus and rectum are typically narrow.

Diagnosis

Diagnosis includes plain radiography of the abdomen showing bowel loops of variable size with a soap-bubble appearance of the bowel contents. Calcifications on the abdominal radiograph usually indicate meconium peritonitis, resulting from an intrauterine intestinal perforation. Microcolon is a highly reliable finding for distal bowel obstruction that may be intraluminal from inspissated meconium or atresia due to intrauterine volvulus. A contrast enema demonstrates a microcolon with inspissated meconium proximally. A contrast enema is contraindicated if the plain film shows calcification.

Treatment

The initial treatment is nonsurgical and begins with a Gastrografin enema. Under fluoroscopic control, a 50% solution of Gastrografin and water is infused into the rectum and colon through a catheter. Gastrografin is hyperosmolar, and, therefore, the infant must be hydrated and have a running IV line before, during, and after the study. The enema usually results in a rapid passage of semiliquid meconium that continues during the next 24 to 48 hours. Follow-up KUB studies are taken at 12 and 24 hours to evaluate the progress of the Gastrografin. Several Gastrografin enemas are frequently required. Mucomyst® (*N*-acetylcysteine) can also be used as enemas or PO/PG to assist in cleaning out the thick meconium (dilute 20% solution to 5% by adding sterile water).

Indications for Surgery

Surgery is indicated if the Gastrografin enema fails to relieve the obstruction, there are calcifications in the abdominal cavity, the infant appears too ill to delay operation, or the diagnosis of meconium ileus is in doubt.

Cystic Fibrosis

Given the frequent association, infants diagnosed with meconium ileus should receive a sweat test to assess for CF. This test is usually not practical prior to surgery because the child has to be at least 2 kg and 2 weeks old (ideally, and at an absolute minimum, 3 days old). At least 100 mg of sweat is collected, and a concentration of sodium chloride above 60 mEq/L is diagnostic. If the test is performed when a baby is < 2kg or < 2 weeks of age, it can generate:

- a false-positive result: due to relatively high NaCl levels in newborns) or
- a false-negative or uninterpretable result (due to inadequate volume of sweat, in which case, test should be repeated when 3 to 4 weeks of age).

A buccal smear detects CF with only 80 to 90% sensitivity, because it looks for only the most common genetic mutations. When oral feedings are begun, pancreatic enzyme preparation is given. Pulmonary and GI follow-up should be arranged.

Meconium Ileus and the Low Birth Weight Infant

Meconium ileus can also occur in extremely low birth weight infants, those weighing < 1 kg. This presents with abdominal distention and may lead to bowel ischemia and necrosis. This condition is thought to be related to immaturity of the bowel myenteric plexus. Treatment is Gastrografin enema, as with meconium plug. Early treatment prevents the complication of necrosis and perforation. Prognosis is excellent, with nearly a 100% survival rate.

MECONIUM PLUG SYNDROME

Meconium plug syndrome occurs secondary to colonic dysmotility. Meconium in the left colon becomes firm, producing a distal obstruction. Any condition that can cause dysmotility in the newborn may produce this syndrome. Specifically, it is associated with maternal eclampsia, diabetes mellitus, transplacental magnesium sulfate exposure, prematurity, hypothyroidism, and sepsis.

Symptoms

The newborn may initially pass small bits of meconium, but then develops abdominal obstruction with vomiting. Differentiating this from Hirschsprung's disease and meconium ileus is difficult.

Diagnosis

A plain abdominal radiograph usually shows dilated loops of bowel and few air fluid levels. A rectal examination may produce normal stool output, but these infants still require a contrast enema.

Treatment

A contrast enema is diagnostic and therapeutic. Affected infants should be tested for CF and hypothyroidism.

IMPERFORATE ANUS

Evaluation of the child with imperforate anus requires careful inspection of the perineum. In 80 to 90% of cases a fistula is found.

Signs and Symptoms

It may take 24 hours for a fistula to declare itself.

Males   A fistula is present in 80 to 90% of males.
- A perineal fistula can be seen as meconium in the perineum and may be hidden under a "bucket-handle" deformity.
- A rectourethral fistula may present with meconium in the urine.
- A rectovesical fistula connects to the bladder neck and is rare.
- If there is no fistula, the risk of Down syndrome is increased.

Females   In 95% of females, there is a fistula.
- A perineal fistula can be seen as meconium in the perineum and may be hidden under a "bucket-handle" deformity.
- Vestibular (posterior fourchette) fistula is just posterior to the hymen.
- The cloaca presents as small external genitalia with a single opening connecting the rectum, vagina, and urethra.

Other Anomalies

Of patients with imperforate anus, 50 to 60% have other anomalies included in the VACTERL association, which is summarized as follows:

- V: vertebral anomalies, tethered cord. Evaluation requires plain spine radiography and ultrasonography ± magnetic resonance imaging.
- A: imperforate anus
- C: cardiac (12 to 22%), including tetralogy of Fallot and VSD. An echocardiogram is necessary for these patients prior to surgery.
- TE: tracheoesophageal fistula
- R: renal and GU anomalies, including vesicourethral reflux, undescended testicle, and hypospadias. A careful GU examination and renal ultrasonography are required.
- L: radial limb abnormalities

Treatment

- A colostomy is unnecessary if a fistula can be dilated (perineal in males, perineal or vestibular in females). If a dilatable fistula is present, the parents can be taught to perform dilations twice a day. Dilation up to a 9 to 12 Hegar is acceptable.
- All others require a colostomy. If a colostomy is necessary, the baby will need a distal colostogram to clarify the GU and rectal anatomy before definitive repair.

INTUSSUSCEPTION

Intussusception usually occurs in the age range of 3 months to 2 years. If the patient is younger, one should suspect a lead point, such as a Meckel's diverticulum or intestinal polyp.

Symptoms

Symptoms are classically a triad of colicky abdominal pain, a sausage-like mass, and currant-jelly stools. These are relatively late findings and are not always present. The ileocecal valve is the most common location for intussusception.

Diagnosis

Diagnosis starts with a KUB study to look for air or stool in the cecum. If the KUB is suspicious, the next step is an air-contrast enema.

Treatment

This enema is usually both diagnostic and curative. The patient is given Unasyn® (ampicillin/sulbactam, 50 mg ampicillin/kg/dose) prior to the air-contrast enema. The physician must have a 14-gauge angiocatheter available in case of massive pneumoperitoneum due to a perforation and subsequent respiratory and circulatory collapse. Reduction is not considered successful unless there is reflux of air or contrast into the ileum. Attempts may be repeated if the baby's condition permits. If the infant has peritoneal signs, the air contrast enema is skipped and the infant is taken directly to surgery.

Postoperative Care

Postoperative care includes admission for 24 hours of observation. The infant is kept NPO for the first 8 hours, and then the diet is advanced. If symptoms recur, a repeat enema is performed. Surgery is essential if reduction cannot be accomplished.

Complications

Recurrence after surgery or enema reduction occurs in approximately 5% of cases. Postoperative intussusception may occur. Postoperative small bowel to small bowel intussusception is particularly difficult to diagnose and is treated surgically.

GASTROINTESTINAL DUPLICATIONS

Duplications are cystic or tubular and contain GI mucosa and smooth muscle in the wall. They can occur anywhere in the GI tract and often share a common wall with part of the GI viscera. One-third of duplications will present in newborns and two-thirds before age 2 years.

Symptoms

The symptoms depend on the level of obstruction. Duplications usually present as bowel obstruction or an enlarging mass. The enlarging mass may compromise adjacent intestinal vasculature producing necrosis and bleeding and/or perforation. If gastric mucosa is present, the cyst may erode into adjacent bowel producing bleeding.

Diagnosis

Ectopic gastric mucosa can be diagnosed with a technetium-99m pertechnetate scan. Chronic bleeding may present as anemia. Ultrasonography is the most useful test to confirm abdominal duplications, while a computed tomography (CT) scan with contrast is the most useful for esophageal lesions.

Treatment

Surgical treatment is resection of the duplication itself, resection of the normal short section of bowel adjacent to the cyst, stripping of the mucosa only, or occasionally the marsupialization into adjacent bowel and anastomosis of the common walls.

HERNIA

Any infant with signs of obstruction must undergo a complete physical examination to evaluate for an incarcerated or strangulated hernia. If present, it must be repaired.

POSTOPERATIVE ADHESIONS

Postoperative adhesions are a common cause of obstruction in the newborn. This can result from any operation that includes entry into the peritoneal cavity. Adhesions occur in up to 5% of major abdominal resections. Early uncomplicated obstructions may be treated with bowel rest, IV hydration, and nastrogastric suction. Postoperative obstructions may occur any time after the operation, although the vast majority occur in the first 2 years. All bowel obstructions require surgical consultation. The decision to treat without surgery must be made by the surgeon.

Functional Obstructions

Bowel motility may be impaired by medications, including magnesium sulfate and narcotics. Sepsis, intra-abdominal abscess or inflammation, hypothyroidism, hypokalemia, and other electrolyte and metabolic disorders may cause an ileus that can be difficult to distinguish from a mechanical bowel obstruction.

Recommended Readings

Adzick NS, Wilson JM, Caty MG, et al, editors. Children's hospital department of surgery house officer manual. Boston (MA): Children's Hospital.

Aschraft KW, Holder TM, editors. Pediatric surgery. 3rd ed. Philadelphia (PA): WB Saunders; 2000.

Baily PV, Tracy TF Jr, Connors RH, et al. Congenital duodenal
    obstruction. A 32-year review. J Pediatr Surg 1993;28: 92–5.

Escobar MA, Ladd AP, Grosfeld JL, et al. Duodenal atresia and
    stenosis: long-term follow-up over 30 years. J Pediatr Surg
    2004;39:867–71.

Greenholz SK, Perez C, Wesley JR, et al. Meconium obstruction
    in the markedly premature infant. J Pediatr Surg 1996;
    31:117–20.

Hajivassiliou CA. Intestinal obstruction in neonatal/pediatric sur-
    gery. Semin Pediatr Surg 2003;12:241–53.

Holschneider AM, Pfrommer W, Gerrescheim B. Results in the
    treatment of anorectal malformations with special regard to
    the histology of the rectal pouch. Eur J Pediatr Surg
    1994;4:303.

Janik JS, Ein SH, Filler RM, et al. An assessment of the surgical
    treatment of adhesive small bowel obstruction in infants and
    children. J Pediatr Surg 1981;16:225–9.

Keinhaus S, Boley SJ, Sheran M, et al. Hirschsprung's disease.
    A survey of the members of the surgical section of the
    American Academy of Pediatrics. J Pediatr Surg 1979;14:588.

Krasna IW, Rosenfeld D, Salerno P. Is it necrotizing enterocolitis,
    meconium of prematurity, or delayed meconium plug?
    A dilemma in the tiny premature infant. J Pediatr Surg
    1996;31: 855–8.

Part 5: Gastrointestinal Bleeding

Karen McAlmon, MD, FAAP, and
Mark Puder, MD, PhD

Introduction

Gastrointestinal (GI) bleeding is a common reason for pediatric surgical consultation. In most cases, the bleeding is not a cause for grave concern. In approximately 50% of cases of GI bleeding in neonates, the cause is never explained. In most cases, urgent surgical intervention is not required.

Definitions

- Hematemesis: bright red or coffee-ground emesis
- Hematochezia: bright red or maroon blood per rectum
- Melena: dark, tarry stools
- Upper GI bleed (UGI): bleeding above the ligament of Treitz (junction of the duodenum and jejunum), associated with hematemesis or melena. In neonates, blood can pass very quickly through the GI tract, and UGI bleeding can sometimes still appear as bright red blood per rectum.
- Lower GI bleed: bleeding beyond the ligament of Treitz, associated with hematochezia.

General Presentation and Management

The presentation ranges from the stable infant, who is asymptomatic with minimal blood loss detected only by analysis of GI secretions or stool, to the rare infant who presents in shock secondary to extensive hemorrhage.

Diagnosis and Management

If there is any doubt about whether blood is present, a heme test should be performed on the specimen.

The diagnosis and management of the infant with GI bleeding includes the following:

- Resuscitation and stabilization, if needed
- Verification that a GI bleed has occurred
- Differentiation between upper and lower GI bleed determined by placing an NGT and aspirating. Recovery of blood is diagnostic of an UGI bleed.
- Identification of the specific disorder causing the bleed
- Treatment of the specific condition.

Differential Diagnosis of Gastrointestinal Bleeding

UPPER GASTROINTESTINAL BLEEDING

Swallowed Maternal Blood

- Signs and symptoms: the presence of hematemesis that can be coffee ground or bright red. Sometimes hematochezia is also seen.
- Diagnosis: made using the Apt-Downey alkali denaturation test – Grossly bloody, not tarry, stool or gastric fluid is mixed with sodium hydroxide. Conversion of oxyhemoglobin to alkaline globin hematin yields a color change from pink to brown-yellow. Adult (maternal) hemoglobin is more sensitive to conversion than fetal (infant's) hemoglobin. Therefore, any color change indicates maternal blood.
- Treatment: no treatment is needed.

Gastritis

Gastritis is usually seen in sick premature infants or infants with perinatal depression. It is also associated with corticosteroid treatment.

- Signs and symptoms: blood, bright red or coffee ground, in gastric aspirate
- Treatment: use nasogastric suction, saline lavage, and H2 blockers (ranitidine) and/or proton pump inhibitors to keep gastric pH > 5. These are usually sufficient treatment. Usually gastritis resolves without the need for surgical intervention.

Hemorrhagic Disease of the Newborn

This is generally caused by a deficiency of vitamin K–dependent clotting factors. Hemorrhagic disease is seen in infants, who have not received vitamin K at birth or whose mothers took medications that interfere with vitamin K (eg, sulfa drugs or phenobarbital).

- Signs and symptoms: it is manifested by generalized bleeding, including hematemesis, hematuria, and prolonged bleeding at venipuncture sites and into the skin. There is a prolonged PT out of proportion to PTT.
- Treatment: vitamin K, 1 mg daily for 5 days, preferably given IV, especially in the setting of active bleeding.

Lower Gastrointestinal Bleeding

ANAL FISSURE

Anal fissure is the most common cause of lower GI bleeding.

- Signs and symptoms: bright red blood visible on the surface of the stool occurs in small spots on the diaper.
- Physical examination: examine the anus to confirm the diagnosis. Use of a nasal speculum or glass test tube may facilitate physical exam.
- Treatment: ensuring that stools are soft and applying ointment for a protective barrier will allow healing with time.

NECROTIZING ENTEROCOLITIS

See "Chapter 8, Genitourinary Disorders." NEC usually affects premature neonates, although 10% of infants with NEC are full term.

- Signs and symptoms: abdominal distention, gastric residuals (sometimes bilious), and GI bleeding (stools positive for occult blood or grossly bloody)
- Diagnosis: the hallmark radiologic finding is pneumatosis intestinalis (submucosal air) on the KUB study.
- Treatment: treatment consists of bowel rest with nasogastric decompression, NPO, nutritional support, and broad-spectrum

antibiotics (gram-positive and gram-negative coverage ± anaerobic coverage depending on degree of severity).

1. Early surgical consultation is recommended.
2. Pneumoperitoneum indicates bowel perforation and the need for surgical intervention.

INTUSSUSCEPTION

Rarely symptomatic before age 3 months

- Signs and symptoms: there are usually signs of intermittent abdominal pain. The infant may draw up his or her legs to the abdomen. There may be vomiting and progressive lethargy. The stool may initially become tinged with blood and later dark red mucoid clots (currant jelly) may be passed.
- Diagnosis: made using plain abdominal radiography, ultrasonography, and/or air-contrast enema. No contrast studies should be performed if there are signs of peritonitis. An air-contrast enema may be therapeutic for ileocolic intussusception. Small bowel to small bowel intussusceptions requires surgical treatment.
- Treatment: all cases of suspected intussusception should be evaluated by a surgeon to determine diagnostic studies and therapy.

MECKEL'S DIVERTICULUM

Rarely symptomatic in the infant.

- Signs and symptoms: the patient presents with bleeding or obstruction. Bleeding is due to heterotopic gastric mucosa producing ulceration or due to ischemia from intussusception or volvulus.
- Diagnosis: made using a Meckel's scan
- Treatment: surgical with either bowel resection or simple diverticulectomy

MALROTATION AND MIDGUT VOLVULUS

Malrotation is a failure of the intestines to rotate counterclockwise as they return to the abdomen during embryologic formation. Secondary volvulus may result in infarction of part or all of the midgut due to obstruction of mesenteric blood supply.

- Signs and symptoms: bilious emesis in an otherwise healthy baby without abdominal distention suggests malrotation with midgut volvulus. The onset of melena, in association with bilious emesis and abdominal tenderness, suggest vascular compromise due to volvulus.
- Diagnosis: UGI series confirms the diagnosis showing malplacement of the ligament of Treitz.
- Treatment: laparotomy with lysis of Ladd's bands and derotation of the bowel is required. An appendectomy is also performed to avoid later difficulties in diagnosing appendicitis due to the atypical location of the appendix. The presence of melena with bilious emesis and abdominal tenderness requires immediate surgical intervention.

ALLERGIC COLITIS

The prevalence of allergic colitis is between 0.2 and 7.5%.

- Signs and symptoms: vomiting, abdominal pain, persistent diarrhea with blood in the stools, and failure to thrive. Hematochezia indicates frank colitis.
- Diagnosis: endoscopy can show erythematous and friable colonic mucosa with biopsies showing polymorphonuclear cells, plasma cells, and eosinophils in the lamina propria. Peripheral eosinophilia and hypoalbuminemia can be seen.
- Treatment: The treatment is removal of cow's milk protein, either by conversion to casein hydrolysate formula or, in breast fed infants, removal of cow's milk from the mother's diet. The bloody stool may take several days to resolve.

Upper or Lower Gastrointestinal Bleeding

GASTROINTESTINAL DUPLICATIONS

Duplications are cystic or tubular and contain GI mucosa and smooth muscle in the wall. They can occur anywhere in the GI tract and often share a common wall with part of the GI viscera. One-third will present as newborns and two-thirds by age 2 years.

- Signs and symptoms: upper or lower GI bleeding usually is due to bowel obstruction or an enlarging mass. The enlarging mass may compromise adjacent intestinal vasculature, producing necrosis, bleeding, and/or perforation. If gastric mucosa is present, the cyst may erode into the adjacent bowel, producing bleeding. Chronic bleeding may present as anemia.

- Diagnosis: ultrasonography is the most useful test to confirm abdominal duplications, whereas CT scan with contrast is the most useful for esophageal lesions. Ectopic gastric mucosa can be diagnosed using a technetium-99m pertechnetate scan.
- Surgical Treatment: The options for surgical treatment are the following:
  1. Resection of the duplication itself
  2. Resection of the normal short section of bowel adjacent to the cyst
  3. Stripping of mucosa
  4. Marsupialization into adjacent bowel and anastomosis of the common walls (rare).

Postoperative Intestinal Bleeding

Bleeding during GI intestinal anastomosis usually occurs, and, therefore, the newborn's stool will test positive after such surgery. The anastomosis can bleed significantly in the postoperative period, sometimes requiring reoperation. The surgeon must evaluate any suspicion of ongoing bleeding.

Coagulopathy

A patient with a coagulopathy due to disseminated intravascular coagulation, thrombocytopenia, liver disease, or any other etiology may present with, or develop, GI bleeding. Treatment is to hold feedings, support intravascular volume, and focus on correcting the coagulopathy and treating its underlying etiology.

Recommended Readings

Adzick NS, Wilson JM, Caty MG, et al, editors. Children's Hospital Department of Surgery House Officer Manual. Boston (MA): Children's Hospital; 2005.

Aschraft KW, Holcomb GW, Murphy JP, editors. Pediatric surgery. 4th ed. Philadelphia (PA): WB Saunders; 2005.

Part 6: Short Bowel Syndrome

Y. Avery Ching, MD Melanie Connolly, MSc, RD, CNSD, Biren P. Modi, MD Tom Jaksic, MD, PhD, and Christopher Duggan, MD, MPH

Introduction

Short bowel syndrome (SBS) is a disorder characterized by decreased gastrointestinal mucosal surface area and fast transit time. This can lead to malabsorption of macro- and micronutrients, electrolyte abnormalities, dehydration, and ultimately malnutrition. A functional definition of SBS in children would be dependent on parenteral nutrition (PN) and/or hydration for at least 90 days because of congenital intestinal malformation and/or acquired diseases leading to intestinal resection. Table 1 lists common etiologies of SBS in children.

Factors Affecting Prognosis

LENGTH OF SMALL BOWEL RESECTED

1. Normal small intestine length is approximately 217 ± 24 cm in infants 27 to 35 weeks gestational age and 304 ± 44 cm in infants ≥ 35 weeks (Figure 1). At term, mean length is reported to be 250 to 300 cm. Another 2 to 3 meters is added to its length during growth to adulthood. The large intestine is 30 to 40 cm at birth, growing to 1.5 to 2 meters in adult life.[1]

2. Loss of intestinal length can limit digestion by reducing exposure of nutrients to brushborder hydrolytic enzymes as well as to pancreatic and biliary secretions.

3. Many studies have examined the relationship between the length of residual small intestine and the success of weaning from PN. It appears that infants require approximately 10 to 30 cm of small intestine, with intact ileocecal valve (ICV), or 30 to 50 cm without ICV to avoid lifelong dependence on PN.[2]

TABLE 1 Common Causes of Short Bowel Syndrome in Infants and Children

- Necrotizing enterocolitis
- Intestinal atresia
- Gastroschisis
- Midgut volvulus
- Inflammatory bowel disease
- Tumors
- Radiation enteritis
- Ischemic injury
- Intestinal pseudo-obstruction
- Total intestinal aganglionosis

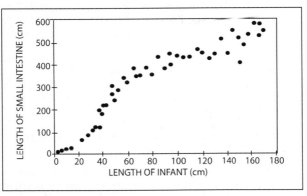

Figure 1 Small intestine length from conception to maturity. Adapted from Weaver L.[1]

PORTION OF SMALL BOWEL RESECTED

1. Duodenal resection may result in iron, folate or calcium malabsorption.
2. The jejunum, with long, large villi, extensive absorptive surface area, highly concentrated digestive enzymes, and many transport carrier proteins, is the primary digestive and absorptive site for

most nutrients. Loss of jejunum is also associated with reduction of cholecystokinin and secretin levels, which secondarily impairs pancreatic and biliary secretions.[3]

3. Loss of the terminal ileum results in malabsorption of bile acids. Steatorrhea, malabsorption of fat-soluble vitamins, and the formation of lithogenic bile may ensue. The terminal ileum is the primary site for vitamin B12 absorption. The ileum also secretes hormones, such as peptide YY, which slows gastrointestinal motility in response to fat malabsorption.

4. Ileal resection reduces intestinal transit time more than duodenal resection.

5. Colonic resection reduces transit time and impairs fluid and electrolyte absorptions.[4]

PRESENCE OR ABSENCE OF ILEOCECAL VALVE

1. The ICV serves to regulate the flow of enteric contents from the small bowel into the colon. The absence of ICV shortens gastrointestinal transit and increases fluid and nutrient losses.

2. In the absence of the ICV, colonic bacteria may contaminate the small intestine, causing an inflammatory response that damages small bowel mucosa, resulting in an exacerbation of the malabsorptive state.[4] Bile salts and vitamin B12 may be deconjugated by the bacteria, further contributing to fat and B12 malabsorptions.[3]

ADAPTIVE AND FUNCTIONAL CAPACITY OF THE REMAINING SMALL BOWEL

1. Intestinal adaptation refers to the gross anatomic and histo-logic changes that occur after significant intestinal resection. In the small bowel, these changes include increased bowel circumference, bowel wall thickness, bowel length, villus height, crypt depth, cell proliferation, and migration to villus tip.[5]

2. These adaptive changes begin 12 to 24 hours after massive intestinal resection and continue for more than 1 year after resection.[3]

3. Younger infants have an increased capacity for intestinal adaptation over time when compared with adults.

4. Enteral nutrition is an important stimulant of intestinal adaptation, and much research is focused on examining whether specific nutrients promote adaptation more than others.

HEALTH OF OTHER ORGANS THAT ASSIST WITH ABSORPTION AND DIGESTION

1. Cholestasis and liver dysfunction can occur in patients with SBS, thereby affecting the absorption and the utilization of nutrients.
2. The major cause of death in children with SBS is PN-associated liver disease.
3. The relationship between PN use and cholestasis is likely multifactorial, and includes the risk factors of sepsis, mucosal atrophy, and bacterial overgrowth. Every effort should therefore be made to reduce the risk of PN-associated cholestasis (Table 2).
4. Other potential factors associated with more severe cholestasis include bacterial overgrowth,[6] less enteral nutrition in the postoperative period,[7] and length of time with diverting ostomy.[8]
5. Preliminary data exist to suggest that the fat source of PN may have an effect on the natural history of PN-associated cholestasis,[9] but more data are needed.

TABLE 2   Steps to Reduce the Risk of PN-associated Cholestasis

Method	Comments
Avoid overfeeding	80 to 100 kcal/kg average parenteral energy requirement among infants
Cycle PN off at least 2 to 6 hours per day	Promotes cyclic release of GI hormones
Aggressively treat and prevent infections	Meticulous CVL care; treat bacterial overgrowth of small bowel
Reduce or modify parenteral fat intake	1 g/kg/day of omega 3 fatty acids
Encourage enteral nutrition	The ultimate goal of therapy

GI = gastrointestinal; CVL = central venous line.
Adapted from Utter SL, Duggan C. Short Bowel Syndrome. In: Hendricks KM, Duggan C, Walker WA, editors. Hamilton: BC Decker Inc; 2000. p. 529–41.

Nutrition Therapy in Short Bowel Syndrome

The goal of nutrition therapy in SBS is to maintain normal growth, promote intestinal adaptation, and avoid complications associated with intestinal resection and PN.

FLUID, ELECTROLYTES AND PARENTERAL NUTRITION

1. During the early postoperative phase, fluid and electrolyte balance is the goal of therapy. Large fluid losses are common and tend to be high in sodium content. Parenteral solutions with at least 80 to 100 mEq/L of sodium are often required to maintain sodium balance.

2. Meticulous attention needs to be paid to the fluid and electrolyte status of SBS patients. This includes daily weights, careful measurement of urine, stool and ostomy losses, and laboratory monitoring of serum electrolytes.

3. Parenteral nutrition is indicated in the management of SBS until small bowel growth and adaptation permit growth with enteral nutrition alone.

   • Day to day variations in fluid loss is common, so it is often advantageous to place the patient on a standard PN solution with fluid and electrolytes appropriate for age, size, and metabolic considerations, and subsequently replace excessive losses with a separate solution based on measurement of actual fluid losses. For example, ostomy fluid can be measured for sodium content and replacement fluid prescribed accordingly.

   • When losses have stabilized, the additional fluid and electrolytes can be added to the PN.

ENTERAL FEEDINGS

1. Enteral nutrition has been shown to stimulate intestinal adaptation in the patient with SBS. Evidence suggests that enteral feedings stimulate mucosal hyperplasia by increasing nutrition to enterocytes and increasing locally secreted trophic factors; stimulate regeneration of the intestinal mucosa following injury; and maintain mucosal mass and normal glucose transport.[4]

2. Common contraindications to enteral feeding
   - paralytic or drug-induced ileus
   - bilious and/or persistent vomiting (defined as more than 3 episodes of emesis in 12 hours)
   - shock/poor perfusion due to cardiac or respiratory insufficiency and/or radiological changes of intestinal ischemia
   - clinical suspicion of obstruction or ileus (severe abdominal distension, decreased ostomy or stool output, and/or radiologic changes of obstruction or ileus)
   - grossly bloody stools or ostomy output
3. Once the patient's fluid and electrolyte status has stabilized and post-operative ileus has resolved, a slow introduction of enteral feedings should be started by continuous infusion over 24 hours.
4. Mothers of newborns with SBS should be referred to a lactation consultant to encourage continued breast milk production. Breast milk's immunologic and anti-infective properties are especially advantageous to the infant having undergone intestinal resection. Breast milk contains growth factors, nucleotides, glutamine, and other amino acids that may play an important role in assisting intestinal adaptation.[8] Breast milk from mothers of premature infants with SBS may need protein and caloric fortifications.
5. If breast milk is unavailable, the selection of enteral formula is somewhat controversial. On the one hand, studies suggest that complex nutrients that require more work for digestion and absorption tend to stimulate adaptation more effectively.[10] On the other hand, the limited mucosal surface area can lead to lactose, protein, and long-chain fatty acid (LCFA) malabsorption with the use of intact formulas. Fluid, electrolyte and metabolic balance can be difficult to achieve if this malabsorption is severe. There are also data to suggest improved outcomes with the use of amino acid-based formula.[11] Therefore, our current practice is to use breastmilk when it is available, but to use amino acid-based formulas when it is not, and/or when supplementation is needed.
6. Medium-chain triglycerides (MCTs) are more water-soluble than long-chain triglycerides (LCTs) and are better absorbed in the presence of bile acid or pancreatic insufficiency. However, MCT fats have a slightly lower caloric density and exert a greater osmotic load in the small intestine. Although fat tends

to be poorly absorbed in SBS, it is a dense calorie source. In SBS patients with a colon in continuity, it has been shown that a mixture of an MCT and LCT diet can improve energy and fat absorption.[12]

7. Carbohydrates may be poorly tolerated as they are broken down by gastrointestinal bacteria into small, osmotically active organic acids that can exert a major osmotic load in the distal small intestine and colon. Glucose may be absorbed without hydrolysis, but its small molecular weight increases solution osmolality. Carbohydrate can be given as glucose polymers to decrease the osmotic load.

8. Fiber supplementation may be helpful in the child with SBS, because some fermentation will occur producing trophic short-chain fatty acids (SCFAs), which are an important fuel for the colonocyte. In addition, fiber can lead to bulkier stool output, which may help with hydration and perineal skin care.

HOW TO FEED

1. Especially in the early refeeding period, continuous enteral feedings via a nasogastric or gastrostomy tube is advantageous in the patient with SBS, because they permit constant saturation of carrier transport proteins, thus taking full advantage of the absorptive surface area available. Older children and adults have an improved capacity to regulate gastric emptying and therefore tolerate gastric bolus or oral bolus feedings better than infants do.

2. Enteral feedings are slowly increased by volume, then by concentration, whereas parenteral calories are decreased by number of hours infused or rate of infusion to maintain optimal nutritional status, control fluid losses, and ensure intestinal adaptation.

3. Small quantities of oral feedings should be introduced in infants two or three times a day to stimulate sucking and swallowing and decrease the risk of oral feeding aversion.

4. The rate of advancement of enteral feeds should be determined by multiple factors, including stool or ostomy output, gastric residuals, and signs of malabsorption (Table 3).

5. Enteral feedings may eventually be transitioned to oral /bolus feedings or a combination of oral/bolus feedings and continuous nocturnal feedings to allow some freedom from the feeding pump.

6. Oral feedings should be small and frequent.

TABLE 3 Suggested Guidelines for Enteral Feeding Advancement in the Infant with Short Bowel Syndrome

Feeding Advancement Principles

- Quantify feeding intolerance primarily by stool or ostomy output and secondarily by reducing substances. Reducing substances should be measured twice daily.

- Assess tolerance no more than twice per 24 hours. Advance no more than once per 24-hour period.

- Ultimate goals: 130 to 200 mL/kg/d
                          100 to 140 kcal/kg/d

- If ostomy/stool output precludes volume advancement at 20 cal/oz for 7 days, then increasing caloric density of the formula can be performed.

- As feedings are advanced, PN should be reduced such that weight gain velocity is maintained.

Guidelines for feeding advancement

Stool output:

If < 10 g/kg/d or < 10 stools/d ------------->advance rate by
                                            10 to 20 mL/kg/d

If 10 to 20 g/kg/d or 10 to 12 stools/d ---> no change

If > 20 g/kg/d or > 12 stools/d -----------> reduce rate or hold
                                            feeds*

Ostomy output:

If < 2 g/kg/h ------------------->   advance rate by 10 to 20
                                      mL/kg/d

If 2 to 3 g/kg/h ---------------->   no change

If > 3 g/kg/h ------------------->   reduce rate or hold feeds*

Stool reducing substances:

If < 1% ------------------------->   advance feeds per stool or
                                      ostomy output

If 1% --------------------------->   no change

If > 1% ------------------------->   reduce rate or hold feeds*

Continued

TABLE 3 *Continued*

Signs of dehydration:	
If absent ------------------------>	advance feeds per stool or ostomy output
If present ---------------------->	reduce rate or hold feeds*
Gastric aspirates:	
< four times previous hour's infusion ------> advance feeds	
> four times previous hour's infusion ------> reduce rate or hold feeds*	

NB: Oral feeds may be offered as follows:

1. Infant is developmentally able to feed by mouth (PO).

2. One hour's worth of continuous feeds may be offered PO BID-TID after 5 days of continuous feeds. During this time, tube feeds should be held.

3. More than 1 hour's worth of continuous feeds may be offered PO once the infant has reached full volume of feeds by continuous route and is demonstrating weight gain at least 7 days have passed on the feeding advancement protocol.

*Feeds should generally be held for 8 hours, then restarted at 75% of the previous rate.
From Utter SL, Duggan C. Short bowel syndrome. In Hendricks KM, Duggan C, Walker WA, editors. Hamilton: BC Decker Inc, 2000. p. 529–41.

7. Excess fluid and electrolyte losses may continue to complicate the management of SBS patients receiving enteral feedings, particularly patients with high output jejunostomies. Oral rehydration solutions with a sodium concentration of 75 to 90 mEq/L should be used to replace losses.

Experimental Therapies in SBS

1. The role of glutamine in gut adaptation in humans remains unconfirmed. A small randomized trial of enteral glutamine has not shown any positive effects,[13] and larger trials of parenteral glutamine have also not confirmed benefit among low birthweight infants.[14]

2. Glutamine in combination with growth hormone has been evaluated as a therapy for adults with SBS.[15,16] Growth hormone causes hypertrophy of the GI tract and increases body weight, distal ileal weight and mucosal weight in rats undergoing 75% resection of SB.[17] Studies of GH in humans have shown mixed results, and no effect was seen in a trial among children.[18]

3. Other hormones (such as epidermal growth factor and IGF-1) may also have a role to play in optimizing intestinal adaptation. Promising results have been shown in animals treated with glucagon-like peptide 2 (GLP-2).[19] A GLP-2 analog has been used in adults with SBS.[20] Studies in children are awaited.

Metabolic Complications of SBS

1. In patients with steatorrhea, LCFA combine in the distal small bowel with magnesium and calcium contributing to a deficiency of these minerals. Calcium becomes unavailable for the formation of calcium oxalate, and bile salts in the colon are thought to increase mucosal permeability to oxalate. These two factors together increase enteric oxalate absorption, which in turn increases the risk of oxalate renal stones.[3]

2. There is an increased incidence of gallstones among both patients with a jejunostomy and those with short bowel in continuity with the colon. It is assumed that precipitation of cholesterol occurs due to the low concentration of bile salts in bile as a consequence of ileal resection, causing an interruption of entero-hepatic circulation of bile.[21]

3. Gastrin secretion is increased, probably due to the loss of the normal feedback mechanism. This results in excess gastric acid which alters luminal pH of the small bowel and adversely affects pancreatic lipase or trypsin activity.[3] Excess acid secretion impairs carbohydrate and protein digestion and absorption, micellar formation, and fat lipolysis, often resulting in malabsorption and diarrhea.[22] Acid blockers can be used to decrease gastric acid and improve absorption.

4. In SBS, overgrowth of bacteria in the small intestine results in deconjugation of bile acids and maldigestion. Bacterial overgrowth should be suspected whenever patients with SBS experience an exacerbation of gastrointestinal symptoms, require additional calories, or lose weight.[23] An additional complication

of bacterial overgrowth is a neurological syndrome associated with D-lactic acidosis. Patients may develop headache, drowsiness, stupor, confusion, behavioral disturbance, ataxia, blurred vision, ophthalamoplegia, or nystagmus. This should be suspected when there is an acidosis with an unexplained anion gap. Bacterial overgrowth can be treated with intermittent courses of antibiotics given orally (eg, metronidazole 20 to 40 mg/kg/d divided q8h, augmentin 20 to 40 mg/kg/d divided q8h, each given for 5 to 7 days, sometimes once per month).

5. Once patients are off PN, vitamin replacement is usually necessary, especially fat-soluble vitamins. Oral requirements may be several times the dietary reference intakes. Trace element status should be monitored closely. In SBS patients, especially those with intestinal stomas, deficiencies of zinc and copper are common.[3] Iron deficiency can result from loss of duodenal-jejunal absorptive area. Calcium supplementation may be required to minimize oxalate absorption.

The Surgical Management of Short Bowel Syndrome

The surgical management of SBS may be divided into three phases, the initial operative strategy, therapy for established disease, and bowel rehabilitation.

INITIAL OPERATIVE STRATEGY

The key element of the initial surgical approach to the multiple causes of SBS is an early recognition of a potential ischemic process, such as intestinal volvulus. Bilious vomiting always mandates emergent surgical consultation. Complete midgut necrosis can occur within 6 hours of volvulus. At laparotomy the major surgical principle, regardless of the cause of intestinal damage, is small intestinal preservation. In necrotizing enterocolitis all major segments of potentially viable bowel (particularly small bowel) should be conserved and often this entails a "second look" operation where marginally viable bowel must be re-evaluated. Similarly in the case of ischemic insult such as that from midgut or segmental volvulus, a second look procedure is often indicated. As a rule only frankly dead intestine should be removed. There is no substitute for an experienced pediatric surgeon in determining the viability of a segment of bowel. Often disease processes involve the terminal ileum and care must be taken to preserve this portion of bowel due to its specialized absorptive capabilities. Unfortunately, the bowel segment immediately adjacent to the ICV may be subject to delayed stricture formation. At each operation, the operative surgeon must carefully measure the small intestine length along the antimesenteric margin as this is the single most important prognostic factor in determining whether small intestinal insufficiency will ensue.

ESTABLISHED SHORT BOWEL SYNDROME

The most important aspects of the treatment of established SBS are the establishment of bowel continuity and the institution of early enteral feeding. Although it is often prudent to wait 6 to 12 weeks after initial surgery to close all stomas in an effort to obviate vascular adhesions, waiting longer than this is generally contraindicated. If there is concern that an operation cannot be done safely after this interval in a particular neonate, transfer to a specialized center should be instituted. The most frequent error in the surgical management of SBS is a delay in the establishment of bowel continuity. Although the colon contributes little to nutrient absorption, its water absorptive capabilities alone are very helpful in establishing effective enteral nutrition. Technical errors, such as leaking or obstructed intestinal anastomoses, should not occur and are vanishingly rare complications in pediatric surgical practice. The creation of gastrostomies to facilitate supplemental enteral feeding should be considered early in the disease process. If gastroesophageal reflux is severe, fundoplication is indicated. The use of tunneled, cuffed, central lines is also of great utility in the treatment of children requiring long-term parenteral nutritional support. It is important to note that techniques that preserve major blood vessels to allow for repeated cannulation are preferred. The placement of these lines via a percuateous subclavian approach under direct fluoroscopic guidance is our usual approach.

BOWEL REHABILITATION

Again the establishment of effective enteral nutrition is the major goal of the chronic management of SBS. It is axiomatic that enterally fed children with SBS are protected from PN-associated hepatic injury. Over the first 6 months of SBS, the small intestine will adapt by increasing considerably in diameter. Although this does increase the effective absorptive capacity of the intestine, it may inhibit effective peristalsis and facilitate bacterial overgrowth. At 6 months, if a child has not been weaned from PN, we will consider a bowel lengthening procedure. There are two such operations utilized.

1. Longitudinal intestinal lengthening and tapering, or the "Bianchi procedure," involves splitting the bowel lengthwise between the leaves of the mesentery and effectively halving its diameter and nearly doubling its length. It does require bowel anastomoses and the procedure cannot be repeated on the same bowel segment at a later date due to the risk of vascular insufficiency.

2. The serial transverse enteroplasty (STEP) procedure is a novel technique in the surgical management of SBS. Using a series of alternating staple firings, the intestine is lengthened and tapered.[24,25] Preliminary studies demonstrate increased intestinal length and improved nutritional indices following the STEP procedure.[26] Furthermore, unlike the Bianchi procedure, patients can undergo repeat STEP operations. At our institution, this operation has become the primary approach to lengthen and taper bowel in SBS patients.

TRANSPLANTATION

Short bowel syndrome patients who have irreversible failure of intestinal function associated with failure of PN therapy (ie, severe hepatic injury, multiple line infections, repeated episodes of dehydration, loss of central access) are candidates for transplantation. Depending on patient pathology and organ availability, patients can receive either an isolated small intestine, liver-small intestine, or multivisceral transplantation. Recent results demonstrate improving short-term patient and graft survival,[27] although more long-term outcomes are still not established.

Summary

The management of SBS is a multistage process that may take years. Aggressive use of enteral nutrition to stimulate intestinal adaptation, carefully selected surgical intervention, and recognition and treatment of possible complications can significantly improve prognosis. A multidisciplinary team effort facilitates and enhances intestinal rehabilitation. Our team is composed of surgeons, gastroenterologists, neonatologists, pharmacists, nutrition physicians, dietitians and nurse practitioners, and has resulted in an improvement in SBS survival rates from 70% to 90%.[28]

References

1. Weaver L. Anatomy and embryology. In: Walker W, editor. Pediatric gastrointestinal disease. Philadelphia (PA): BC Decker, Inc; 1991. p. 195–215.

2. Kurkchubasche AG, Rowe MI, Smith SD. Adaptation in short-bowel syndrome: reassessing old limits. J Pediatr Surg 1993;28:1069–71.

3. Ziegler MM. Short bowel syndrome in infancy: etiology and management. Clin Perinatol 1986;13:163–73.

4. Kamin D, Corleto. Intestinal failure, short bowel syndrome and intestinal transplantation. In Duggan C, Watkins JB, Walker WA, (eds). Nutrition in pediatrics. Hamilton (ON): BC Decker, Inc, 2008.

5. Buchman AL. Etiology and initial management of short bowel syndrome. Gastroenterology 2006;130(2 Suppl 1):S5–S15.

6. Kaufman SS, Loseke CA, Lupo JV, et al. Influence of bacterial overgrowth and intestinal inflammation on duration of parenteral nutrition in children with short bowel syndrome. J Pediatr 1997;131:356–61.

7. Sondhcimer JM, Cadnapaphornchai M, Sontag M, Zerbe GO. Predicting the duration of dependence on parenteral nutrition after neonatal intestinal resection. J Pediatr 1998;132:80–4.

8. Andorsky DJ, Lund DP, Lillehei CW, et al. Nutritional and other postoperative management of neonates with short bowel syndrome correlates with clinical outcomes. J Pediatr 2001;139:27–33.

9. Gura KM, Duggan CP, Collier SB, et al. Reversal of parenteral nutrition-associated liver disease in two infants with short bowel syndrome using parenteral fish oil: implications for future management. Pediatrics 2006;118:e197–201.

10. DiBaise JK, Young RJ, Vanderhoof JA. Intestinal rehabilitation and the short bowel syndrome: part 1. Am J Gastroenterol 2004;99:1386–95.

11. Bines J, Francis D, Hill D. Reducing parenteral requirement in children with short bowel syndrome: impact of an amino acid-based complete infant formula. J Pediatr Gastroenterol Nutr 1998;26:123–8.

12. Jeppesen PB, Mortensen PB. The influence of a preserved colon on the absorption of medium chain fat in patients with small bowel resection. Gut 1998;43:478–83.

13. Duggan C, Stark AR, Auestad N, et al. Glutamine supplementation in infants with gastrointestinal disease: a randomized, placebo-controlled pilot trial. Nutrition 2004;20:752–6.

14. Poindexter BB, Ehrenkranz RA, Stoll BJ, et al. Parenteral glutamine supplementation does not reduce the risk of mortality or late-onset sepsis in extremely low birth weight infants. Pediatrics 2004;113:1209–15.

15. Byrne TA, Morrissey TB, Nattakom TV, et al. Growth hormone, glutamine, and a modified diet enhance nutrient absorption in patients with severe short bowel syndrome. JPEN J Parenter Enteral Nutr 1995;19:296–302.

16. Scolapio JS, Camilleri M, Fleming CR, et al. Effect of growth hormone, glutamine, and diet on adaptation in short-bowel syndrome: a randomized, controlled study. Gastroenterology 1997;113:1074–81.

17. Shulman, DI, Hu CS, Duckett G, Lavallee-Grey M. Effects of short-term growth hormone therapy in rats undergoing 75% small intestinal resection. J Pediatr Gastroenterol Nutr 1992;14:3–11.

18. Lifschitz CH, Duggan CP, Langston C, et al. Growth hormone therapy in children with short bowel syndrome: a randomized, placebo controlled trial. Gastroenterology 2003;124:A64.

19. Liu X, Nelson DW, Holst JJ, Ney DM. Synergistic effect of supplemental enteral nutrients and exogenous glucagon-like peptide 2 on intestinal adaptation in a rat model of short bowel syndrome. Am J Clin Nutr 2006;84:1142–50.

20. Jeppesen PB, Sanguinetti EL, Buchman A, et al. Teduglutide (ALX-0600), a dipeptidyl peptidase IV resistant glucagon-like peptide 2 analogue, improves intestinal function in short bowel syndrome patients. Gut 2005;54:1224–31.

21. Lennard-Jones JE. Review article: practical management of the short bowel. Aliment Pharmacol Ther 1994;8:563–77.

22. Lifschitz CH. Enteral feeding in short small bowel. In: Baker SB, Baker RD, Davis AD, editors. Pediatric enteral nutrition. New York: Chapman & Hall; 1994. p. 280–90.

23. Dibaise JK, Young RJ, Vanderhoof JA. Enteric microbial flora, bacterial overgrowth, and short-bowel syndrome. Clin Gastroenterol Hepatol 2006;4:11–20.

24. Kim HB, Lee PW, Garza J, et al. Serial transverse enteroplasty for short bowel syndrome: a case report. J Pediatr Surg 2003;38:881–5.

25. Kim HB, Fauza D, Garza J, et al. Serial transverse enteroplasty (STEP): a novel bowel lengthening procedure. J Pediatr Surg 2003;38:425–9.

26. Javid PJ, Kim HB, Duggan CP, Jaksic T. Serial transverse enteroplasty is associated with successful short-term outcomes in infants with short bowel syndrome. J Pediatr Surg 2005;40:1019–23; discussion 23–4.

27. The Intestinal Transplant Registry. http://www.intestinal-transplant.org (accessed June 30, 2007).

28. Modi BP, Langer M, Ching YA, et al. Improved survival in a multi-disciplinary short bowel syndrome program. J Pediatr Surg 2008;43:20–24.

Part 7: Inguinal Hernia

Arin K. Greene, MD, Sang Lee, MD and
Mark Puder, MD, PhD

Anatomy

The processus vaginalis is a peritoneal diverticulum that extends through the internal inguinal ring. As the testicle descends during the final trimester from its intra-abdominal position into the scrotum, it brings a portion of the processus down with it. The portion surrounding the testes becomes the tunica vaginalis. The remaining processus in the inguinal canal usually obliterates. This eliminates the communication between the peritoneal cavity and the scrotum. A communication may persist asymptomatically. If fluid communicates with the abdomen to the testicle, a hydrocele is present (Figure 1). If intra-abdominal contents are present, then a hernia is present (indirect most common) (Figure 2). A inguinal hernia never spontaneously resolves and always requires surgery.

Epidemiology

- One-third of children with inguinal hernias present in the first 6 months of life.
- For full-term infants, the incidence is 0.5 to 1% but increases with lower gestational age, rising to 16 to 25% in the premature population.
- The male:female ratio is approximately 6:1.
- Sixty percent are on the right, 30% on the left, and 10% are bilateral in both sexes.
- Of groin hernias in infants, 98.6% are indirect inguinal, 1.2% are direct inguinal, and 0.2% are femoral hernias.
- Twins and individuals with a family history have a higher incidence of inguinal hernia.
- The younger the infant, the higher the risk that the hernia will become incarcerated. The incidence of incarcerated hernia is 12% for boys and 17% for girls. Thirty-one percent of incarcerated hernias occur in infants < 2 months of age.

Pathogenesis

- The processus vaginalis develops as an out-pouching of the peritoneal cavity through the internal inguinal ring during the third trimester. The processus accompanies the testicular descent into the scrotum and is then obliterated. The distal processus remains as the tunica vaginalis.
- Although the timing of the obliteration of the processus is unknown, it likely obliterates shortly after birth because studies have found that 57 to 94% are patent at birth.
- A patent processus vaginalis is a risk for hydrocele or hernia formation. When the processus contains peritoneal fluid alone, a hydrocele results. When it contains abdominal viscera, a hernia results.
- Risk factors for converting an asymptomatic processus into an inguinal hernia include chronic respiratory disease (chronic lung disease, cystic fibrosis), increased intra-abdominal pressure (ascites, repair of omphalocele or gastroschisis, ventriculoperitoneal shunts, and peritoneal dialysis), exstrophy of the bladder, and connective tissue disorders.

Diagnosis

PHYSICAL EXAMINATION

- Hernias often present as a smooth and firm mass lateral to the pubic tubercle in the inguinal canal. The mass may extend into the scrotum and will enlarge with increased intra-abdominal pressure (crying or straining).
- The hernia may be expressed in a quiet infant by laying the infant supine with extended arms and legs to increase intra-abdominal pressure.
- If a hernia is not clearly expressed with an increase in intra-abdominal pressure, the spermatic cord may be palpated where it crosses the pubic tubercle (silk glove sign).
- An incarcerated hernia cannot be returned to the abdominal cavity. Symptoms suggesting an incarcerated hernia include pain, emesis, and irritability. The mass is usually well defined and does not reduce spontaneously. Incarcerated hernias in

children can rapidly evolve into strangulation and gangrenous hernia contents.

- Strangulation is suspected with intense pain, bilious or feculent emesis, bloody stools, fever, tachycardia, edema and erythema in the region of the hernia, tender mass and distended abdomen. The testes may be swollen secondary to impaired venous blood return.

RADIOGRAPHIC STUDIES

- Plain radiographs will show intestinal contents within the scrotum. It may show intestinal obstruction or gas in the intestinal wall, if intestinal strangulation is present. This is rarely used or necessary for diagnosis.
- Ultrasonography may be used to differentiate a hydrocele from a hernia.

Differential Diagnosis

TESTICULAR TORSION

- The patient presents with an acute onset of pain often without a history of an inguinal hernia.
- The testes are very tender and often retracted upward (high riding).
- The swelling does not involve the external ring and inguinal canal.
- All suspected cases of incarcerated and strangulated hernias or testicular torsion must be urgently seen by a surgeon. There is a very high incidence of testicular death within 6 hours (see Chapter 9, "Neurological Disorders").
- In utero, testicular torsion usually presents as a painless mass and is diagnosed by physical examination in the newborn. The overlying skin may be ecchymotic or edematous. Distinguishing neonatal torsion from an incarcerated hernia may require an urgent operation.

LYMPHADENITIS

- There is a history of infection in the area of the inguinal or femoral lymph nodes.

- Multiple tender and fixed masses are palpable lateral to the external ring.

HYDROCELE

- Peritoneal fluid is located in a patent processus vaginalis.
- It is often present since birth and may be bilateral.
- The swelling is translucent, non-tender, smooth, and moveable.
- Fluid usually surrounds the testis. However, a hydrocele involving the spermatic cord will be located in the upper scrotum of the inguinal canal separate from the testis.
- Palpation sometimes reveals narrowing at the external inguinal ring.
- It trans-illuminates brightly.
- Most resolve during the first 2 years of life as the patent processus vaginalis closes. High ligation of the processus vaginalis is indicated for a persistent hydrocele after 2 years of age.

Management of Incarcerated Hernias

As with all inguinal hernias, this condition is age related and occurs most often in infants during the first year of life. Most can be reduced manually, which obviates the need for emergency surgery.

REDUCTION TECHNIQUES

- Occasionally, simply holding the baby in steep Trendelenburg's position reduces the hernia owing to the gravitational pull on the mesentery.
- Sedation may be necessary (see Chapter 15, "Health Maintenance/Discharge Planning"). After sedation, have an assistant hold the infant above the knees in a frog leg position to relax the abdominal wall. Use one hand to fix the hernia, while the other hand should press the incarcerated mass upward toward the canal. Apply a considerable length of steady pressure (five minutes may be required to produce the desired reduction). Try to milk the bowel contents out of the incarcerated bowel until it "pops" back into the abdomen. Some hernias reduce easily, whereas others require several attempts. After reduction, ensure that the testes are lying in the scrotum. Surgical consultation should be obtained for all possible incarcerated hernias.

POST-REDUCTION MANAGEMENT

- If reduction is successful, admit the patient and repair the hernia electively within 24 to 48 hours, allowing edema to resolve.
- During this time, the infant should have serial examinations to rule out re-incarceration.

THE UN-REDUCIBLE HERNIA

- Emergency surgical intervention is required if the hernia cannot be reduced.
- Persistent intestinal obstruction may lead to vascular compromise and necrosis.
- If small bowel is frankly necrotic, resection is necessary, either via the groin incision or by a separate abdominal incision.
- Incarcerated inguinal hernias in girls are usually sliding hernias containing ovary and fallopian tube. These can be repaired on a semi-elective basis, provided that there is no compromised bowel involved. The blood supply to the ovary is not usually impaired, however, there are reports of ovarian strangulation.

Non-incarcerated Hernias in Premature Infants

- There is an increased rate of testicular atrophy, vas deferens injury and recurrence after repair.
- Timing of repair weighs risks of incarceration and more difficult repair due to the thin hernia sac against risks of anesthesia, possibility of increased complications and recurrence. It can depend on patient co-morbidities, age, and weight.
- The non-incarcerated hernia in a premature infant with multiple other problems may be repaired just prior to discharge. If repair cannot be easily facilitated prior to discharge, operation soon thereafter is acceptable, provided that parents have been fully educated regarding the diagnosis and urgency of incarceration.

Postoperative Management

- At our institution, babies < 60 weeks post-menstrual age with a history of prematurity (< 37 weeks gestational age) are admitted for apnea monitoring overnight after hernia repair.
- Local anesthetic is usually placed into the surgical wound in the operating room.
- Infants are treated with acetaminophen as needed.
- The sutures are usually under the skin and are absorbable.
- There are usually no activity limitations.

Bilateral versus Unilateral Repair

Fifty to sixty percent of infants under 2 years of age with a unilateral inguinal hernia have a contralateral patent processus. Of these, only 10 to 15% will develop a clinical contralateral hernia. The incidence of patent processus falls to 40% after 2 years of age. Most surgeons decide on selective contralateral exploration based on risk factors for the presence of a contralateral hernia including age < 2 years, history of incarceration, gender (F > M), prematurity, presence of associated disorders, or increased abdominal pressure.

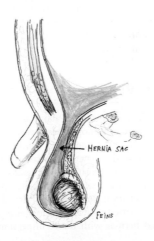

Observational data on metachronous (simultaneously occurring) hernias reveal that clinically evident hernias requiring repair occur in 8 to 31% of patients following initial hernia repair. Because the large majority of patients will not develop a clinically evident contralateral hernia, many surgeons elect not to perform contralateral exploration. Conversely, those surgeons who do routinely explore the contralateral side cite the risks and consequences of incarceration as justification enough. The primary benefit is decreased rates of incarcerated hernia and its potentially highly morbid sequelae verses potential injury to the vessels or vas deferens.

Techniques of contralateral inspection include ultrasonography and direct evaluation via laparoscope, either through an infraumbilical port or through the ipsilateral hernia sac. Herniography, probing and insufflation of the contralateral hernia are seldom performed. Ultrasound can be performed with > 90% sensitivity and specificity, but is operator dependent and measurement criteria for hernias are arbitrary. Direct evaluation can be done via the hernia sac using a 70-degree scope with > 99% sensitivity and specificity.

Open Repair

The standard and most frequently used approach to repairing an inguinal hernia is through a small incision in the natural inguinal crease. The vas deferens and the vascular supply are separated from the hernia sac and the sac is ligated (Figure 3). Absorbable sutures are used for the closure and the wound is covered with dermabond (Ethicon) or sterile dressing.

Laparoscopic Repair

Laparoscopic repair is becoming a viable option, with improvement in technique and technology. Previously, recurrence rates and longer operative times were cited as contraindications to this approach, but recent studies have shown complication rates similar to the open approach. The advantages of laparoscopic repair, both pro-peritoneal and intra-abdominal, are facile investigation of the contralateral side and immediate repair of any discovered hernia, improved cosmesis with smaller incisions, ability to reduce and repair incarcerated hernias with direct inspection of incarcerated contents, and potentially less manipulation of the vas deferens and testicular vessels. For surgeons who do not routinely perform contralateral inspection, the laparoscopic technique provides fewer advantages. Larger series of patients with more analysis of recurrence rates are still necessary.

Complications

RECURRENCE

- The incidence is < 1% for uncomplicated hernias and up to 20% for incarcerated hernias.
- Risk factors for recurrence are the same as those for development of the original hernia (see above).
- Some indirect hernias result from failure to ligate the hernia sac high enough at the internal ring or other technical errors.
- A direct or femoral hernia noticed after the repair of an indirect hernia was either a concomitant hernia that was missed during the original hernia repair or resulted from damage to the inguinal canal during the initial operation.

SCROTAL SWELLING

- Swelling is very common.
- A hydrocele may result from fluid located in the distal hernia sac, whereas a hematoma may result from the excision of the distal hernia sac.
- Both hydroceles and hematomas usually resolve spontaneously.

TESTICULAR COMPROMISE, CYANOSIS, OR ATROPHY

- Incarcerated or strangulated hernias may impair testicular blood flow by compression of the testicular vessels.
- Diagnosis is made by histological examination or reduced size on follow-up.
- The incidence of testicular compromise or cyanosis is 2.6 to 5% for incarcerated hernias and 11 to 29% for testicles examined during emergency operation. The incidence of atrophy is only 1%.
- Unless clearly necrotic, a compromised (cyanotic) testicle is generally left in place and usually survives.

SPERMATIC CORD INJURY

- Incidence is 1%.
- This injury is often only recognized with bilateral injury when the patient reaches adulthood.
- Unilateral injury may contribute to infertility secondary to loss of the blood–testis barrier with the production of anti-spermatozoa antibodies.

INTESTINAL INJURY

- A strangulated hernia containing intestine may lead to intestinal ischemia.
- Less than 1.5% of strangulated hernias require intestinal resection.
- The mortality rate ranges from 0 to 9% and occurs most often in premature infants with associated cardiac disease.

IATROGENIC UNDESCENDED TESTES

- Incidence is approximately 0.2%.
- It results from either failure to return the testes to the scrotum after the hernia repair or secondary to subsequent retraction.
- It requires orchidopexy.

Recommended Readings

Jona JZ. The incidence of positive contralateral inguinal exploration among preschool children – a retrospective and prospective study. J Pediatr Surg 1996;31:656–60.

Weber TR, Tracy TF. Groin hernias and hydroceles. In: Ashcraft KW, Murphy JP, Sharp RS, et al, editors. Textbook of peditric surgery. Philadelphia (PA): WB Saunders; 2000. p. 654 p. 208–62.

Lau ST, Lee YH, Caty MG. Current management of hernias and hydroceles. Semin Pediatr Surg 2007;16:50 p. 208–7

Part 8: Umbilical Hernia

Camilia R. Martin, MD, MS, FAAP, and
Steven J. Fishman, MD, FACS, FAAP

Embryology

For formation of the anterior abdominal wall, refer to "Part 2: Omphalocele."

FORMATION OF THE UMBILICAL RING

- The umbilical ring is at the center of the four somatic folds comprising the abdominal wall.
- Final contracture and closure of the umbilical ring occurs after the umbilical cord is ligated and the umbilical vessels thrombose.
- Failure of the umbilical ring to completely close results in an umbilical hernia.

Incidence of Umbilical Hernia

- The true incidence is unknown, but it is estimated to be 18% in white infants[1] and 42% in black infants.[2]
- The incidence is increased with prematurity and low birth weight.[3,4]
- The frequency is equal in boys and girls.

Prenatal Diagnosis and Treatment

An umbilical hernia is usually not diagnosed in the prenatal period. However, in rare circumstances an umbilical hernia can be detected with prenatal ultrasonography.[5]

Postnatal Presentation

- An umbilical hernia is generally a lesion of no concern, often noted in the newborn period as a protrusion of the umbilicus during straining and crying.

- The fascial defect is usually < 2 cm in diameter.
- Rarely, complications may occur including incarceration and spontaneous rupture.[4]

   The risk of incarceration increases with increasing age and with defects of medium size (0.5 to 1.5 cm in diameter). However, incarceration has been reported for umbilical hernia of all sizes.[6,7]

   Spontaneous rupture is associated with increased abdominal pressure, umbilical trauma, and umbilical infection. Some instances have no clear predisposing factor.[8,9]

- The majority close spontaneously by 3 years of age. Spontaneous closure is less likely after 3 years of age, for hernias > 1.5 cm in diameter for hernias with excessive redundant skin, and for hernias that are associated with an underlying condition, such as hypothyroidism, Down syndrome, and Beckwith–Wiedemann syndrome.[3,4,10]
- Surgical correction is recommended for hernias that have not spontaneously closed by 4 or 5 years of age because of the diminished chance of spontaneous closure and the initiation of body image awareness.

Postnatal Diagnosis

- Umbilical hernias are easily diagnosed based on the umbilical protuberance, palpable fascial defect, and redundant umbilical skin.
- Rarely associated disorders include trisomy 21, congenital hypothyroidism, and Beckwith–Wiedemann syndrome.[3]

Differential Diagnosis

- It is important to distinguish an umbilical hernia from supraumbilical and epigastric hernias. The latter hernia types are due to defects along the linea alba, are more likely to be symptomatic, and do not close spontaneously. As a result, surgical closure is indicated.[11]
- Another defect of the umbilical region to consider in the differential diagnosis is a small omphalocele.

Preoperative Management

No special preoperative management is recommended. Routine procedures should be followed.

Anesthesia

- The hernia repair is conducted under general anesthesia using inhalational agents and bag and mask ventilation.[12]
- The depth of anesthesia must be closely monitored to prevent sudden increases in abdominal pressure and resultant evisceration through the open umbilicus.

Surgical Management

- This operation is usually performed as an outpatient procedure.
- The approach is by an infra- or intraumbilical incision.
- The hernia sac is excised, and the fascial defect is sutured.
- A dressing is applied. For uncomplicated umbilical hernias, a pressure dressing may be unnecessary. In a recent randomized study, pressure dressings were not shown to reduce wound infection, hematoma formation, or hernia recurrence rate compared with using no wound dressings.[13]

Postoperative Management

- Pain is controlled with oral analgesics.
- There are no activity restrictions.
- If applied, the dressing can be removed after 5 to 7 days.

Complications and Outcome

Complications are uncommon and outcomes are favorable.

References

1. Woods GE. Some observations on umbilical hernia in infants. Arch Dis Child 1953;8:450–62.

2. Crump EP. Umbilical hernia: occurrence of the infantile type in negro infants and children. J Pediatr 1952;40:214–23.

3. Garcia VF. Umbilical and other abdominal wall hernias. In: Ashcraft KW, editor. Pediatric surgery. WB Saunders Company; 2000. p. 639–49.

4. O'Donnell KA, Glick PL, Caty MG. Pediatric umbilical problems. Pediatr Clin North Am 1998;45:791–99.

5. Richards DS, Kays DW. Prenatal ultrasonographic diagnosis of a simple umbilical hernia. J Ultrasound Med 1998;17:265–67.

6. Chirdan LB, Uba AF, Kidmas AT. Incarcerated umbilical hernia in children. Eur J Pediatr Surg 2006;16:45–8.

7. Lassaletta L, Fonkalsrud EW, Tovar JA, et al. The management of umbilicial hernias in infancy and childhood. J Pediatr Surg 1975;10:405–9.

8. Durakbasa CU. Spontaneous rupture of an infantile umbilical hernia with intestinal evisceration. Pediatr Surg Int 2006;22:567–9.

9. Weik J, Moores D. An unusual case of umbilical hernia rupture with evisceration. J Pediatr Surg 2005;40:E33–5.

10. Palazzi D, ML B. Care of the umbilicus and management of umbilical disorders. In: Rose B, editor. UpToDate. Waltham (MA); 2007.

11. Keshtgar AS, Griffiths M. Incarceration of umbilical hernia in children: is the trend increasing? Eur J Pediatr Surg 2003;13:40–3.

12. Davis PJ, Hall S, Deshpande JK, Spear RM. Anesthesia for neonates and premature infants. In: Motoyama EK, Davis PJ, editors. Smith's anesthesia for infants and children. Mosby; 1996. p. 572.

13. Merei JM. Umbilical hernia repair in children: is pressure dressing necessary. Pediatr Surg Int 2006;22:446–8.

Part 9: Feeding Tubes

Debora Duro, MD, MS, Athos Bousvaros, MD, and Mark Puder, MD, PhD

Reasons for Placing a Feeding Tube in an Infant

An infant is fed through a feeding tube for any of the following reasons:

- To adequately nourish and promote growth and development in an infant with insufficient oral intake
- To protect against aspiration in an infant who cannot protect his or her airway during swallowing
- To allow a route to administer medications in infants who cannot take them orally (eg, children with seizure disorders)
- To decrease orally aversive behavior in infants resistant to feeding
- To reduce excessive amounts of time spent feeding an infant, thus allowing caretakers to focus on the infant's other medical and developmental needs, as well as the needs of their other children

Illnesses and Conditions in which Feeding Tubes Are Placed

OROPHARYNGEAL DYSPHAGIA

Dysphagia is the inability to adequately swallow. It can occur in the following setting:

- Immature swallow
- Cerebral palsy
- Facial palsies (ie, Möbius' syndrome)
- Muscle weakness syndromes (eg, botulism, myasthenia, or spinomuscular atrophy)

GASTROINTESTINAL MALFORMATIONS AND MOTILITY DISTURBANCES

- Esophageal atresia and tracheoesophageal fistula (TEF)
- Diaphragmatic hernia

- Microgastria
- Short-bowel syndrome
- Gastroschisis and omphalocele
- Decompression for expected prolonged ileus after major abdominal operation
- Chronic intestinal pseudo-obstruction

OTHER CHRONIC ILLNESSES

Other chronic illnesses where nutrition may be impaired include the following:

- Bronchopulmonary dysplasia
- Cystic Fibrosis
- Cyanotic or acyanotic congenital heart disease
- Chronic renal failure
- Seizure disorders
- Other progressive neurologic or metabolic disorders (ie, Leigh disease)

BEHAVIORAL AND FUNCTIONAL DISORDERS

- Hyperactive gag that limits nutrition
- Severe oral aversion and food refusal that is unresponsive to behavioral therapy

Evaluation of a Child With a Feeding or Nutritional Disorder

CHART REVIEW

- Weight, height, weight-for-height Z score, growth curve
- Documentation of underlying illnesses (eg, congenital heart disease)
- Documentation of prior respiratory events (eg, aspiration pneumonia, apnea)
- Documentation of vomiting or reflux
- Calculation of fluid and caloric intake (by mouth and by tube)

HISTORY FROM CARETAKER

The infant's history should be obtained (eg, from a parent or a nurse in the NICU). The following information should be obtained about the infant:

- Ability to suck
- Any gagging, choking, or apnea during feeding
- Amount of liquid the infant can take in at one time (eg, 45 mL per feeding)
- Duration of a feeding (eg, 45 min). The single most important question to ask parents is How long does it take you to feed your baby?

PHYSICAL EXAMINATION

The physical examination should focus on assessing any palatal and tongue abnormalities, overall muscle tone, and signs of chronic lung or heart disease. Ideally, the physician assessing the patient should feed the baby, but this important task is usually relinquished to nurses or feeding therapists.

LABORATORY STUDIES

Findings from laboratory studies are generally normal in infants with malnutrition. On occasion, these tests may provide a clue to diagnosis (eg, anemia in reflux esophagitis, eosinophilia in allergy, hypoalbuminemia in cystic fibrosis). The typical nutritional screen includes complete blood count with differential, electrolytes, calcium, phosphorus, albumin/total protein, and liver function tests.

NUTRITIONAL EVALUATION

Formal anthropometric assessments (eg, triceps skin folds) are rarely done in young infants but may be done in older children. Indirect calorimetry is a very comprehensive test performed at the bed side for 30 minutes. It provides an accurate estimation of basal metabolic rate, which can be used to assess energy expenditure and energy intake.

CHEST RADIOGRAPH

Look for signs of chronic aspiration.

BARIUM SWALLOW

There are two types of barium swallow, the conventional and the modified.

Conventional Barium Swallow

The conventional barium swallow test is performed by a radiologist. This test provides a brief evaluation of the infant's swallow and provides a crude assessment of swallowing dysfunction or oral aspiration. However, it also provides information about esophageal and gastric anatomy including H-type TEF, hiatal hernia, pyloric stenosis, duodenal stenosis, and malrotation. Therefore, conventional barium swallow should always be performed in an infant with significant feeding dysfunction.

Modified Barium Swallow

A modified barium swallow test is also called a videofluoroscopic swallowing study. It is performed by a speech or occupational therapist in conjunction with a radiologist. This test involves feeding an infant with suspected oropharyngeal dysphagia a wide variety of age-appropriate foods of varying textures. For an infant, this typically involves formula mixed with barium, with varying amounts of cereal added as a thickener. The therapist assesses the infant's lip closure, sucking ability, tongue movements, bolus propulsion, and cricopharyngeal relaxation. The therapist also assesses for aspiration into the tracheobronchial tree.

The modified barium swallow is a sensitive assessment of swallowing dysfunction and aspiration but provides no information about esophageal or gastric anatomy.

Choosing a Feeding Tube

- In choosing a feeding tube, the options include the following: nasogastric tube (NGT), a nasojejunal tube (NJT), G tube, a gastrojejunal tube (GJT), and jejunostomy (surgical J tube). Each of these tubes has both advantages and disadvantages (Table 1).
- In most premature or term infants with feeding disorders, placement of an NGT is the first feeding strategy used. Nasogastric feedings allow hydration and nutrition, permitting growth of the infant, as well as a detailed evaluation of the swallowing.

TABLE 1 Advantages and disadvantages of various feeding tubes

Type of tube	Advantages	Disadvantages
NG	Easily placed Useful in short term	May enter lungs Promotes oral aversion
	No anesthesia required	Uncomfortable for patient
NJ	No anesthesia required	Usually requires fluoroscopic placement
	Minimizes vomiting of feedings	Reflux of gastric contents or bile may still occur Easily displaced
		Promotes oral aversion
		Requires continuous feeds
G tube	Permanent access Does not interfere with swallow	Risks of surgery/anesthesia
	Larger bore diameter than nasal tubes	May worsen GE reflux
		Skin rashes/infections around site
		Social stigma
GJ tube	Same as with G tube PLUS	Requires Fluoroscopic placement
	Decreased risk of GE reflux/vomiting	J tube may flip back into stomach, requiring tre quent replacement
		Bilious reflux may occur
		Risk of intestinal I intussusception around J. tube Requires continuous feeds

Continued

TABLE 1 *Continued*

Type of tube	Advantages	Disadvantages
Surgical jejunostomy	Semi-permanent intestinal access	Requires a large patient (>10 kg)
	Minimizes risk of GE reflux of food	Tube may dislodge
	Requires continuous feeds	Severe skin rashes

GE = gastroesophageal; GJ = gastrojejunostomy; G = gastrostomy; J = jejunostomy; NG = nasogastric; NJ = nasojejunal.

- In infants with severe gastroesophageal (GE) reflux, transpyloric NJTs may allow feeding while protecting the airway.
- If patients require a feeding tube for longer than 2 months, consideration should be given to a gastrostomy or other permanent tube to minimize the development of complications of long-term NGT placement (especially worsening oral aversion).
- Gastrostomies are most commonly placed in children with cerebral palsy, other neurologic conditions, severe bronchopulmonary dysplasia, uncorrected congenital heart disease and for improvement of nutritional status (eg, cystic fibrosis).

Placement of a Gastrostomy Tube

Gastrostomy tubes are usually placed by surgeons in conjunction with other pediatric subspecialists. Given the potential for rare but serious intra-abdominal complications of gastrostomy placement, it is recommended (at a minimum) that a surgeon be consulted and be aware of any patient undergoing a G-tube placement. Ideally, a surgeon should be participating in the actual tube placement. Depending on an institution's resources and personnel, gastrostomies have been placed by surgeons alone, surgeons in conjunction with gastroenterologists, gastroenterologists alone, or interventional radiologists.

SURGICAL TECHNIQUES

Gastrostomy Tube Placement

Percutaneous endoscopic gastrostomy (PEG) is the most common approach at our institution and involves the Gauderer (pull) technique. Gastromy can also be performed using the following techniques:

- Push technique
- Stamm (open) gastrostomy
- Laparoscopic gastrostomy
- Interventional radiology (Seldinger technique)

EVALUATION OF THE INFANT FOR PEG PLACEMENT

- Documentation of specific indication for the feeding tube
- Documentation why short-term (ie, nasogastric) feeding is insufficient or inadequate for this patient
- Identification of factors that may increase the risks of the procedure or be relative or absolute contraindications to PEG tube placement

RELATIVE CONTRAINDICATIONS TO PEG TUBE PLACEMENT

1. Small size (less than 2 kg) may put a child at risk of esophageal perforation from attempting to pull a PEG tube down the esophagus
2. Extensive prior abdominal surgery with adhesions
3. Ventriculoperitoneal shunt (fluoroscopy may be needed to place the tube)
4. Cardiac pacemaker (may require fluoroscopy to place the tube)
5. Severe reflux with history of aspiration or inability to swallow (may require transpyloric tube or fundoplication)
6. Bleeding disorder (hemophilia)
7. Neutropenia or immunodeficiency

The absolute contraindication to PEG placement is the inability to bring the anterior gastric wall in apposition to the anterior abdominal wall (eg, patients with severe ascites or if the colon is directly fixed to the anterior wall of the stomach from adhesions).

PEG USING THE PULL (GAUDERER) TECHNIQUE

The endoscopist (gastroenterologist) inserts an endoscope into the stomach and insufflates the stomach. Concurrently, the surgeon and endoscopist localize an appropriate site for placement by transillumination. The surgeon then cleans the abdominal skin and inserts an angiocatheter through the skin into the stomach. A guidewire is passed through the angiocatheter and into the stomach. The endoscopist then pulls the guidewire out of the mouth. The gastrostomy tube is then tied to the guidewire at the mouth end, and the guidewire and tube are pulled down the mouth and into the stomach. Figures 1 and 2 illustrate this technique.

THE STAMM (OPEN) GASTROSTOMY TUBE PROCEDURE

The Stamm procedure is often performed during an open abdominal operation or as a separate operative procedure. General anesthesia is used, and either a midline or a transverse incision is made. Double purse-string sutures are placed into the stomach around the G tube. These sutures plus four more encircling sutures are placed and secured to the abdominal wall to prevent leakage of feeds and gastric contents. The tube is secured to the skin with sutures and tape. Recovery and management are similar to the PEG tube technique.

LAPAROSCOPIC GASTROSTOMY TUBE PLACEMENT

The laparoscopic technique is performed using one or two trocar sites. One site is used as the G-tube exit site. This technique is often used during concomitant laparoscopic antireflux surgery (fundoplication). The primary advantage of the laparoscopic technique is that direct visualization of the stomach eliminates the risk of inadvertent hollow viscous injury. Another advantage is the applicability of the technique to small infants (< 2 kg). Finally, the ability to place a button gastrostomy as a primary procedure obviates the need for a second procedure for tube conversion to a button.

PLACEMENT BY INTERVENTIONAL RADIOLOGY

Image guided percutaneous gastrostomy insertion is considered to be a safe technique to secure access to the alimentary tract in neonates,

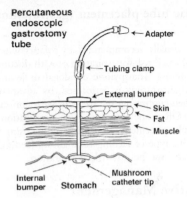

Figure 1 Schematic representation of the percutaneous gastrostomy tube.

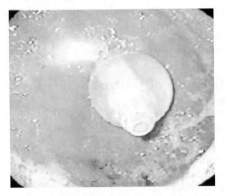

Figure 2 Endoscopy view of the gastrostomy from the stomach.

especially in patients with esophageal atresia. In this situation, the abdomen might be gasless therefore difficult to access the stomach wall. This technique does not require laparotomy and can be performed in an experienced radiology hands easily with low rate of complications.

Transpyloric tube placement (gastrojejunal tube [GJ])

A GJ tube is usually recommended in infants with severe GE reflux with increased risk for aspiration or with documented delay of gastric emptying. Transpyloric duodenal or jejunal tubes are placed after a gastrostomy is performed, by advancing the tube further and then confirming the position with contrast. This can be done in the OR as one procedure or by interventional radiology. Transpyloric tube placement can be achieved by using fluoroscopic techniques. This type of feeding tube allows feeding while protecting the airway for increase risk of aspiration.

Postoperative Management

- Control pain with acetaminophen or morphine.
- Consider additional antibiotic prophylaxis (for 24 hours).
- Feeding regimens will vary. Many patients can be fed orally or via tube 6 to 8 hours after tube placement, but physicians often hold feedings until the day after placement to improve pain control and decrease vomiting.

Complications of Gastrostomy Tube Placement

Complications encountered within the first two weeks include the following:

- Wound infections (cellulitis, occurring in 10% of patients)
- Colonic perforation
- Duodenal hematoma
- Bleeding
- Necrotizing fasciitis
- Gastric outlet obstruction from the tube

Late complications include the following:

- Cellulitis
- Gastrocolic fistula

- Worsening GE reflux
- Catheter dislodgement or perforation
- Granulation tissue

Care and Management

FEEDING REGIMEN

The infant's feeding regimen should be determined in conjunction with the parents, nutritionist, neonatologist, and gastroenterologist. Whether to choose full-tube feeding or combined oral and tube feeding depends on underlying illness and degree of dysphagia. Patients with an inability to protect the airway and recurrent aspiration (eg, infants with severe cerebral palsy) will probably need to receive all their calories by tube. In contrast, babies who can successfully suck and swallow (including most babies with congenital heart disease and bronchopulmonary dysplasia) will receive tube feedings in addition to what they take by mouth.

TYPE AND CONCENTRATION OF MILK

Unless an infant has milk or soy allergy, breast milk, conventional cow's milk infant formula (eg, Enfamil or Similac) is appropriate for tube feeding most infants who are less than one year. Milk concentration will range from 20 to 30 kcal/ounce, and it can be varied according to the infant's fluid requirements. Unless an infant has fluid restrictions, as in infants with bronchopulmonary disorder, 20 kcal/ounce formula is acceptable for tube feedings. Four scoops of Enfamil powder in eight ounces of water give 20 kcal/ounce formula; five scoops in eight ounces give 25 cal/ounce formula. Concentrations above 25 kcal/ounce should be given in consultation with a nutritionist, with the addition of carbohydrates or oil.

METHOD OF FEEDING

Tube feedings may be given using gravity (ie, pouring the formula into the tube), bolus feeding delivered by a pump (eg, 6 ounces delivered over 1 hour given four or five times a day), or continuously (eg, 40 mL per hour given for 20 hours). Nighttime feeds are usually given continuously.

Continuous feedings may be better tolerated by infants with reflux. However, bolus intermittent feedings are more physiologic and allow the infant to be disconnected from machinery for most of the day. Because of the small volume capacity of the jejunum, all jejunal feedings must be continuous.

ASSESSMENT OF FEEDING

Depending on their underlying condition, infants may require as little as 80 kcal/kg/d or as much as 150 kcal/kg/d to grow. Therefore, babies who are tube fed should be seen frequently, every 2 to 4 weeks initially, and the feedings adjusted to promote a normal growth velocity. Electrolytes, calcium, magnesium, phosphorus, albumin, vitamin A and D levels should be checked at a minimum once a year.

SKIN CARE OF GASTROSTOMY

- Daily washes with soap and water around the gastrostomy site are usually adequate to prevent infection. Gauze should not be kept under the tube as it will trap secretions and irritate the skin.
- Granulation tissue, overexuberant wound healing, may occur around the gastrostomy site. This tissue may be unsightly and sometimes bleed.
- Cellulitis may occur around the gastrostomy site. It is usually treated with either amoxicillin/clavulanate (Augmentin), cephalexin, or clindamycin given orally or intragastrically.

TUBE REPLACEMENT

- The initial tube usually can be changed to a low-profile gastrostomy device (eg, Mic-Key, AMT low profile gastrostomy device, BARD button) after the gastrostomy tract has matured. At our institution, we like to allow the tract to mature for approximately 6 months before changing the tube.
- Depending on the patient and the type of device, the tube may be either removed percutaneously or changed endoscopically.
- The principal complication of the initial tube replacement is inadvertent insertion of the replacement device into the

peritoneum instead of the stomach, causing peritonitis if the patient is fed. For this reason, we perform a barium contrast study after the initial gastrostomy change to document intragastric tube placement. Subsequent tube changes after the first may be performed without a contrast study.

- Early inadvertent dislodgement of a tube must be dealt with promptly. The gastrostomy site will often close within 6 hours, requiring a second operative procedure. A flexible well-lubricated catheter that has a smaller diameter than the original tube is placed into the G-tube site opening. The infant is taken to the fluoroscopy department to place the proper tube and confirm its intragastric position. Water-soluble contrast, NOT barium, should be used.

GE REFLUX

- A subset of patients (approximately 20%) will develop significant vomiting and GE reflux after gastrostomy tube placement. This is particularly true in patients with congenital heart disease and neurologic impairment. Most of these patients can be managed medically with H2 blockers (eg, famotidine or ranitidine), proton pump antagonists (eg, omeprazole), and prokinetics (eg, metoclopramide).
- For this reason, we do not routinely perform Nissen fundoplications in infants undergoing gastrostomy tube placement unless there is a history of severe reflux unresponsive to medical therapy. However, some infants (especially those with neurologic impairment) may fail medical therapy and require a fundoplication in the future.

TRANSITION TO ORAL FEEDINGS

- Tube-fed infants may have a significant decrease in their oral intake after a gastrostomy tube is placed; this is very disconcerting to parents. In most infants, as the underlying illness improves, and the infant continues to develop, interest in oral feedings gradually increases. However, this process may take years.
- Intensive speech and occupational therapy may be helpful in decreasing oral aversion and improving swallowing skills.

Recommended Readings

Aziz D, Chait P, Kreichman F, Langer JC. Image-guided percuta-
    neous gastrostomy in neonates with esophageal atresia. J Pediatr
    Surg 2004;39:1648–50.

Burd A, Burd RS. The who, what, why, and how-to guide for gas-
    trostomy tube placement in infants. Adv Neonatal Care
    2003;3:197–205.

Fox VL, Abel SD, Malas S, et al. Complications following percu-
    taneous endoscopic gastrostomy and subsequent catheter
    replacement in children and young adults. Gastrointest Endosc
    1997;45:64–71.

Gauderer MW. Percutaneous endoscopic gastrostomy: a 10 year
    experience with 220 children. J Pediatr Surg 1991;26:288–94.

Rothenberg SS, Bealer JF, Chang JH. Primary laparoscopic place-
    ment of gastrostomy buttons for feeding tubes. A safer and
    simpler technique. Surg Endosc 1999;13:995–7.

Part 10: Gastroesophageal Reflux

Anees Siddiqui, MD, Thomas Hamilton, MD, and Samuel Nurko, MD, MPH

Gastroesophageal reflux (GER) is the retrograde movement of stomach contents into the lumen of the esophagus. It occurs normally in the vast majority of healthy neonates. When this is accompanied by clinical or histological pathology, then it is known as gastroesophageal reflux disease (GERD). GER is common in both premature and full-term babies and may lead to esophagitis, difficulty with weight gain, irritability, or respiratory symptoms.

Pathophysiology

The esophagus serves as a conduit between the oral cavity and the stomach. Its lumen is generally kept patent. The downward movement of boluses through the esophagus is facilitated by high amplitude peristaltic waves. At the distal end of the esophagus is the lower esophageal sphincter (LES), which is both tonically contracted and kinked by the hiatal crura to prevent to return of gastric contents into the stomach. Therefore, there is a pressure barrier that separates the stomach from the esophagus, preventing free reflux of gastric contents into the esophagus. Contrary to initial publications, recent studies have confirmed that premature and term newborn infants have competent LES pressure.

During each swallow, the LES relaxes to allow the passage of food into the stomach. There are also transient lower esophageal sphincter relaxations (TLESR), which occur without swallowing. These relaxations are increased in patients with GERD and seem to be the main pathophysiological process by which GER occurs. Recent studies have shown that the TLESR in premature babies have the same characteristics as those described in older children and adults. TLESR are stimulated in response to meals. Studies in prematures have shown that their TLESR are more often associated with liquid reflux, and that TLESR trigger 50 to 100% of the reflux episodes. The other episodes may be associated with increased intragastric pressure.

The use of xanthines may also be associated with an exacerbation of reflux. The mechanism that has been postulated is an increase in TLESR.

FACTORS THAT INCREASE REFLUX EVENTS

- Esophageal
  - Esophageal dysmotility
  - Increased TLESR
  - Hiatal Hernia
- Gastric
  - Extrinsic Pressure
  - Impaired accommodation (eg, microgastria)
  - Delayed gastric emptying
  - Medications
  - Xanthines
- Nasogastric (NG) tube feedings

SURGICAL CONDITIONS WHICH PREDISPOSE TO GERD

- History of esophageal or gastric surgery
  - TEF status post-repair
  - Esophageal atresia status post-repair
  - Congenital diaphragmatic hernia
  - Gastrostomy tube placement

Incidence

- No studies have established the incidence of GERD in a neonatal population, but regurgitation is very common.
- By using impedance testing, it has been reported that otherwise healthy premature infants may have ~70 reflux episodes (both acid and nonacid) in a 24-hour period.
- Studies in older infants show that 50% of those who are less than 3 months of age have regular regurgitation events.
- NG feedings have been shown to increase the amount of reflux events in preterm infants.

Signs and Symptoms

The following are the most common symptoms that have been associated with GER:

- Feeding intolerance
- Recurrent vomiting/ regurgitation
- Failure to thrive
- Fussiness/irritability
- Apnea/choking/recurrent pneumonia
- Posturing and arching back
- Gastrointestinal bleeding/anemia

The chronic exposure of esophageal mucosa to refluxate predisposes to the development of esophagitis, which results in many of the signs and symptoms of GERD. Esophagitis is readily identifiable on biopsy and, at times, gross inspection. Vomiting and regurgitation are typical symptoms that are associated with GER. Irritability and arching can be the most prominent clinical symptoms, although recent studies using impedance technology have suggested that there does not seem to be a correlation between GER and those symptoms.

Other symptoms of GERD are thought to arise from the presence of material in the oropharynx and resultant aspiration (apparent life-threatening events [ALTE]: apnea, stridor, pneumonia, and respiratory distress). These are considered as the atypical symptoms associated with reflux. Even though apnea and ALTE can be associated with GER, recent studies have shown that in the majority of patients, apnea and GER are not associated.

There are different techniques to establish an association between symptoms and GER. The most cost effective, particularly when atypical symptoms are present, is the administration of empiric therapy, but in those cases in which there is no response or the symptoms are life threatening, further evaluation is necessary.

Diagnostic Modalities

Tests are done to either exclude anatomic malformations (radiography, endoscopy), factors that predispose to worse reflux (radiography, scintigraphy), to asses for complications (radiography, endoscopy), or to establish the presence of pathologic reflux (pH probe, impedance monitoring or endoscopy)

- Radiography: the upper gastrointestinal series is the study of choice to exclude anatomic causes of reflux and vomiting (ie, obstruction). It is not used to establish the presence of reflux.

- Endoscopy/Histology: rarely needed in the premature or neonate as long as there is no evidence of GI bleeding. Endoscopic evaluation with biopsy and histology will elucidate the degree of esophageal mucosal damage caused by reflux and allows the exclusion of other inflammatory conditions. This modality may also be used to estimate the integrity of the LES and investigate the presence of a Hiatal Hernia.

- Esophageal pH Monitoring: pH monitoring involves the placement of a catheter from the nares into the stomach. Monitoring generally takes place over a 24-hour period. A port, or ports, on the probe measure the pH of esophageal contents. A pH of less than 4 is generally felt to be acid reflux. There are reference norms published as to the number of acid reflux events that are thought to be within normal limits. The advantage of this test is that it is easily available and easy to interpret. The main draw back is that most of the reflux events in prematures is nonacidic, and therefore, not detected by pH monitoring.

- Esophageal Intraluminal Impedance with pH: this technology measures changes in impedance value between different sensors along a catheter. A reflux episode is characterized by a precipitous retrograde drop in the resistance brought about by the catheter coming in contact with an electrolyte containing solution. The extent of the reflux episodes can also be measured. Impedance monitoring is similar to pH monitoring in that a catheter is placed from nares to the distal esophagus. The benefit of this study is in that it will record both acid and nonacid events, which is important in prematures and neonates in whom most of the reflux is non-acid, as it occurs after feedings. Impedance also allows the study of patients while continuing feedings. Its limitations lie in the need for nasal intubation (this term implies endotracheal intubation, I would rather say nasal catheter placement) for catheter placement and the length and complexity of study interpretation. There are normal standards for prematures babies, and the test is becoming more available. Its main indication is to establish a correlation between symptoms and reflux.

- Nuclear medicine: gastric emptying measure by scintigraphy is useful to detect abnormalities in gastric motility. A delayed gastric emptying may predispose a patient to have reflux.

Treatment

The commonly referenced step-up or step-down approaches to the medical management of reflux in the adult literature have not been validated in NICU patient populations. However, it is useful to think of GERD treatment in terms of escalating interventions. On the other hand, in cases with severe GERD or its complications, aggressive therapy is needed form the beginning.

CONSERVATIVE MANAGEMENT

Conservative management will generally be sufficient in addressing the majority of infants' reflux and regurgitation symptoms. Because many infants have an easier time keeping down small meals, it is a good idea to try smaller, more frequent feedings. However, common sense is needed as some infants do not tolerate this approach. Thickening the milk (may be expressed breast milk) also helps. Adding rice cereal makes the liquid less likely to reflux up out of the stomach into the esophagus. Studies show that although the total amount of reflux may not change, the symptoms improve with thickened milk feedings. Keeping the baby upright before and after feedings will also decrease the amount of reflux. Specific recommendations are as follows:

- Keep the child upright for 30 minutes after a meal: in a NICU setting this will often times not be possible. However, it is recommended to afford the baby the longest possible time upright after feeding to facilitate esophageal clearance and gastric emptying.
- Incline the head of the bed: the head of the bed or bassinet may be inclined to 30 degrees to facilitate esophageal clearance and gastric emptying.
- Positioning: several recent studies using pH-impedance have addressed the effect of positioning on reflux. They have shown that the amount of reflux is less if the child is positioned in the right lateral decubitus (right side down) position for the first

30 minutes after a feeding; then switch to left lateral decubitus (left side down) for the interval period.

- Thickening the milk: this may be done in term children who do not have a malabsorptive process or compromised intestinal mucosa as part of their pathology. Thickened milk has been shown to improve reflux symptoms in several studies. There are several thickeners available on the market, all with similar efficacies. Rice cereal and Carob bean are commonly used. Dry rice cereal may be mixed, 4 gm (1 tablespoon) to 30 mL of formula, to achieve a viscosity of 170 cps at neutral pH. Note: it may be necessary to increase nipple patency to facilitate proper flow.

- Decrease feeding volume and other feeding adjustments: the volume of the feedings may be decreased, with a concurrent increase in frequency to maintain total volume delivered. This maneuver holds a theoretic value, but no studies have adequately shown decrease in symptomatic GERD. The caloric density of the milk may be increased, although gastric emptying is slowed by increased calories, in particular if they are provided by fat. In some cases, continuous intragastric feedings may be necessary. In severe cases, the use of nasojejunal feedings may be necessary as a way to bypass the stomach and provide enteral feedings

- Formula Change: milk protein intolerance often leads to colitis, a primary manifestation of which may be vomiting. It is reasonable to switch to a hypoallergenic formula and monitor for clinical response if the child's nutritional requirements can be met.

MEDICAL MANAGEMENT

Pharmacotherapy may be prescribed when conservative therapy has not resolved the symptoms and when the diagnosis of GERD is reasonably certain. At times, medications are used as a diagnostic tool. There are 4 categories of pharmacotherapy geared towards the treatment of GERD: antacids, H_2 receptor antagonists, proton pump inhibitors, and prokinetic agents.

- Antacids: liquid antacids can be used to neutralize the acid present in the stomach. They may be useful in cases of mild symptoms and as a diagnostic tool (for example to see whether an episode of irritability responds to acid suppression). Care should be given not to overdose as they contain magnesium and aluminum.

- Histamine$_2$ Receptor Antagonists: these drugs competitively inhibit histamine receptors on the basolateral membrane of parietal cells, thereby decreasing gastric acid production. These are the only drugs that have been studied (in randomized controlled groups) for the treatment of erosive esophagitis in pediatric populations.
- Proton pump inhibitor (PPI): These drugs irreversibly inhibit the H$^+$/K$^+$-ATPase located on the apical aspect of parietal cells. Therefore, their duration of effect is related to the turnover of the proton pump. Numerous adult studies have shown their superiority to H$_2$-blockers in the treatment of erosive esophagitis. No studies have reproduced this data in neonates. They are, however, very frequently used and are often considered first-line therapy.
- Prokinetic Agents: Prokinetic agents are used to increase gastric emptying and thereby decreasing reflux events. There are no randomized studies that have shown that the use of a prokinetic in prematures or neonates is beneficial. The most commonly used include metoclopramide and erythromycin. Erythormycin has been shown in several randomized trials in prematures and neonates that it does not seem to have a significant effect in those whose primary symptom of GERD is feeding intolerance. Concern about the possibility of infants exposed to erythromycin developing pyloric stenosis has been raised. Metoclopramide is associated with irritability in a significant number of patients and can be associated with dystonic reaction and tardive dyskinesia. It has not been shown to be effective in infants. Side effects of prokinetic agents can be catastrophic (cisapride, cardiac arrythmias; metclopropamide, tardive dyskensia).

Dosing Considerations

- PPIs should be dosed approximately 30 minutes before a meal and not in the presence of H2-blockers or antacids. It may be given with the TPN.
- Patients on a PPI will often have a nocturnal acid breakthrough, which can be treated with qHS administration of an H2-blocker.
- In patients with a feeding device (G-tube, NG) effectiveness of acid blockade can be measured by testing gastric pH.

Adverse Effects of Acid Blockade

Gastric acidity is part of the innate immune response of the body. In that it serves as an excessively caustic environment for potential invading pathogens. Several studies in both adult and pediatric literature have demonstrated increased colonization and the potential for bacterial translocation in patients who are on acid blockade. Both PPI and H2-blocker use has been shown to increase the risk of gastroenteritis and community acquired pneumonia. Recent data suggests that Ranitidine use in the neonatal intensive care unit may predispose to the development of late onset sepsis. Therefore, it should be noted that although there are potential benefits to aggressive acid blockade, there are potential adverse effects that cannot be taken lightly.

SURGICAL MANAGEMENT

When clinical symptoms fail to respond to maximal medical management, surgical treatment is considered. The vast majority of neonates will not require surgical intervention. The long-term effects of medical therapy must be weighed against the risk of operative intervention. If a trial period of postpyloric feeding is tolerated, intervention is deferred. It is possible that reflux of the child may be controlled medically as the patient gets older. Surgical intervention is strongly considered only when other underlying conditions have been ruled out (eg, metabolic problems, allergy). In particular, anatomic studies (UGI) are needed to exclude: extrinsic compression (ie, vascular rings) or intrinsic obstruction (ie, pyloric stenosis, esophageal web, or malrotation) as the cause for recurrent emesis.

Indications for Antireflux Procedure After Medical Therapy has Failed:

- Severe reflux in patients with impaired swallowing from central or peripheral neurologic disorders. In many instances, a G-tube may be the only intervention that may be needed. Therefore, a trial of NG feedings is recommended before a fundoplication is performed.
- Failure to thrive because of vomiting, despite maximal medical management

- Recurrent respiratory events or ALTE associated with gross emesis, oral regurgitation, or evidence of pathologic reflux and symptom association by testing
- Patients with esophageal atresia are at particular risk for severe GERD given the underlying intrinsic esophageal dysmotility and the obligatory anatomic cephalad migration of the distal foreshortened esophageal segment into the thoracic cavity postoperatively. However, they are also at a major risk of developing dysphagia postoperatively.

Operations

Antireflux surgery works by the principle of lengthening the intraabdominal portion of the esophagus. This uses positive intraabdominal pressure to maintain intraluminal gastric contents in the stomach.

Open Nissen Fundoplication   This surgical technique involves mobilization of the distal esophagus and a 360 degree wrap of the anterior fundic fold around the esophagus.

Laparoscopic Nissen Fundoplication   Advances in instrumentation and technique have allowed for laparoscopic techniques to be used safely in many neonates. Primary advantages are shorter recovery, improved cosmesis and a trend toward less adhesive, small bowel obstructions.

Choice of surgical technique and operation is dependent on the experience and preference of the surgical team. Some surgeons prefer an anterior wrap or Toupet. The idea is to provide less long-term dysphagia but at the cost of more recurrent reflux in most series. No prospective randomized trials have shown clear advantages to a specific surgical technique.

Concomitant Placement of Gastrostomy

- Essential for neonates with impaired swallowing.
- Necessary when it is anticipated that the patient may be at risk of gas bloat syndrome.
- For some patients, G-J tubes (gastro-jejunostomy) may be acceptable in place of fundoplication. The most common problem with

G-J tubes is frequent migration with recurrent need for tube repositioning.

Postoperative Care

- Most neonates post fundoplication can resume enteral feeds safely within 24 hours.
- Some surgeons routinely perform a postoperative UGI to check for leak and position of the fundoplication. This serves also as a baseline for future comparative study.
- Parents need to be aware that depending on how tight the fundoplication is, it may be impossible or very difficult for the patient to vomit after the operation. If a patient subsequently develops gastroenteritis, a nasogastric tube may be required to achieve gastric decompression when a gastrostomy is not present.

Complications of Antireflux Surgical Procedures

- Early complications: operative risk from anesthesia, atelectasis, pneumonia, perforation, or early disruption of the wrap from technical failure
- In the early postoperative period, a high index of suspicion for any unexpected clinical symptoms should prompt an immediate UGI to look for leak or disruption of the fundoplication.
- Late complications: dysphagia, gas bloat, breakdown of the fundoplication, recurrent reflux, dumping syndrome, or esophageal stricture
- As with early complications, complete history and an UGI are the first line to evaluate postoperative problems. The UGI may identify a stricture, migration, disruption, or herniation of the fundoplication. It is important to administer barium both orally and by G-tube (if present) with adequate volumes to fill the stomach.
- The use of pH probe or impedance is indicated to evaluate the functional status of the fundoplication.
- Dysphagia because of tightness of the wrap or from esophageal strictures often responds well to esophageal dilatation, whereas migration or disruption of the fundoplication may lead to a need for reoperation.
- Outcomes that are long term are excellent in properly selected patients.

References

1. Omari T. Lower esophageal sphincter funftion in the neonate. Neoreviews 2006;7:e13.

2. Bianconi SM. Gudavalli, et al. Ranitidine and late-onset sepsis in the neonatal intensive care unit. J Perinat Med 2007; 35:147–50.

3. Canani RB, Cirillo, P et al. "Therapy with gastric acidity inhibitors increases the risk of acute gastroenteritis and community-acquired pneumonia in children." Pediatrics 2006;117: e817–20.

4. Colletti RB, Di Lorenzo C. Overview of pediatric gastroesophageal reflux disease and proton pump inhibitor therapy. J Pediatr Gastroenterol Nutr 2003;37(Suppl 1): S7–S11.

5. Dinsmore JE, Jackson RJ et al. The protective role of gastric acidity in neonatal bacterial translocation. J Pediatr Surg 1997; 32:1014–6.

6. Hament JM, Bax NM, et al. Complications of percutaneous endoscopic gastrostomy with or without concomitant antireflux surgery in 96 children. J Pediatr Surg 2001;36: 1412–5.

7. Lopez-Alonso M, Moya MJ, et al. Twenty-four-hour esophageal impedance-pH monitoring in healthy preterm neonates: rate and characteristics of acid, weakly acidic, and weakly alkaline gastroesophageal reflux. Pediatrics 2006; 118:e299–308.

8. Nelson SP, Chen EH, et al. Prevalence of symptoms of gastroesophageal reflux during infancy. A pediatric practice-based survey. Pediatric Practice Research Group. Arch Pediatr Adolesc Med 1997;151:569–72.

9. Su W, Berry M, et al. Predictors of gastroesophageal reflux in neonates with congenital diaphragmatic hernia Journal of Pediatric Surgery 2007;(42):5.

10. van Wijk MP, Benninga MA, et al. Effect of body position changes on postprandial gastroesophageal reflux and gastric emptying in the healthy premature neonate. J Pediatr 2007;151:585–90, 590 e1-2

TABLE 1   Differential Diagnosis of Symptoms That may be Gastroesophageal Reflux Disease

Vomiting	Feeding intolerance	Failure to Thrive	Irritability/ Fussiness	Apnea/Choking/ ALTE	Posturing	GI Bleeding
Obstruction	Systemic diseases	Lack of caloric intake	Colic	Chronic lung disease	Seizure disorder	Gastritis
Tracheo-Esophageal fistula	Protein allergy and intolerance	Malabsorption	Food allergy	Prematurity syndrome	Sandifer	Ulcers
Esophageal atresia	Vascular ring	Metabolic disorders	NEC	Sepsis	Colic	Vascular malformations
Malrotation	Infections	Pancreatic insufficiency	Pancreatitis	Seizure disorder or other neurologicproblems	Neurologic problems	Allergy
Duodenal web	Malab-sorption	Chromosomal problems	Cardiac disease	Laryngeal cleft	Metabolic problems	
Pyloric stenosis	Motility disorders	Cardiac disease	sepsis	Cardiac disease		

Continued

TABLE 1 Continued

Vomiting	Feeding intolerance	Failure to Thrive	Irritability/Fussiness	Apnea/Choking/ALTE	Posturing	GI Bleeding
Annular pancreas	Medications that slow GI motility			Choanal atresia		
Hirschsprung disease				Swallowing problems		
Motility disorders						
Others				H-type tracheo-esophageal fistula		
Protein intolerance				Metabolic problems		
Metabolic disorder (RTA)						
Increased ICP						
Sepsis						
Necrotizing enterocolitis						

ALTE = apparent life-threatening events; ICP = ; RTA = .

TABLE 2 Commonly Used Antireflux Pharmacotherapy

Class	Medication	Dosage	Notes
Antacids	Antacids	1 to 2 mL/kg/dose after meals	Several available formulations (aluminum hydroxide, magnesium hydroxide); side effects:electrolyte abnormalities, constipation, diarrhea
Histamine$_2$ antagonists	Ranitidine	PO, IV: 2 to 3 mg/kg/d div Q8 to Q12; IV gtt: 0.04 to 0.08 mg/kg/h	side effects: headache, vomiting, diarrhea, elevated transaminases, thrombocytopenia; cytochrome P450 inhibitor; t1/2 = 3.5 to 6.6 h; Peak serum concentration = 1 to 3 h oral
	Cimetidine	5 to 10 mg/kg/d div Q8 to Q12 (Oral, IM, and IV)	side effects: headache, vomiting, diarrhea, pancytopenia, arrhythmias with IV push; cytochrome P450 inhibitor; t1/2 = 3.5 h in neonate
Proton pump inhibitors	Omeprazole	0.7 to 3 mg/kg/d div Q12 to Q24	side effects: headache, diarrhea, abdominal pain; cytochrome P450 inducer; high 1st pass metabolism; will take 3 days to achieve therapeutic effect; paucity of data regarding appropriate dose

Continued

TABLE 2 *Continued*

Class	Medication	Dosage	Notes
	Lansoprazole	0.5 to 1.6 mg/kg/d	Side effects: headache, diarrhea, abdominal pain, fatigue, rash; cytochrome P450 inducer; no studies evaluating safety and efficacy in neonates were found
	Pantoprazole	No available dosing recommendations	Side effects: Headache, diarrhea, abdominal pain, fatigue, rash; cytochrome P450 inducer
Prokinetics	Metoclopramide	0.1 to 0.2 mg/kg/d div QID	Side effects: irritability, extrapyramidal symptoms, tardive dyskinesia, fatigue; dopamine receptor antagonist; improves gastric emptying; recent meta-analysis of available data reported insufficient evidence to support of oppose use in neonatal GERD
	Erythromycin	3 mg/kg/dose q8h (PO)	Side effects: there may be a higher incidence of hypertrophic pyloric stenosis (> 2weeks of use and use in first 2 weeks of life), cardiac arrhythmias (IV formulation),

Continued

TABLE 2 Continued

Class	Medication	Dosage	Notes
			abdominal cramping, vomiting, diarrhea, bacterial overgrowth; Mechanism is by acting as a motilin analogue.
	Cisapride	0.1 to 0.2 mg/kg/dose	Side effects: associated with prolonged QTc, and sudden death. Available in the United States only under the Limited Access Program.

GERD = gastroesophageal reflux disease.

Part 11: Ostomy Diversions and Management

Sandy Quigley, MS, CPNP, CWOCN, Anne R. Hansen, MD, MPH, and Mark Puder, MD, PhD

Ileostomy, colostomy, and urostomy diversions are commonly used in the management of congenital and acquired surgical diseases in neonates, infants, and older children. The primary goal in GI surgery is the preservation of as much bowel as possible. When the urinary tract is affected, the primary goal is preservation of renal function and decompression of the upper tracts, with future reconstructive efforts directed toward the establishment of continence.

The surgically created stoma is defined by the portion of the bowel or urinary tract involved. A stoma does not have nerve endings to transmit pain. It is very vascular and may bleed slightly when rubbed or irritated. Fortunately, many of these stomas are temporarily placed to allow the affected area to heal and/or grow, with few patients requiring a permanent ostomy.

Selection of Stoma Site

- Preoperative site selection is preferable when feasible.
- Placement of the stoma within the rectus abdominus muscle reduces the risk of prolapse.
- Avoid the umbilicus, skin folds, scars, waistline, and any bony prominence (such as anterior iliac crest or ribs) whenever possible to have a smooth skin surface to which the ostomy wafer can adhere.
- An adequate adhesive surface must be created. Ideally, at least 1.5 or 2 cm of smooth peristomal skin is required for a pouching system to adhere. When two stomas are required, a 1.5 to 2 cm separation is necessary to facilitate pouch adherence.
- Select a site away from the incision whenever possible to reduce the risk of contaminating the incision with stool.

Preparation of the Bowel

Refer to Chapter 1.2, "General Surgical Considerations."

Options for Surgical Stoma Construction

Various options are available for surgical construction of a stoma. Among them are the following methods.

GASTROINTESTINAL DIVERSIONS

One theoretical advantage to an ostomy is that it reduces intraluminal pressure to that of atmospheric, thereby reducing the perfusion pressure needed to supply the bowel .

End Stoma

- An end stoma is constructed by dividing a portion of the small or large intestine, bringing out the proximal end, then turning it back on itself like a cuff, as a single stoma sutured onto the abdominal surface (Figure 1).
- A distal segment may be surgically removed, based on the disease entity, with the remaining bowel oversewn.

Mucous Fistula

If the distal bowel segment is brought out onto the abdominal surface as a separate stoma, it is called a "mucous fistula" (Figure 2), thus named because of the mucous discharged from this nonfunctional bowel. The ostomy itself should appear as pink, viable mucosal tissue. For the first few postoperative days, it should be covered with a nonadherant dressing such as Xeroform or Vaseline

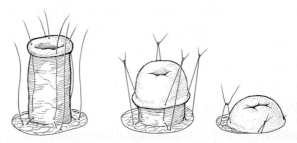

Figure 1   End stoma construction.

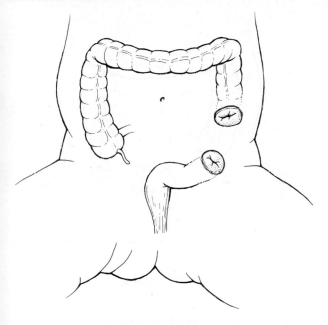

Figure 2   End stoma with Mucous fistula.

covered with gauze. Once the mucous production has started, generally one week postopertive, an absorptive gauze is sufficient.

Hartmann's Pouch

- When the distal (or defunctionalized) intestine is oversewn and left in the abdominal cavity rather than removed, it is known as a Hartmann's pouch (Figure 3).
- This section of distal large intestine, whose proximal end is sutured, closed, and left within the peritoneal cavity is contiguous with the rectum and anus.
- If the distal bowel remains left in place intact and oversewn, the bowel may be reconnected to the stoma at a later date. This procedure is known as a "takedown."

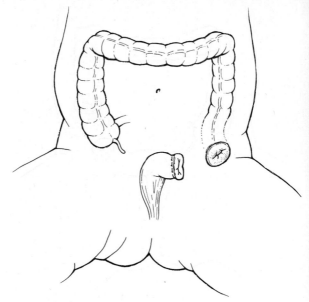

Figure 3   End stoma with Hartmann pouch.

Loop Stoma

This is a loop of bowel brought out through the abdominal wall providing fecal diversion (Figure 4). This is commonly constructed when a temporary diversion is needed, and a minimal surgical procedure is desired.

- The loop of bowel may be opened transversely or longitudinally. This is temporarily held in position for approximately 10 to 14 days on the abdominal surface by a support device such as a red rubber catheter.
- There is one stoma with two openings: a proximal (functional) end that discharges stool and a distal (nonfunctional) end that discharges mucus.

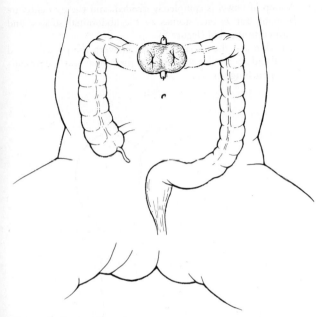

Figure 4 Loop stoma.

- Although bowel contents exit through the proximal region, the proximal bowel remains in continuity with the distal bowel. This stoma is not completely diverting as some stool will enter the distal stoma.
- Failure to support the loop of intestine until complete healing occurs may result in retraction of the stoma to an intraabdominal position.
- The surgeon should be notified immediately if the support device is dislodged.

Double-Barrel Stoma

This is constructed when complete diversion of the fecal stream is indicated.

- A loop of bowel is completely divided, and the two ends are brought out as end stomas to the abdominal surface and sutured to the skin (Figure 5).
- The skin and the fascia are closed between the proximal and distal ends to provide separation of the stomas and a more suitable pouching surface.

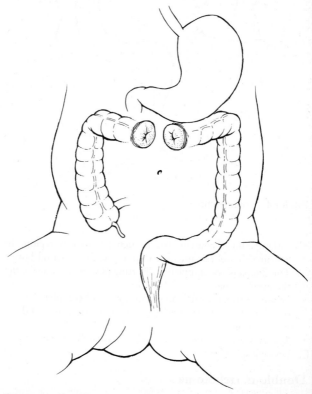

Figure 5   Double-barrel stoma.

Necrotizing Enterocolitis

See Chapter 7, "Part 3: Necrotizing Enterocolitis" of this chapter. NEC with bowel perforation is a surgical emergency usually requiring laparotomy and examination of the entire bowel from stomach to rectum.

- Commonly, multiple areas of necrotic or gangrenous bowel will be separated by viable segments of bowel.
- To preserve as much bowel length as possible, multiple marginally viable end stomas are constructed.
- Based on the clinical status of an individual patient, surgical options are to either exteriorize stomas through a separate incision adjacent to the laparotomy incision or to bring stomas out through the incision.
- Fluid losses from the section of bowel exteriorized must be monitored closely and may be challenging to replace.
- In some circumstances, a jejunostomy or proximal ileostomy will result in excessive output because the gastric, pancreatic, and biliary secretions are not absorbed. Surgically placing the bowel back in continuity allows for increased surface area for absorption of these secretions as well as enteral feedings.
- Anastomotic strictures are common in the distal defunctionalized bowel.
- Prior to ostomy closure, preoperative radiographic contrast studies are imperative to determine intestinal caliber and continuity.
- Many factors determine the timing of stoma closure. In infants, the amount of stool output, weight gain, and presence of parenteral nutrition associated liver injury are particularly important. Other coexisting medical or surgical conditions may affect the timing of ostomy closure.
- Secretory diarrhea may develop following restoration of bowel continuity in patients with inadequate distal bowel segments.
- In addition to surgically created stomas, some babies develop spontaneous entero-cutaneous fistulas involving ischemic, inflamed, or perforated bowel. These are managed with high-absorbency dressings or pouching systems to protect the surrounding skin. Once the ischemic or inflammatory process has completely resolved, these fistulas must be resected.

URINARY TRACT DIVERSION

Urinary tract diversion may be created at almost any level of the urinary system. Diversions are usually named for the structures involved in the diversion.

Urinary diversions are most commonly performed to promote healing of fistulous tracts involving the bladder when a condition or disease necessitates relief of obstructive uropathy or when the bladder must be removed because of malignancy.

Ureterostomy

This is a diversion at the ureteral level when the distal ureter(s) is obstructed or when the bladder is nonfunctional or removed.

- The ureter is divided at the most distal point possible, brought out through the abdominal wall, and anastomosed to the skin.
- It may be unilateral or bilateral depending on whether one or both kidneys are functional.
- Ureteral stents are usually sutured in place for 10 to 14 days to support the ureters and to maintain patency.
- The cutaneous location of skin level ureterostomy stomas is variable, depending on the length and mobility of the involved ureters.
- Ureterostomies often are not pouched because the anatomic location near the costal margin is not suited for pouch adherence. In these cases, the ureterostomies drain freely into the diaper.
- Peristomal skin irritation is uncommon, and minimal skin care is required.
- Ureterostomies are often temporary diversions in neonates.

Ileal Conduit

An ileal conduit is constructed when the ureters are drained into a small segment of ileum (referred to as a "conduit") that is used to discharge urine.

- One end of the conduit is sutured closed in the abdominal cavity and the other end is brought out as a stoma onto the abdominal surface (Figure 6).
- Compared with ureterostomies, the two major advantages are
  1. the surgeon is able to construct a protruding stoma in a location that allows pouch adherence and
  2. it significantly reduces the risk of stoma stenosis.

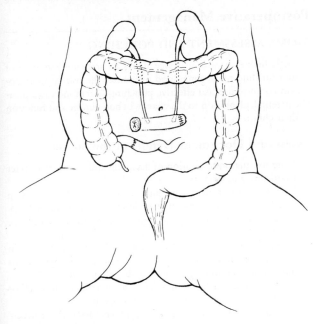

Figure 6 Ileal conduit.

Vesicostomy

This is diversion at the bladder level used to provide temporary bladder drainage.

- Vesicostomy is performed through an incision between the umbilicus and symphysis pubis.
- The dome of the bladder is mobilized and the wall of the bladder is secured to the rectus fascia.
- The bladder mucosa is then sutured to the abdominal skin opening as an ostomy.

Postoperative Management

STOMA ASSESSMENT AND POUCHING

Properly fitting an ostomy device allows accurate measurement of output for fluid replacement and minimizes the risk of peristomal skin compromise. An effective pouching system increases positive parental adaptation to the change in body image and function of their child.

Assess and Document Details of the Stoma

- Note the anatomic location of diversion and stoma type (refer to operative report).
- Document the mucosal viability at least every 6 hours with specific attention to mesenteric blood flow. Maroon or black discoloration or excessive bleeding is a concern and should be brought to the immediate attention of the surgeon.
- Assess the height of the stoma, ideally 1 to 2 cm above skin level. It can be challenging to provide a tension-free anastomosis when mobilizing the stoma above skin level.
  1. Stomas can be below skin level (retracted), at skin level, or protruding beyond skin level (prolapsed).
  2. Adaptations to basic pouching procedures may be necessary, if one is unable to maintain pouch adherence for at least a 24-hour period.
  3. If the stoma has prolapsed, the perfusion should be assessed, and the length of the prolapse should be documented, measuring from the abdominal surface.
  4. The prolapse should be assessed twice daily and as needed.
- Measure the stoma at its base using a stoma measuring guide to determine the opening size of the pouch wafer.
- Note the location of the stomal opening (by clock hour) and whether it is at skin level or not. Due to the details of how the bowel can be attached to the abdominal wall, as well as the differential healing of the ostomy tissue, some stomal opening are not located in the center of the ostomy. The location of the bowel lumen within the ostomy will determine the direction in which stool exits. Pouching modifications may be necessary if the stomal opening is not central.

- There is only minimal stool production immediately postoperatively. Therefore, a pouch is not applied for the first 24 to 48 hours. This allows for assessment of stoma viability. Apply Xeroform gauze over the stoma, and change it twice daily until the first stool output appears. Xeroform maintains the moisture of the stoma and is not traumatic to the mucosal surface when removed.
- Measure the effluent volume. Less than 2 mL/kg/h is expected. Volume in excess of this should be replaced. The surgeon should determine the replacement solution and the ratio of output to replacement. (See Chapter 1, "General Considerations.")
- Assess and document the condition of the abdominal suture line. Note any signs of infection. Cover the suture line with nonadherent gauze and a transparent film dressing (eg, Bio-occlusive or Tegaderm) to protect the wound from stool contamination.

"REFEEDING"

Anecdotally, it is known that collecting stool output from the proximal bowel diversion and refeeding it via a catheter into the distal bowel limb improves mucosal absorption and enhances bowel adaptation. Particularly, if proximal diversion is relatively high in the small bowel, refeeding allows patients to have improved absorption of special nutrients that are only absorbed in the terminal ileum. Furthermore, it may decrease total parenteral nutrition cholestasis.

Premature Infants

Compared with term infants, there are several characteristics particular to preterm infants' skin that must be taken into consideration when choosing techniques and products for the application of an ostomy pouch.

- Premature infants have more permeable skin as well as a higher ratio of surface area to body weight, allowing a relatively higher concentration of chemicals to be absorbed. Therefore, minimize skin sealants, adhesives, and adhesive removers.
- There is decreased cohesion between the epidermis and the dermis leaving the epidermis relatively vulnerable to trauma. Minimize the use of tape and adhesives. Use nonalcohol sealants and pectin-backed barriers. Moisten wafers and remove them slowly while supporting the skin.

Pouch Application Instructions

- Use only transparent one-piece pediatric pouches. Two-piece pouches do not provide adequate flexibility and contouring for the neonatal abdominal surface.
- If there is no peristomal skin compromise, apply a protective, nonalcohol skin barrier wipe (eg, 3M Cavilon No Sting) to the surface area where the wafer will adhere. Monitor closely for signs of skin inflammation resulting from contact with stool. The epidermis may or may not be intact. If peristomal skin is denuded due to exposure to stool, apply a layer of Stomahesive powder to denuded areas only, then "seal" powder with barrier wipe.
  1. Peristomal skin compromise may be characterized by any of the following: erythema, maceration, erosions, or a candidal (monilial) rash.
  2. Clinical features of topical candidal rash are erythema with satellite papules and pustules.
  3. If a rash exists, apply a layer of antifungal powder to the area and seal with a barrier wipe.
  4. Change the pouch in 24 hours to reassess and reapply antifungal powder. If the skin is improved, change the pouch every 48 hours.
- Cut the aperture in the wafer to fit around the stoma without exposing excess skin. Do not circumferentially constrict the stoma.
  1. If the stoma is prolapsed (telescoped out), assess perfusion, then measure and document the length of prolapse from the abdominal surface for reassessment twice daily and as needed.
  2. Cut "snips" in the wafer aperture 1/2 cm long at 12, 3, 6, and 9 o'clock to fit around base of the stoma. This allows unrestricted movement of the stoma without compromising the blood supply by increasing the diameter of the opening in the wafer to accommodate the additional length of bowel.
- Apply a thin line of Stomahesive paste via a 5 mL syringe around the wafer opening.
- Apply the wafer to the skin. Mold and contour onto the skin exerting gentle pressure for 2 to 5 minutes to maximize adherence.

- It is extremely important to place cotton balls inside the ostomy pouch to wick the watery effluent into the bag rather than allowing it to leak underneath the ostomy wafer. This both increases wear time by improving pouch adherence and enabling the accurate measurement of the effluent volume by weighing the cotton balls as one would a wet diaper.

Pouch Emptying

The pouch must be emptied when it is one-third full, otherwise it may pull away from the abdomen due to the increased weight. Empty the pouch into a basin or use a syringe. Clean the inner lip of the end of the pouch with gauze to decrease odor and eliminate clothes staining. It is not recommended to clean the pouch by squirting water inside with a syringe because it often decreases adherence of the pectin wafer to the skin and results in leakage.

Pouching Challenges

PERISTOMAL SKIN COMPROMISE

Mechanical

Epidermal stripping occurs if one pulls up on the wafer causing "tenting" of the skin with inadequate counterpressure to support the underlying skin. This presents as patchy erythema.

- Treatment is careful attention to minimize trauma to skin during wafer removal.

Fungal Infection

Patients at risk are those on antibiotics and with stool directly on the skin under the wafer. This presents as a macular or papular rash with satellite lesions. However, presentation may be atypical in patients with darker skin tones due to the difficulty in appreciating erythema.

- Treat with an antifungal powder, then seal with a nonalcohol barrier wipe (eg, 3M Cavilon No Sting), and proceed with the steps outlined above.

Allergic Reaction

An allergic reaction may occur from product sensitivity. This presents as erythema and pruritus.

- Treat by patch testing an alternative product elsewhere on the body for at least 24 hours. Then substitute with the nonreactive product.

Irritant Dermatitis

Inflamed peristomal skin may result from direct contact with enzymatic fecal drainage. When the epidermis is denuded, it should be managed with astringent soaks (eg, Domeboro) that help to constrict blood vessels, and soothe the inflammation to promote healing.

- Domeboro is available in more than one form. For a 1:20 dilutional ratio dilute two crushed Domeboro tablets in 12 oz. (360 mL.) or 2 powdered packets in 16 oz. (480 mL.) tepid water and apply. Then apply powder and sealant as instructed above.

Mucocutaneous Separation

This presents as a visible "trough" between the stoma and abdominal skin, leaving a defect that must heal by scar formation. Patients at particular risk are those with poor nutrition, receiving corticosteroids, or whose stoma is poorly perfused. Separation may be circumferential or involve only a portion of the stoma.

- Measure and document the size (eg, 1 cm wide at 3 to 9 o'clock) to assess the interval change. Treat by filling in the trough with methylcellulose powder (Stomahesive) and sealing with a nonalcohol barrier wipe. After the initial seal, a repeat application may be needed to completely fill the trough.
- Then proceed with the pouching as above. Cut an opening in the wafer to accommodate the base of the stoma. Excess exposure of skin around stoma often results in peristomal skin compromise.

Poor "Wear Time" (< 24 Hours)

- Assess skin integrity and look for candidal yeast rashes that may require treatment with antifungal powder sealed with nonalcohol barrier wipe. Discontinue the Stomahesive paste (because it contains undesirable levels of alcohol for the newborn population) and replace it with a piece of moldable pectin ring (Eakin Cohesive Seal or Hollister Adapt Barrier Rings). Mold the ring around the stoma base and apply the pouch directly over the ring.

- Do not use tincture of benzoin. This is unacceptably caustic to skin.

SCARS, CREASES, AND FOLDS

These may result in leakage or poor adhesion due to an uneven abdominal surface. Fill in these areas with a Stomahesive paste to create a seal. If wear time is less than 24 hours, adjust the amount of paste used.

LIFTING

Urine may undermine the outer borders of the wafer and cause lifting. This is generally more of an issue with boys than girls because of the projection of the urinary stream up onto the abdominal surface.

- Waterproofing the wafer borders with a transparent film dressing (eg, Bioclusive) may increase wafer integrity.

Stomal Complications

STOMA BLEEDING

A small amount of bleeding from the capillaries at the mucosal surface is common and should be expected. An improperly sized pouch opening (too small) may injure the mucosa and lead to bleeding. Extensive bleeding is not normal and should be brought to the immediate attention of the surgeon.

NECROSIS

Normally, stomas are moist, well perfused, and beefy red or pink. Evaluating stoma viability is particularly important during the early postoperative period when necrosis is most likely to occur.

- Ischemia and necrosis may occur from excessive tension on the mesentery compromising blood flow, or from interruption of blood supply to the stoma, such as from an embolus or sutures tied too snugly around the stoma.

- Necrosis may be scattered or circumferential on the mucosa; the depth may be superficial or deep at the fascial level or below.
- Necrosis of the stoma may require a second laparotomy and should be brought to the attention of the surgeon.

PROLAPSE

This is a telescoping of the bowel out through the stoma. It occurs most frequently in the distal limb of loop stomas. In infants, it may result from poorly developed fascial support. Other factors may include inadequate fixation of bowel to the abdominal wall, an excessively large opening in the abdominal wall, or increased abdominal pressure associated with crying or tumors.

- When a prolapse first occurs, it must be evaluated by a surgeon to determine if there is a component of ischemia or obstruction, either of which requires surgical intervention.
- After the initial surgical assessment, the prolapsed stoma should be assessed regularly for perfusion, length, and function (eg, are feedings well tolerated).
- If it is not associated with ischemia or obstruction, it can be managed conservatively by cutting extra "snips" in the wafer at 12, 3, 6, and 9 o'clock to accommodate the stoma base and avoid circumferential constriction.

RETRACTION

This refers to a stoma that retracts below skin level, resulting in a concave defect in the abdomen where the stoma is located. It is often preceded by a necrotic stoma and/or mucocutaneous separation. This presents a challenge in maintaining adequate pouch adherence.

- The use of flexible, one-piece pouches and barrier pastes are critical determinants of successful pouch adherence.

LACERATION

A stomal laceration is usually a shallow, linear discoloration in the stoma mucosa and often is due to the pouching technique.

- Assess whether the pouch opening is too small or if a prolapsed stoma is rubbing against the plastic ring (flange) of a two-piece pouching system.

INCISION DEHISCENCE

Dehiscence needs to be evaluated by a surgeon. The extent of tissue loss and viability of tissue in wound base, as well as the presence of a wound infection, are factors taken into consideration in determining the clinician's course of action. Depending upon the patient's history and coexisting morbidities, options include surgery or debridement of devitalized, necrotic tissue followed by topical dressings daily with close observation of the wound bed healing status. Optimizing the patient's oxygenation and nutritional status are imperative to ensure adequate wound healing occurs.

STENOSIS

This is caused by tight fascia or skin. Stenosis may present as a bowel obstruction or a decrease in stool output.

- The initial treatment is drainage and usually requires surgical revision.

ANASTOMOTIC LEAK

This presents with abdominal pain and sepsis. It requires surgical management and new stomas may be needed for diversion.

BOWEL OBSTRUCTION

This presents with abdominal distention, vomiting, and pain.

- Initial management includes surgical evaluation and decompression using nasogastric suctioning.
- Surgical repair is sometimes necessary.

HERNIA

The bowel enters a fascial defect around the stoma and presents as a bulge under the subcutaneous tissue. This is a frequent complication in the very thin abdominal wall of the premature newborn.

- Repair is at the discretion of the surgeon.
- Strangulation is a surgical emergency.

Ostomy teaching should begin as soon as possible to allow adequate time for parents to develop confidence and skill in ostomy care. Whenever possible, two providers should be taught ostomy care to offer support and respite to one another. Family education literature is available on the Children's Hospital, Boston (MA), internal Web site "Patient Care: Info Sheets: Ostomies: A patient's guide to ileostomies and colostomies and home care instructions for pouch change."

Recommended Readings

Borkowski S. Pediatric stomas, tubes, and appliances. Pediatr Clin North Am 1998;45:1419–35.

Craven DP, Fowler JS, Foster ME. Management of a neonate with necrotizing enterocolitis and eight prolapsed stomas in a dehisced wound. J Wound Ostomy Continence Nurs 1999; 26:214–20.

Doughty D. Complex ostomy care: pediatric stomas, high output stomas and difficult pouching situations. World Council of Enterostomal Therapist Journal 2006;26:26–31.

Erwin-Toth P. Teaching ostomy care to the pediatric client: a developmental approach. J Enterostomal Ther Nurs 1988;15:126–30.

Garvin G. Wound and skin care for the PICU. Crit Care Nurs Q 1997;20:62–71.

Irving V. Wound care for preterm neonates. Infants 2006;2:102–6.

Malloy MB, Perez-Woods R. Neonatal skin care: prevention of skin breakdown. Pediatr Nurs 1991;17:41–8.

McGarity WC. Gastrointestinal surgical procedures. In: Hampton BG, Bryant RA, editors. Ostomies and continent diversions: nursing management. St. Louis: Mosby Year Book; 1992. p. 349–73.

Pallija G, Mondozzi M, Webb A. Skin care of the pediatric patient. J Pediatr Nurs 1999;4:80–7.

Rogers V. Managing preemie stomas: more than just a pouch. J Wound Ostomy Continence Nurs 2003;30:100–110.

EIGHT

Genitourinary Disorders

Part 1: Obstruction of the Urinary Tract, Including Hydronephrosis

John T. Herrin, MBBS, FRACP, and
Richard S. Lee, MD

Embryology

- Development of the pronephros (nonfunctional in human) at 3 weeks is quickly followed between 4 and 6 weeks by the development of the mesonephros—a series of craniocaudal tubules developed from the anterior mesoderm, which drain into the mesonephric (wolffian) duct and then into the allantois. At 6 weeks, the ureteric bud develops from the lower mesonephric duct and grows into the mesoderm, stimulating division of the (ureteric) metanephric duct and formation of the metanephros.[1–4]

- Sequential divisions form the ureter and pelvis (divisions 2 to 3), major and minor calyces (divisions 3 to 6), papillary ducts, and the collecting ducts and nephrons from subsequent divisions at 15 to 22 weeks. Lack of development of pronephros prevents development of the mesonephros and subsequently lack of metanephric development, causing renal agenesis or marked renal dysplasia and absence of the ipsilateral testis in the male.

- Parallel development of the lower urinary tract occurs with opening of the mesonephric duct to the allantois and cloaca at 5 weeks. Approximately 1 week later, the urorectal fold forms as a septum dividing the posterior gastrointestinal tract from the anterior urogenital sinus (UGS)/genitourinary system.

- By 7 weeks, separate vesicoureteral openings form and the allantois degenerates to a cord, which becomes the urachus and the upper bladder, whereas the trigone develops from the wolffian duct remnant. Müllerian system development produces a ureterovaginal cord, which opens into the UGS caudal to the development of the mesonephric duct. In the female, the Müllerian duct forms the vaginal vestibule and lower vagina, and the median septum becomes the vagina and uterine cervix. In the male, Müllerian system regression leads to the prostatic urethra.
- Ureteral ectopia, vesicoureteric reflux, and paraureteral diverticulae arise because the ureteral bud forms more cranial or caudal than normal.
- Ureteroceles form if (1) the ureteral bud is abnormal or (2) Chwalle's membrane at the distal ureter persists beyond the time when urine flow is established.
- Prune-belly syndrome occurs as a result of faulty mesodermal development at 6 to 12 weeks. Several mesodermal elements are involved (abdominal wall, ureter, bladder, and testes). Other theories of development in prune-belly syndrome include the following: (1) the deformed abdominal wall results from distended viscera or increased intra-abdominal pressure and (2) the abdominal wall defect is primary and the decreased intra-abdominal pressure causes a urinary abnormality.
- Hydronephrosis occurs if there is obstruction at any level of the urinary tract.

Hydronephrosis: Classification

FUNCTIONAL

- Obstructive hydronephrosis—wide spectrum of severity
- Nonobstructive hydronephrosis—diuresis induced[1,7]
   1. Hydronephrosis associated with vesicoureteric reflux

ANATOMIC

- Urethral/bladder neck
   1. Posterior urethral valves

   2. Urethral atresia

   3. Vaginal dilation owing to UGS or cloacal anomaly

- Bladder
  1. Neurogenic bladder
  2. Clot
  3. Tumor
- Ureter
  1. Ureterocele (may also cause bladder outlet obstruction)
  2. Megaureter
  3. Ectopic ureter
- Ureteropelvic junction—ureteropelvic junction obstruction

Incidence

- The incidence is 3.8% (3.9% males, 3.6% females) in autopsy series.
- Antenatal hydroncphrosis occurs in -- 1 to 5% of patients on routine antenatal ultrasonography.[5] Approximately, 60% will resolve spontaneously.[5]

Prenatal Diagnosis/Treatment

- Antenatal ultrasonography may demonstrate unilateral or bilateral hydronephrosis, ureteral dilation, and/or an enlarged bladder. Such findings require postnatal follow-up. It is important that the antenatal ultrasonography ascertain the degree of dilation, presence of calyceal dilation, character of renal parenchyma, and ureteral dilation as these influence postnatal evaluation.[7] Several grading systems have been developed to diagnose and grade the severity of antenatal hydronephrosis. There is a lack of consensus between grading systems, however in general the more severe the hydronephrosis and bilateral hydronephrosis carry a worse prognosis.[6,7]
- Oligohydramnios may be detected clinically or by ultrasonography in the presence of severe bilateral obstruction. This can be associated with pulmonary hypoplasia.
- Patients with severe bladder outlet obstruction but with evidence of salvageable renal function can be considered for in utero diversion. Selection of patients is controversial.[9–12]

- Obstruction may be associated with other syndromes, Down syndrome, caudal regression syndrome, which may be diagnosed antenatally. Features of these syndromes should be sought postnatally.

Postnatal Presentation

- Many patients are asymptomatic, and the diagnosis is made by an abnormal sonogram obtained as follow-up of antenatal findings.[13]
- Early urinary tract infection or sepsis is common if there is significant obstruction.
- Electrolyte abnormalities (hypo- or hyperkalemia, hypocalcemia, acidosis) can occur if the obstruction is significant enough to interfere with functional tubular development.
- Renal failure will occur if the obstruction is severe and bilateral. Blood urea nitrogen (BUN) and, to a lesser degree, serum creatinine are elevated as a result of obstruction. BUN rise will be blunted if the protein intake is low or late in being established. Small muscle mass affects creatinine measurement.
- High degrees of obstruction may cause urinary ascites.[14]

Postnatal Diagnosis

- Renal ultrasonography defines unilateral versus bilateral disease, site of obstruction, and the nature of change in renal tissue—medical renal disease versus obstruction.[15,16]
  1. Early renal ultrasonography (days 1 to 2) should be performed if there is a suggestion of high-grade obstruction or urethral valves on antenatal studies.
  2. Later, renal ultrasonography (days 4 to 10) is more appropriate for less severe anomalies because it avoids errors in interpretation caused by relatively low urine flow in the immediate newborn period, particularly with variations in degree of hydration.
- Renal radionuclide scan—dimercaptosuccinic acid—for definition of functional tissue (presence or absence of kidneys and relative percentage function) or MAG 3 for assessment of

function and to help define the degree of obstruction—
enhanced with diuretic washout. Diuretic-enhanced renal
scanning allows stratification of hydronephrosis.

- Voiding cystourethrography (VCUG) should be performed
  because vesicoureteric reflux occurs in approximately 25% of
  patients with renal anomalies or hydronephrosis.[15] VCUG may
  not be necessary in babies with isolated mild dilation on postnatal ultrasonography. VCUG is necessary to diagnose posterior urethral valves, ureterocele, and to define bladder anatomy.

Differential Diagnosis

- Multicystic dysplasia produces a cystic nonfunctioning mass
  that is usually unilateral.
- True obstruction:
  1. Posterior urethral valves: Congenital obstructive membrane
     just above the pelvic diaphragm; thought to be a remnant
     of migration of the ureteral bud. Wide spectrum of sever-
     ity; can produce severe renal and bladder dysfunction.
  2. Ureteropelvic junction obstruction: Anatomic or func-
     tional obstruction at the proximal ureter. Intrinsic (fibrous
     dysplasia of ureter; absence of normal musculature) or
     extrinsic (crossing vessel to lower pole of ureter; may pro-
     duce variable obstruction). Wide spectrum of severity and
     renal effects; controversy as to how to determine the need
     for intervention.
  3. Primary megaureter: Intrinsic (owing to atretic or stenotic
     amuscular segment) or extrinsic (crossing vessel or fibrous
     bands)
  4. Secondary megaureter:
     a. Prune-belly syndrome (triad syndrome, Eagle-Barrett
        [prune-belly] syndrome) is characterized by (1) absence or
        marked thinning of abdominal muscles producing the
        wrinkled appearance resembling a "prune" skin, (2) unde-
        scended testes, and (3) renal or ureteral abnormalities.
     b. Neurogenic bladder, usually associated with
        meningomyelocele.
  5. Ectopic ureter: Abnormal insertion of the ureter into the
     bladder neck, urethra, prostate, seminal vesicles, and

vagina. Often associated with a poorly functioning kidney or upper pole of duplex system.

6. Ureterocele: Dilated distal segment of the ureter within the bladder; may involve the bladder neck. Single system more common in boys, with variable obstruction. Duplex system: upper pole associated with ureterocele and lower pole potentially with reflux and/or obstruction secondary to ureterocele.

7. UGS/cloacal anomaly: Vagina filled with urine obstructs the bladder neck. May have hydronephrosis, ascites, and oligohydramnios.

- Vesicoureteral reflux: May produce hydronephrosis without obstruction. Potential for spontaneous resolution. Greater male incidence. Many have evidence of renal impairment without infection.[17] May be an element of poor drainage that is secondary to dilation and kinking of refluxing ureter. Combination of reflux and obstruction very risky owing to infection. Megacystis-megaureter syndrome with massive bilateral reflux with large bladder.[18]

- Nonobstructed (hydronephrosis) megaureter: Distinction between "obstructive" and "nonobstructive" hydronephrosis is controversial.[19] Idiopathic nonrefluxing megaureter may result from polyuric syndromes (rare in neonatal period apart from neonatal Bartters syndrome or diabetes insipidus following anoxia), later in life nephrogenic diabetes insipidus or renal dysplasia with a significant concentrating defect or "salt-losing" nephropathy with a solute diuresis. Urosepsis can produce marked transient ureteral and renal dilation that resolves with treatment of the sepsis; may need reevaluation to define functional anatomy accurately.[20]

- Neonatal ascites produces abdominal distention, which can be confused clinically with bilateral hydronephrosis. The ascites may, in fact, follow severe obstruction with potential rupture at the caliceal fornix.

- Renal mass, such as a renal tumor—mesoblastoma or nephroblastoma

- Other abdominal masses[21]: Bowel duplication cysts, ovarian masses, or neuroblastoma

- Renal ultrasonography and radionuclide scan are able to differentiate between masses and obstructive lesions.

Preoperative Management: Therapy and Diagnosis Proceed Together

- Careful attention to fluid and electrolyte balance because of acidosis, hyperkalemia, and decreased concentrating ability may result from impaired tubular function.[21] Profound electrolyte and water losses may follow postobstructive (release) diuresis. It is important to place an intravenous line before catheterization.[22]
- Antibiotic coverage: Prophylaxis until time of surgery with ampicillin or cephalexin. This is instituted because urinary tract infection is approximately 12 times that seen in a normal urinary tract, occurs most commonly under 6 months of age and is slightly higher in females or in the presence of lower ureteral obstruction.[6] Urinary tract infection should be controlled and appropriate antibiotic coverage continued until drains and catheters are removed postoperatively.
- Timing for surgery:
  1. Control infection with antibiotics: Third-generation cephalosporin or ampicillin/gentamicin (avoid if concerns regarding renal function) together with urinary tract drainage if necessary. Catheter or nephrostomy drainage may be necessary if there is high-grade obstruction and difficulty in clearing infection despite appropriate antibiotic therapy.
  2. Restore circulating volume and correct electrolyte and acid-base abnormalities.
  3. Supplement to provide for ongoing losses.
- Exclude neurologic dysfunction of the bladder as a cause of obstruction with a spinal ultrasound (performed at the same time as the initial renal ultrasound if appropriate), voiding cystourethrogram and/or urodynamic study.
- Response to urinary catheter drainage is important because it allows assessment of the effect of emptying on renal function. A trial of continuous drainage or clean intermittent catheterization may achieve emptying and decompression without the need for surgery. Anticipate and replace postobstructive (release) diuresis. Replace urinary losses as measured initially with a 2.5% dextrose-based solution to prevent

dextrose-induced diuresis if infusion volume is high. Add 40 mEq/L NaCl and 30 to 40 mEq/L NaHCO$_3$ (or 0.45% saline), and potassium replacement depending on losses (usually 20 to 30 mEq/L KCl).

- Full assessment of structure and function:
  1. Exclude neurologic dysfunction of the bladder as a cause of obstruction with a spinal ultrasound, voiding cystourethrogram and/or urodynamic study.
  2. Determine the degree and site of obstruction to allow planning for the appropriate relief of obstruction and optimal drainage.
- Medical regimen appropriate for the degree of renal function:
  1. Fluid balance: Best guided by providing insensible losses (400 mL/m2/24 h) and mL for mL replacement of measured losses. Patient should be weighed daily or twice daily depending on the magnitude of the losses.
  2. Electrolyte balance:
     a. Calcium/vitamin D supplementation should be started preoperatively if the baby is hypocalcemic.
     b. Adjust phosphate load: Choose a low-phosphate formula (eg, Similac PM 60/40, together with calcium carbonate binders if reduced renal function).
     c. Potassium load may need formula adjustment. Sodium polystyrene sulfonate (Kayexalate) administration or loop diuretic may also be necessary to control potassium before relief of obstruction. Kayexalate carries extra risk in the immature infant and suspension should be diluted in dextrose solutions rather than sorbitol aiming at a reduced mixture osmolality to reduce the risk of necrotizing enterocolitis, Kayexalate plugging or bezoar.
  3. Nutrition: Enteral feedings are preferable preoperatively if tolerated. Consideration of specific formula (Similac PM 60/40, etc). Caloric density should be adjusted to provide adequate calories (100 to 120 kcal/kg) with tolerable potassium and phosphate loads adjusted for renal function. Caution must be taken not to exceed the limits of renal output for patients in an oliguric state. Added calories as polycose or medium chain triglyceride will allow an increase in calories without an increase in potassium and phosphate load.

4. Correction of acid-base abnormalities: Bicitra (sodium citrate-citric acid) to control sodium loading; dilute with formula or water to reduce the gastrointestinal osmolar load and prevent osmotic diarrhea.

Anesthesia

- Careful attention must be paid to fluid and electrolyte balance. Start intravenous fluid when made nil by mouth preoperatively to avoid dehydration.
- A prophylactic antibiotic such as cephalosporin should be administered preoperatively.

  Intraoperatively, it is important to avoid high solute load and bolus administration, which may produce a solute diuresis and cause or exacerbate dehydration. Measured urine losses should be replaced starting in the operating room.

Surgical Management

- Relief of obstruction: Defined by anatomic etiology of obstruction.
  1. Posterior urethral valves
     a. Transurethral valve ablation using infant cystoscope (6.9 French [F]): Usually leave the urethral catheter for 1 to 3 days.
     b. Low birth weight (< 3 kg): Vesicostomy may be needed because a small urethral caliber may make endoscopic valve ablation unfeasible.
     c. Significant controversy as to management of the severely azotemic patient with valves: Primary valve ablation versus temporary supravesical diversion.
     d. Early complete reconstruction has been advocated by some but remains controversial.[21]
  2. Megaureter
     a. Indications for surgery controversial; usually reduced function or infection.[23-25]
     b. Often requires ureteral reconstruction (excisional tapering) and reimplantation into the bladder.
     c. Needs bladder catheter (4 to 7 days) and ureteral stents (4 to 7 days) if ureter is tapered.

3. Ureteropelvic junction obstruction
   a. Indications for surgery controversial; usually reduced function or infection.[26,27] Studies have shown little or no improvement in renal function despite improvement in drainage.

      Emergency therapy to establish drainage may be necessary in the face of obstruction with deteriorating renal function, urinary tract infection with urosepsis, or in the face of a giant hydronephrosis with mass effect interfering with feeding.
   b. Pyeloplasty: excise obstructed segment and anastomose the pelvis and the ureter
   c. If crossing vessel, need to transpose ureter to opposite side in most cases
   d. Bladder catheter and wound drain (2 to 4 days)
   e. Usually no need for stent or nephrostomy tube unless a solitary kidney or other compromising situation.
4. Reflux
   a. Prophylactic antibiotics regardless of degree of reflux
   b. Indications for surgery controversial; continued renal functional impairment, infection, and acid-base imbalance
   c. May be high grade in newborn boys, some with functional renal impairment
   d. Can be associated with element of bladder dysfunction
5. Ectopic ureter
   a. Surgical repair needed
   b. If affected kidney functions, it may be salvaged with ureteral reimplantation and ureteroureterostomy (in duplex system).
   c. If nonfunctioning, remove kidney along with ureter; partial nephrectomy in duplex.
6. Ureterocele
   a. Endoscopic incision for initial decompression may be curative in some cases.[29]
   b. Partial nephrectomy of upper pole when no function
   c. Ureterocele excision and reimplantation of ureters if function present in upper pole and reflux into lower pole

7. UGS/cloacal anomaly
   a. Catheter drainage (intermittent) of vagina to decompress bladder[30]
   b. Delayed reconstruction of the UGS/cloaca
8. Establish adequate postoperative drainage
   a. If there are any questions as to adequacy of repair, proximal drainage of reconstructed system
   b. Bladder drainage facilitates healing of bladder and proximal repairs.
   c. If urine leak is likely, drain surgical site.

Postoperative Management

- Weigh patient at baseline and then daily or twice daily (if losses are high) to maintain meticulous fluid balance.[22,23]
- Replace fluid and electrolyte losses; postobstructive (release) diuresis may lead to large losses of sodium, potassium, chloride, bicarbonate, phosphorous, and magnesium (calcium?).[22,23]
- Avoid routine potassium and phosphorous replacement; it is preferable to replace measured losses. In the presence of a tubulopathy, such as Fanconi's syndrome, inherited forms of renal tubular acidosis (RTA), replacement of potassium is necessary. However, the RTA of obstructive uropathy is associated with hyperkalemia; supplemental potassium is not appropriate.[22,23]
- Continue prophylactic antibiotic coverage for the urinary tract until the stents and catheter drains have been removed and healing has taken place.[22,23]

Complications/Outcome

- Common complications of obstructive uropathy include the following:
  1. Oligohydramnios in utero if bilateral—Potter's syndrome
  2. Urosepsis
  3. Secondary renal dysplasia—decreased renal function
  4. Postobstructive (release) diuresis with profound fluid and electrolyte losses

5. Concentrating defects/polyuric syndromes—nephrogenic or central diabetes insipidus or associated renal dysplasia are a rare cause of dilated ureter and bladder in neonatal period and produce changes in later life.
6. Persisting renal tubular abnormalities
   a. RTA
   b. Sodium-losing nephropathy
7. Transient renal tubular abnormalities
   a. Pseudohypoaldosteronism has been described with clearing after relief of obstruction and treatment of the infection
   b. Concentrating abnormalities
8. Recurrent flank pain and acute pelvic obstruction
9. Hematuria after minimal trauma

- Outcome
  1. Early survival is excellent.
  2. With bladder obstruction, anticipate ongoing bladder dysfunction despite relief of obstruction.
  3. Inadequate decompression increases risk of infection.
  4. Late renal failure occurs as a result of renal maldevelopment and/or scarring.
  5. If the patient has associated neurologic abnormalities (myelodysplasia, tethered cord, spina bifida), this will be a major determinant of long-term outcome.

References

1. Stephens FD, Cook WA. Congenital urologic anomalies. In: Gotschalk SA, editor. Diseases of the kidney. Boston (MA): Little, Brown and Co; 1988. p. 691–714.
2. Woolf AS. Embrology. In: Barratt TM, Avner E, Harmon WE, editors. Pediatric nephrology. Baltimore (MD): Lippincott, Williams and Wilkins; 1998. p. 1–20.
3. Cuckow PM, Nyirady P, Winyard PJ. Normal and abnormal development of the urogenital tract. Prenat Diagn 2001; 21:908–16.
4. Kaplan GW. Embryology of the genitourinary tract. In: Retik AB, Cukier J, editors. Pediatric neurology. Vol 14. p. 96–113.

5. Scott JE, Renwick M. Urological anomalies in the Northern Region fetal abnormality survey. Arch Dis Child 1993; 68:22–6.

6. Lee RS, Cendron M, Kinnamon DD, Nguyen HT. Antenatal hydronephrosis as a predictor of postnatal outcome: a meta-analysis. Pediatrics 2006;118:586–93.

7. Peters CA. Obstruction of the fetal urinary tract. J Am Soc Nephrol 1997;8:653–63.

8. Sidhu G, Beyene J, Rosenblum ND. Outcome of isolated antenatal hydronephrosis: a systematic review and meta-analysis. Pediatr Nephrol 2006;21:218–24.

9. Harrison MR, Golbus MS, Filly RA, et al. Fetal hydronephrosis: selection and surgical repair. J Pediatr Surg 1987; 22:556–8.

10. Johnson MP, Bukowski TP, Reitleman C, et al. In utero surgical treatment of fetal obstructive uropathy: a new comprehensive approach to identify appropriate candidates for vesicoamniotic shunt therapy [discussion]. Am J Obstet Gynecol 1994;170:1770–6.

11. Manning FA, Harrison MR, Rodeck C. Catheter shunts for fetal hydronephrosis and hydrocephalus. Report of the International Fetal Surgery Registry. N Engl J Med 1986;315:336–40.

12. Freedman AL, Johnson MP, Gonzalez R. Fetal therapy for obstructive uropathy: past, present, future? Pediatr Nephrol 2000;14:167–76.

13. Mandell J, Blyth BR, Peters CA, et al. Structural genitourinary defects detected in utero. Radiology 1991;178:193–6.

14. Adzick NS, Harrison MR, Flake AW, deLorimier AA. Urinary extravasation in the fetus with obstructive uropathy. J Pediatr Surg 1985;20:608–15.

15. Herrin JT. Hydronephrosis. In: Burg FDIJ, Wald ER, Pollin RA, editors. Current pediatric therapy. Philadelphia (PA): WB Saunders; 1998. p. 834–7.

16. Zerin JM, Ritchey ML, Chang AC. Incidental vesicoureteral reflux in neonates with antenatally detected hydronephrosis and other renal abnormalities. Radiology 1993;187:157–60.

17. Nguyen HT, Bauer SB, Peters CA, et al. 99 m technetium dimercapto-succinic acid renal scintigraphy abnormalities in

infants with sterile high grade vesicoureteral reflux. J Urol 2000;164:1674–9.

18. Mandell J, Lebowitz RL, Peters CA, et al. Prenatal diagnosis of the megacystis-megaureter association. J Urol 1992; 148:1487–9.

19. Peters CA. Urinary obstruction in children. J Urol 1995;154:1874–84.

20. Pais VM, Retik AB. Reversible hydronephrosis in the neonate with urinary sepsis. N Engl J Med 1975;292:465–7.

21. McVicar M, Margouleff D, Chandra M. Diagnosis and imaging of the fetal and neonatal abdominal mass: an integrated approach. Adv Pediatr 1991;38:135–49.

22. Herrin JT. Preparation of the renal patients for surgery. Int Anesthesiol Clin 1975;13:183–202.

23. Hendren WH. A new approach to infants with severe obstructive uropathy: early complete reconstruction. J Pediatr Surg 1970;5:184–199.

24. Hendren WH. Operative repair of megaureter in children. J Urol 1969;101:491–507.

25. Keating MA, Escala J, Snyder HM III, et al. Changing concepts in management of primary obstructive megaureter [discussion]. J Urol 1989;142:636–40.

26. Peters CA, Mandell J, Lebowitz RL, et al. Congenital obstructed megaureters in early infancy: diagnosis and treatment [discussion]. J Urol 1989;142(2 Pt 2):641–5.

27. Hanna MK. Antenatal hydronephrosis and ureteropelvic junction obstruction: the case for early intervention [editorial]. Urology 2000;55:612–5.

28. Koff SA. Postnatal management of antenatal hydronephrosis using an observational approach. Urology 2000;55:609–11.

29. McAleer IM, Kaplan GW. Renal function before and after pyeloplasty: does it improve? J Urol. 1999;162:1041–4.

30. Coplen DE, Barthold JS. Controversies in the management of ectopic ureteroceles. Urology 2000;56:665–8.

31. Hendren WH. Cloaca, the most severe degree of imperforate anus: experience with 195 cases. Ann Surg 1998;228:331–46.

Part 2: Renal Venous Thrombosis

David A. Diamond, MD, and
John T. Herrin, MBBS, FRACP

Renal venous thrombosis (RVT) is the most frequently detected neonatal vascular anomaly. In this disorder, clotting occurs initially in small intrarenal capillary and venous channels, less commonly extending into the major renal vein or inferior vena cava (IVC)—hence the designation RVT. In 10–20% of cases, there is bilateral renal involvement, and in unilateral cases, there is a slight left-sided predominance.

Mechanisms

Thrombosis occurs as a result of hypercoagulability, which may be attributable to acquired or inherited disorders. Acquired hypercoagulability may occur in the setting of hypovolemia, hypotension, thrombocytosis, hyperosmolality, polycythemia, or rarely, surgery. Inherited abnormalities, such as factor 5 Leiden and gene mutation factor 2, which leads to prothrombin abnormality, are relatively common. Rarer inherited deficits in the coagulation system include antithrombin III and protein S or C deficiency. In some cases, a combination of acquired and inherited disorders may predispose the infant to RVT.

Incidence

RVT is rare in the neonate, with a poorly defined incidence in the range of two in 100,000 live births. As many patients are asymptomatic, the true frequency is likely underestimated.

Prenatal Diagnosis

A number of cases depicting prenatal diagnosis of RVT have been described. Prenatal existence of RVT may be highly suggested by the finding of calcification of the renal vein or IVC in the early postnatal period.

Postnatal Presentation

- Hematuria (usually gross)
- Hypertension
- Palpable abdominal mass (unilateral or bilateral) owing to enlarged kidneys
- Decreased urine output
- Tenderness over the mass—pain and irritability
- Edema of lower extremities (if IVC involvement)
- Renal failure
- Proteinuria which is occasionally massive. Mean time for presentation is day 1 to 2 after onset of hematuria.

  If any of the risk factors outlined in Table 1 is present, careful fluid and electrolyte balance will be required to minimize risk.

Postnatal Diagnosis

- Complete blood count/prothrombin time/partial thromboplastin time (PTT)/fibrinogen/fibrin split products. Thrombocytosis is a risk factor; however, thrombocytopenia develops during the thrombotic process.
- Renal Doppler ultrasonographic study of kidneys, IVC, and renal vessels shows enlarged, diffusely homogeneous hyperechogenic kidney(s), with loss of corticomedullary differentiation. IVC +/− renal vein shows thrombus, increased resistive index, loss of pulsation, or reversal of diastolic flow signals in renal veins or intrarenal vessels.

The kidney length at presentation predicts outcome; there is an inverse correlation between depression of glomerular filtration and renal length. Renal length greater than 6 cm predicts permanent damage.

- Nuclear medicine scan should be done to assess perfusion and function.
- Contrast studies, such as intravenous pyelography or computed tomography, are unnecessary and may precipitate further extension of the process.
- Magnetic resonance angiography is rarely required.

TABLE 1   Risk Factors for Neonatal Renal Venous Thrombosis

1. Clinical correlates

    - Male (2:1 ratio)
    - IDM
    - Birth asphyxia

2. Indwelling catheters

    - Umbilical catheter (arterial or venous)
    - Inferior vena cava catheter

3. Intravascular volume depletion

    - Sepsis
    - Dehydration
    - Hypotension
    - Exposure to hyperosmolar agents (intravenous radiocontrast, hypertonic glucose solutions)

4. Change in blood composition accentuate other factors

    - Thrombocytosis
    - Polycythemia
    - Hypercoagulable states
    - Factor 5 Leiden
    - Prothrombin gene mutations G 20210A
    - Elevated lipoprotein A
    - Protein C and S deficiency

Differential Diagnosis

The classic triad of renal mass, hematuria, and thrombocytopenia occurs in only 13% of cases. Unilateral RVT is the most common form in term infants, whereas bilateral presentation is more common in low gestational age infants

- Renal mass: Renal and abdominal ultrasonography together with a renal scan will differentiate between the following:
    1. Hydronephrosis
    2. Polycystic disease of the kidney
    3. Multicystic dysplasia
    4. Tumor—mesoblastic nephroma, adrenal hemorrhage, or ganglioneuroma, neuroblastoma, or ovarian tumor

- Hematuria
  1. Vitamin K deficiency
  2. Urinary tract infection
  3. Nephrocalcinosis or renal stone
  4. Other coagulation abnormalities—hemophilia, factor IX
  5. Hydronephrosis
- Hypertension
- Sepsis
- Other causes of disseminated intravascular coagulation (DIC)

Medical Management

- Initial therapy should address the predisposing conditions described in Table 1, sections 2, 3, and 4. Consideration of more vigorous treatment in patients with renal length greater than 6 cm at presentation is warranted.
- Meticulous fluid/electrolyte balance—prophylactic hydration is the most effective approach. When symptoms suggest that thrombosis has occurred, hydration, together with electrolyte and acid-based correction, should be continued, whereas diagnostic measures proceed.
- Anticoagulation and thrombolytic therapy are controversial. The risk of cerebral bleeding in the sick neonate, extension of adrenal bleeding (if present), and difficulties in control of peripheral coagulation need to be weighed against the potential for cure of a process in which delivery to the smaller intrarenal venous capillaries is unknown but probably compromised. In addition to bleeding abnormalities, heparin-induced hyperkalemia may pose further danger in an obstructed (venous outflow in the setting of RVT) or abnormal kidney. Treatment with fibrinolytic agents has not been shown to restore circulation in unilateral thrombosis, but can be helpful in restoring circulation in patients with bilateral thrombosis.

Our practice is to individualize therapy based on the gestational age of the infant, the extent of the thrombus, and the degree of coagulopathy. Infants less than 35 weeks' gestation have a significant risk of intraventricular hemorrhage that must be factored into the risk-benefit analysis. If the thrombosis is unilateral and there is no evidence of DIC or underlying coagulation abnormality, we treat with careful fluid-electrolyte balance and monitor to determine that extension is not occurring. If the thrombosis is bilateral or associated with extension into the IVC and/or DIC or underlying inherited coagulation is present, we use systemic heparinization commencing with a loading dose of 50 to 100 U/kg and then continuing an infusion at 25 to 50 U/kg titrated to keep the PTT at 1.5 times normal. This is started after checking antithrombin III activity because this factor is necessary for heparin to work as an anticoagulant. Plasma infusion may be necessary if antithrombin III activity is decreased. We consider thrombolytic therapy with tissue plasminogen activator (TPA), delivered either locally or systemically, if the clotting process extends despite heparinization or if renal failure is present with bilateral RVT. If TPA therapy is required, plasma may be necessary as a source of thromboplastin.

- Hypertension is treated vigorously aiming at low normal blood pressure for gestational age and weight. Initial therapy is with intravenous hydralazine 0.05 to 0.1 mg/kg repeated every 2 to 3 hours as necessary and then every 6 to 8 hours. Change hydralazine to oral dose as soon as practical, 0.25 to 1 mg/kg (or approximately twice the intravenous dose) every 6 to 8 hours. If control is not rapidly attained or the blood pressure is rising, give intravenous enalaprilor oral captopril and titrate to control blood pressure.

Surgical Management

Surgery is very rarely indicated but is most appropriate if IVC thrombosis results from an umbilical venous catheter, causing bilateral venous thrombosis and renal failure. In this setting, presumably the thrombotic process originates in the IVC, not the intrarenal capillaries. Surgery is less likely to be helpful in the context of an umbilical arterial catheter causing a thrombus that originates in the renal parenchyma and extends to the renal vein and IVC.

Anesthesia

- Careful fluid balance
- Continued therapy for hypertension using enalapril if appropriate

Postoperative Management

Postoperative management includes

- meticulous fluid/electrolyte balance,
- vigorous treatment of hypertension, and
- continuation of anticoagulation and thrombolytic therapy if surgery has been necessary.

Complications/Outcome

- Common complications
  1. Hypertension is common at the onset of thrombosis and, although usually transient, may last for as long as 1 to 3 years or even be permanent in 34%. Late scarring commonly leads to adolescent hypertension even in patients who have earlier resolution.
  2. Renal infarction leads to long-term scarring with poor renal growth. During adolescence, this may be associated with hyperfiltration syndrome—progressive hypertension, proteinuria, and renal failure. Permanent long-term depression of GFR occurs in one-third of cases.
- The mortality of RVT is approximately 5%. Survival depends on the etiology of the thrombosis. Secondary RVT carries a better prognosis than primary RVT (eg, sepsis has a good outcome for survival if the infection can be controlled). Renal outcome, however, is variable. Independent of etiology, two-thirds of the kidneys will undergo some atrophy.

Recommended Readings

Chevalier RL. What treatment do you advise for bilateral or unilateral renal thrombosis in the newborn with or without thrombosis of the inferior vena cava? Pediatr Nephrol 1991;5:679.

Diamond DA, Gosalbez R. Neonatal urologic emergencies. In: Walsh PC, Retik AB, Vaughn ED Jr, Wein AJ, editors. Campbell's urology. 7th ed. Philadelphia: WB Saunders; 1998.

Marks SD, Massicotte MP, Steele BT, et al . Neonatal renal venous thrombosis: clinical outcomes and prevalence of prothrombotic disorders. J Pediatr. 2005;146:811–6.

Messinger Y, Sheaffer JW, Mrozek, et al. Renal outcome of neonatal renal venous thrombosis: review of 28 patients and effectiveness of fibrinolytics and heparin in 10 patients. Pediatrics 2006;118:c1478–84.

Morcan H, Bealtie TJ, Murphy AV. Renal venous thrombosis in infancy: long term follow up. Pediatr Nephrol 1991;5:45–9.

Ricci MA, Lloyd MA. Renal venous thrombosis in infants and children. Arch Surg 1990;125:1195–9.

Winyard PJ, Bharucha T, De Bruyn R, et al. Perinatal renal venous thrombosis: presenting length predicts outcome. Arch Dis Child Fetal Neonatal Ed 2006;91:F273–8.

Part 3: Multicystic Dysplastic Kidney

Joseph G. Borer, MD

Definition

HISTORIC ASPECTS

The term "multicystic kidney" was first used by Schwartz in his description of a unilateral process for which the specimen resected and examined was composed of few cysts of varying sizes in which the kidney substance was difficult to recognize and completely lacked any resemblance to a kidney.[1] Spence further highlighted these contrasts to "polycystic kidney" disease and formalized the distinction between the two entities for purposes of clarity and classification.[2]

SUBTYPES

Multicystic kidney, otherwise known as multicystic dysplastic kidney (MCDK) represents a severe form of nongenetic renal dysplasia. Two different subtypes of MCDK have been described: pelvoinfundibular atresia[3] and the hydronephrotic type of MCDK.[4] These designations denote a difference in gross appearance of the kidney and typical histologic findings that do not appear to be of clinical significance.

Etiology

Both the subtypes of MCDK, pelvoinfundibular atresia and the hydronephrotic type, infer in their titles the common etiology of all MCDKs, that of an obstructive process in early embryonic renal development. There is an evidence to support MCDK as representing an active process with some areas of the kidney having increased expression of genes active in nephrogenesis and anti-apoptosis (IGF2, WT1, PAX2, WNT4, BCL2), whereas in other areas, a lack of expression may be associated with increased cell death. Furthermore, the size of the MCDK and its cysts may be a result of the outcome of these competing forces.[5]

Presentation

ABDOMINAL MASS

Historically, the MCDK presented most commonly as a palpable abdominal mass. The finding of an abdominal mass in the newborn has been regarded a urologic emergency as the majority of such masses are genitourinary in origin. Most frequently, the finding of an abdominal mass in the newborn represents a *diagnostic* rather than a surgical emergency, as most entities in this age group do not require immediate surgical intervention.[6]

DIFFERENTIAL DIAGNOSIS (NEWBORN RENAL MASS)

The differential diagnosis of a renal mass in the newborn includes the following:

- MCDK
- Hydronephrosis (Ureteropelvic junction obstruction)
- Hydroureteronephrosis (Ureterovesical junction obstruction)
- Congenital mesoblastic nephroma
- Wilms tumor
- Neuroblastoma
- Polycystic kidney disease (autosomal dominant polycystic kidney disease [ADPKD], autosomal recessive polycystic kidney disease [ARPKD], glomerulocystic disease)

PRENATAL ULTRASONOGRAPHY

The current widespread use of prenatal ultrasonography has changed the manner and greatly increased the frequency with which the diagnosis of MCDK is made, now making the prenatal presentation (presumed ultrasonographic diagnosis) of MCDK the most common presentation. Prenatal ultrasonographic diagnosis of MCDK has also allowed important insight into the natural history of this entity.[7–9]

Imaging

ULTRASONOGRAPHY

MCDK has typical findings on ultrasonographic imaging, and therefore, lends itself to detection on prenatal and postnatal evaluation with a high degree of accuracy. The most useful ultrasonographic criteria for identifying MCDK include (1) the presence of interfaces between the cysts, (2) nonmedial location of the largest cyst, (3) absence of an identifiable renal sinus, (4) multiplicity of oval or round cysts that do not communicate, and (5) absence of parenchymal tissue.[10]

CROSS-SECTIONAL TECHNIQUES

In some cases of cystic renal mass, cross-sectional imaging such as computerized tomography or magnetic resonance imaging may be necessary for clarification of anatomy and diagnosis. Examples include MCDK in one component of a horseshoe kidney,[11] crossed renal ectopia,[12,13] or one pole of a duplex kidney.

RENAL NUCLEAR SCINTIGRAPHY

Renal scintigraphy using technetium-99m (^{99m}Tc) labeled dimercaptosuccinic acid (DMSA) renal scan is the most sensitive means of assessing renal function. Absence of radionuclide uptake on ^{99m}Tc labeled DMSA renal scan confirms the diagnosis of MCDK.

Diagnosis

IMAGING

Characteristic ultrasonographic findings allow for a high degree of confidence in making the diagnosis of MCDK although not foolproof.[14] The diagnosis of MCDK in a cystic renal mass, regardless of presentation, is confirmed by renal scintigraphy. As stated previously, absence of radionuclide uptake on ^{99m}Tc labeled DMSA renal scan confirms the diagnosis of MCDK in a cystic renal mass with typical ultrasonographic findings.

HISTOLOGY

Microscopically, cysts are characteristically lined with low cuboidal epithelium. The cysts are separated by thin septa of fibrous tissue and primitive dysplastic elements, in particular, primitive ducts. Frequently, immature glomeruli, and on occasion, a few mature glomeruli are present.[5]

CLINICAL

MCDK usually presents as a unilateral irregular mass, whereas other cystic diseases are more commonly bilateral; ADPKD with bilateral masses often has an irregular surface, and ARPKD and glomerulocystic disease present as smooth reniform masses.

Management

OBSERVATION

Serial Ultrasonography

In general, routine nephrectomy is not recommended following the diagnosis of MCDK. Although there is a risk of possible deleterious outcome, this risk is small, and observation is by far the most common and recommended mode of management.[15-17] Following a confirmed diagnosis of MCDK, current recommendations from the National Multicystic Kidney Registry are as follows: renal ultrasound every 3 to 6 months for the first year of life, every 6 to 12 months less than 5 years, and annually thereafter.[17]

Spontaneous Resolution Rates

Several studies have roughly estimated spontaneous resolution rates for MCDK.[7-9,17] Over 159 patients with MCDK have been followed for more than 5 years with the help of the National Multicystic Kidney Registry.[17] Glassberg reported updated figures for the status of neonatal MCDK followed for greater than 5 years, and the vast majority become either smaller (38%) or stabilize (38%) in size and only 1.3% become larger.[5]

DELETERIOUS OUTCOMES

Recognized potential unfavorable outcomes include (1) hypertension (HTN),[15] (2) tumor development (a risk which is not eliminated solely by reabsorption of cyst fluid—perhaps similar for HTN),[18,19] and (3) increase in size of cysts to the point of clinical significance. Beckwith estimated the risk of developing Wilms tumor in an MCDK at approximately one in 2,000 based on his experience with histologic review of over 7,500 Wilms tumor specimens, and in his opinion, this did not justify prophylactic nephrectomy.[20]

INTERVENTION

Indications

Not all MCDKs are benign in their presentation or natural history and, therefore, are not appropriate for observation but rather warrant intervention. In the newborn, cases of gastric outlet obstruction and respiratory compromise secondary to a MCDK and requiring early nephrectomy have been reported.[21] Nephrectomy may be preferred when uncertainty surrounds the diagnosis, especially in the presence of unusual or complex anatomy.[11,14] Parental choice for nephrectomy in infancy, to eliminate the possibility of HTN or tumor development in the future, is perhaps the most common reason for resection of the MCDK.

Open Surgical Resection

Open nephrectomy as an outpatient surgical procedure has been described.[22] This approach for nephrectomy is performed through a small subcostal flank incision, produces minimal morbidity and offers an alternative to endoscopic resection and nonsurgical management of the MCDK.

Endoscopic Resection

A minimally invasive laparoscopic or retroperitoneoscopic approach is ideal for resection of the MCDK. This technique is equally effective with potentially less morbidity relative to open surgical and laparoscopic techniques. Instrumentation of 2-mm diameter has facilitated the direct approach to the kidney in its retroperitoneal location in the smallest of patients. Regarding relative cost-effectiveness, early nephrectomy is supported only when observation involves screening with ultrasonography every 3 months until 8 years of age.[23]

Special Considerations

CONCOMITANT VESICOURETERAL REFLUX

A significant incidence of associated vesicoureteral reflux, approximately 18 to 43%, has been identified in the contralateral kidney of infants with MCDK.[17,24–26] The high incidence of vesicoureteral reflux in this population makes voiding cystourethrogram advisable in these children because if present, reflux affects the only functioning kidney.

SOLITARY KIDNEY

Individuals, newborn or otherwise, with a MCDK indeed have a solitary (functioning) kidney and must be aware of important issues such as participation in "collision" or "contact" sports. The individual with a MCDK may choose to partake in such activity but should do so only after awareness of potential significant hazard(s) and possible dire consequences, and after the individual is adorned with appropriate protective gear.

References

1. Schwartz J. An unusual unilateral multicystic kidney in an infant. J Urol 1936;35:259–63.
2. Spence HM. Congenital unilateral multicystic kidney: an entity to be distinguished from polycystic kidney disease and other cystic disorders. J Urol 1955;74:693–706.
3. Griscom NT, Vawter GF, Fellers FX. Pelvoinfundibular atresia: the usual form of multicystic kidney: 44 unilateral and two bilateral cases. Semin Roentgenol 1975;10:125–31.
4. Felson B, Cussen LJ. The hydronephrotic type of unilateral congenital multicystic disease of the kidney. Semin Roentgenol 1975;10:113–23.
5. Glassberg KI. Renal dygenesis and cystic disease of the kidney. In: Wein AJ, Kavoussi LR, Novick AC, Partin AW, Peters CA, editors. Campbell-walsh urology. Philadelphia (PA): Saunders Elsevier; 2007. p. 3334–39.

6. Diamond DA, Gosalbez R. Neonatal urologic emergencies. In: Walsh PC, Retik AB, Vaughan ED Jr, Wein AJ, editors. Campbell's urology. 7th ed. Philadelphia (PA): W. B. Saunders; 1998. p. 1635–38.

7. Avni EF, Thoua Y, Lalmand B, et al. Multicystic dysplastic kidney: natural history from in utero diagnosis and postnatal followup. J Urol 1987;138:1420–4.

8. Hashimoto BE, Filly RA, Callen PW. Multicystic dysplastic kidney in utero: changing appearance on US. Radiology 1986;159:107–9.

9. Rickwood AM, Anderson PA, Williams MP. Multicystic renal dysplasia detected by prenatal ultrasonography. Natural history and results of conservative management. Br J Urol 1992;69:538–40.

10. Stuck KJ, Koff SA, Silver TM. Ultrasonic features of multicystic dysplastic kidney: expanded diagnostic criteria. Radiology 1982;143:217–21.

11. Borer JG, Glassberg KI, Kassner EG, et al. Unilateral multicystic dysplasia in 1 component of a horseshoe kidney: case reports and review of the literature. J Urol 1994;152(5 Pt 1):1568–71.

12. Nussbaum AR, Hartman DS, Whitley N, et al. Multicystic dysplasia and crossed renal ectopia. AJR Am J Roentgenol 1987;149:407–10.

13. Rosenberg HK, Snyder HM III, Duckett J. Abdominal mass in a newborn: multicystic dysplasia of crossed fused renal ectopia—ultrasonic demonstration. J Urol 1984;131:1160–1.

14. Minevich E, Wacksman J, Phipps L, et al. The importance of accurate diagnosis and early close followup in patients with suspected multicystic dysplastic kidney. J Urol 1997;158(3 Pt 2):1301–4.

15. Gordon AC, Thomas DF, Arthur RJ, Irving HC. Multicystic dysplastic kidney: is nephrectomy still appropriate? J Urol 1988;140(5 Pt 2):1231–4.

16. Orejas G, Malaga S, Santos F, et al. Multicystic dysplastic kidney: absence of complications in patients treated conservatively. Child Nephrol Urol 1992;12:35–9.

17. Wacksman J, Phipps L. Report of the multicystic kidney registry: preliminary findings. J Urol 1993;150:1870–2.

18. Birken G, King D, Vane D, Lloyd T. Renal cell carcinoma arising in a multicystic dysplastic kidney. J Pediatr Surg 1985;20:619–21.

19. Homsy YL, Anderson JH, Oudjhane K, Russo P. Wilms tumor and multicystic dysplastic kidney disease [discussion 2259–60]. J Urol 1997;158:2256–9.

20. Beckwith JB. Editorial comment. J Urol 1997;158:2259–60.

21. Triest JA, Bukowski TP. Multicystic dysplastic kidney as cause of gastric outlet obstruction and respiratory compromise. J Urol 1999;161:1918–9.

22. Elder JS, Hladky D, Selzman AA. Outpatient nephrectomy for nonfunctioning kidneys [discussion 714–5]. J Urol 1995;154(2 Pt 2):712–4.

23. Perez LM, Naidu SI, Joseph DB. Outcome and cost analysis of operative versus nonoperative management of neonatal multicystic dysplastic kidneys [discussion 1216]. J Urol 1998;160(3 Pt 2):1207–11.

24. Al-Khaldi N, Watson AR, Zuccollo J, et al. Outcome of antenatally detected cystic dysplastic kidney disease. Arch Dis Child 1994;70:520–2.

25. Atiyeh B, Husmann D, Baum M. Contralateral renal abnormalities in multicystic-dysplastic kidney disease. J Pediatr 1992;121:65–7.

26. Flack CE, Bellinger MF. The multicystic dysplastic kidney and contralateral vesicoureteral reflux: protection of the solitary kidney. J Urol 1993;150:1873–4.

Part 4: Polycystic Kidney Disease

John T. Herrin, MBBS, FRACP

Renal cysts develop as a result of parenchymal maldevelopment and are thus congenital but not necessarily inherited or genetic in origin.[1,2] Primary cystic changes may be seen in the newborn period, whereas secondary cystic change develop in abnormal or damaged tissue—scar, inflammation, or tumor—occurs later in life.

Embryology

* The genetic syndromes autosomal recessive polycystic kidney disease (ARPKD) and autosomal dominant polycystic kidney disease (ADPKD) are marked by genetic potential for the development of cysts. In both ARPKD and ADPKD, an increase in messenger ribonucleic acid, expression of epidermal growth factor, and protein in cyst fluid have been described. Mistargeting or mislocation of enzymes to the apical rather than the basal surface of the cell results in secretion into the cyst lumen rather than return to the circulation. Inhibition of cyst formation by tyrosine kinase inhibitors in vitro and genetic inhibition in vivo suggest that control or prevention of cyst formation and progressive renal disease is likely in the future. Specific defects in biosynthesis and transport of proteoglycans lead to possible interaction between tubular cells and matrix. Cysts develop as the result of a second "hit" or damaging event, either genetic or chemical.[3] The actual cystic change results from hyperplasia (proliferation) of cells, excess tubular secretion, or abnormal extracellular matrix formation.

* Classification of cystic disease in the newborn:
  1. Genetically based[4]
     a. ARPKD
     b. ADPKD
     c. Multicystic disease/familial juvenile nephronophthisis
  2. Glomerulocystic disease (GCD)[1]
     a. Tuberosclerosis ± ADPKD
     b. von Hippel-Lindau disease
     c. Micromulticystic GCD
     d. Pluricystic GCD

3. Hereditary cystic dysplasia, including multicystic dysplasia
4. Cystic change associated with other syndromes
- Genetics
  1. APPKD—short arm chromosome 6 at 6p12[5]
  2. ADPKD
     a. PKD1, short arm chromosome 16[6]
     b. PKD2, long arm chromosome 4
     c. Other PKD syndromes (Meckel-Gruber syndrome; Beckwith-Wiedemann syndrome; Zellweger syndrome; trisomy 13; Inversin abnormalities [chronic tubulointerstitial nephritis, hypertension, early chronic renal failure and NPHP2 abnormality]) and sites are likely to be further differentiated.[7]

Incidence

- ARPKD 1:20,000 (1:10,000 to 1:40,000)[5]
- ADPKD 1:1,000 (1:200 to 1:1,000)[6]

Prenatal Diagnosis/Treatment

- Oligohydramnios may be present in those patients with extensive involvement. These patients are likely to have cardiorespiratory distress, and arrangement for delivery at a center with intensive care unit facilities should be made if families decide to proceed with pregnancy.
- Antenatal ultrasonography shows large echogenic kidneys of varying sizes with a normal pelvis and ureter. (Hydronephrosis or obstructive uropathy results in large kidneys with decreased echogenicity within the collecting system and ureter.)[7–9]
- ADPKD has a good prognosis in childhood. Cyst development and progression usually occur later in adolescents or early adulthood.
- ARPKD patients also show increased echogenicity in the liver.[9,10]
- In patients with very early-onset ADPKD, cyst formation occurs in the third trimester, but oligohydramnios is rare.[6]
- Patients with multicystic dysplasia or severe renal dysplasia may have hyperechogenic kidneys of variable size, with multiple cysts also of variable size.[7]

Postnatal Presentation

- Obstructed labor may rarely occur owing to enlarged kidneys of cystic disease (ADPKD, ARPKD, and GCD).[6,8]
- Abdominal examination reveals a distended abdomen with palpable renal masses. The kidneys of ARPKD and GCD lead to smooth-surfaced reniform masses that are usually bilateral. In ADPKD, the renal surface is irregular.[2,10]
- Patients with ARPKD of extensive involvement (80 to 90%) usually present with cardiopulmonary distress and often need extensive respiratory support.[10]
- Hypertension is common in ARPKD (90%) and affects fewer patients with ADPKD and GCD (20 to 25%).[6,10]
- Renal failure is uncommon in newborns with ADPKD and GCD but is present in some newborns, with extensive involvement of ARPKD. Oliguric renal failure in infancy carries a poor prognosis.[1,10]
- Associated features of syndromes with a renal cystic component—trisomy C, D, and E; Zellweger syndrome (cerebrohepatorenal syndrome); Bardet-Biedl syndrome. Here, the cysts are usually less than 2 mm in size and cortically located. The cystic change is most often not symptomatically significant.[7]
- Urinary tract infection
- Cholangitis occurs even in the newborn period in patients with ARPKD.[8]

Postnatal Diagnosis

- Ultrasonography of both kidneys and liver is necessary to distinguish between ARPKD, ADPKD, and GCD.
  1. In the nursery, ARPKD involvement of both kidneys and the liver is characteristic. The kidneys are enlarged, hyperechogenic, and kidney shaped without discrete cysts.[9,11,12]
  2. ADPKD patients in the very early-onset group can have extensive bilateral cysts in the newborn period. The remainder of ADPKD patients shows a spectrum of enlarged hyperechogenic kidneys, with cysts in only a minority of patients in the newborn period. Early cysts may be unilateral and of variable size. The liver does not show cysts in newborns with ADPKD.[6,8]

3. GCD has hyperechogenic kidneys without liver cystic involvement.
- Radionucleotide studies—MAG3 function and radionuclear nucleotide cystogram to exclude vesicoureteric reflux and multicystic dysplasia as causes of a renal mass. The MAG3 scan also provides information on differential function.

Differential Diagnosis

- Enlarged kidney
  1. Polycystic kidney
  2. GCD may occur as a nonsyndromic (sporadic) isolated disorder as a component of another syndrome—trisomy C, D, and E—or as glomerular cysts as a minor component of abnormal or dysplasic kidney.
  3. Nephroblastomatosis
       Tuberosclerosis—cysts resembling ADPKD or as hamatomas (angiomyolipoma)
- Cyst formation
  1. ARPKD
  2. ADPKD
  3. Meckel syndrome
  4. Bardet-Biedl syndrome
  5. Trisomy C, D, and E
- Hepatic fibrosis
  1. Meckel syndrome
  2. Jeune syndrome
  3. Short-rib polydactyly syndrome
  4. Ivemark syndrome
  5. Caroli's disease
  6. Congenital hepatic fibrosis

Preoperative Management

- Monitor and maintain fluid and electrolyte balance; decreased concentrating ability is common.
- Treat hypertension vigorously with the goal of low normal blood pressure. Therapy is commenced with captopril if renal function is normal and with propranolol if not. Hydralazine may be added for acute control.

- Correct acid–base abnormalities.
- A medical regimen appropriate for the degree of renal function is detailed in the section on hydronephrosis. Briefly,
  1. Maintain fluid and electrolyte balance, including daily weight.
  2. Monitor growth; adjust caloric intake and formula.
  3. Supplement calcium and vitamin D.
  4. Minimize phosphate load with low-phosphate formula.
  5. Minimize potassium load; low-potassium formula and correction of acidosis may be needed. Sodium polystyrene sulfonate administration or loop diuretic may be necessary.
- Prophylactic antibiotic (cephalosporin) preoperatively.

Anesthesia

- Careful fluid balance and sodium replacement.
- Avoid fluid and sodium loading (danger of hypertension).

Surgical Management

- Dialysis catheter placement
- Multicystic dysplasia—conservative management if involution is occurring
- Complications: hemorrhage, infection

Postoperative Management

Conservative therapy rests on careful fluid and sodium balance (see also section on medical regimen appropriate for renal function in section on hydronephrosis).

- Conservative—monitor and maintain fluid balance.
- Treat hypertension—vigorous treatment aimed at low normal blood pressure. Angiotensin-converting enzyme (ACE) inhibitors, plus calcium channel blocker if necessary. ACE inhibitors decrease cyst formation.
- Diet

1. Provide adequate caloric balance.
2. Avoid protein loading long term.
- Correct acidosis.

Surgery may be considered in patients with massive renal enlargement, persistent respiratory compromise, or suboptimal nutrition associated with decreased renal function. In these patients, nephrectomy, peritoneal dialysis, optimization of nutrition is preview to early life transplantation.[13]

Complications/Outcome

- Outcome depends on the type and extent of cystic disease but is usually associated with slowly progressive renal failure and hypertension as cysts increase in number and size and replace normal renal tissue.
- Common complications include the following:
  1. Fluid overload—sensitivity to intravascular volume particularly if oliguria is present.
  2. Hypertension is common in patients with ARPKD, even in the nursery. ADPKD patients become hypertensive with associated LVH and progressive cyst formation after adolescence.
  3. Renal failure depends on the degree of renal involvement in all types of cystic disease.
  4. Cystic complications include hemorrhage into the cyst cavity, infection, hyperreninemia from cyst pressure on surrounding renal tissue, and renal scarring.
  5. ADPKD is a systemic disease with variable timing of symptomatic onset from infancy to adulthood, providing three patterns based on time of symptomatic presentation:
     a. Very early onset (< 12 months)[2,6,8]
     b. Childhood (12 months to 20 years)[6]
     c. Adult (20 years and older)[6]
- Long-term follow-up of ADPKD reveals extrarenal manifestations, suggesting that this is a systemic disease, whereas ARPKD in long-term follow-up shows progressive features of hepatic fibrosis.

References

1. Bernstein J. Glomerulocystic kidney disease—nosological considerations. Pediatr Nephrol 1993;7:464–70.

2. McDonald RA, Watkins SL, Avner ED. Polycystic kidney disease. In: Barratt TM, Avner ED, Harmon WE, editors. Pediatric nephrology. 4th ed. Lippincott, Willliams and Wilkins; p. 459–74.

3. Germino GG. Autosomal dominant polycystic kidney disease: a two-hit model. Hosp Pract 1997;32:81–2, 85–8, 91–2.

4. Calvert JP, Grantham JJ. The genetics and physiology of polycystic disease of the kidney. Semin Nephrol 2001;21:107–23.

5. Guay-Woodford LM, Meucher G, Hopkins SD, et al. The severe perinatal form of autosomal recessive polycystic kidney disease (ARPKD) maps to chromosme 6p21.1-p12: implications for genetic counseling. Am J Hum Genet 1995;56:1101–7.

6. Gabow PA, Johnson AM, Kaehny WD, et al. Factors affecting the progression of renal disease in autosomal dominant polycystic kidney disease. Kidney Int 1992;41:1311–9.

7. Boyer O, Gagnadoux MF, Guest G, et al. Prognosis of autosomal dominant polycystic disease of diagnosed in utero or at birth. Pediatr Nephrol 2007;22:380–8.

8. Cole BR, Conley SB, Stapleton FB. Polycystic kidney disease in the first year of life. J Pediatr 1987;111:693–9.

9. Chilton SJ, Cremin BJ. The spectrum of polycystic disease in children. Pediatr Radiol 1981;11:9–15.

10. Herrin JT. Phenotypic correlates of autosomal recessive (infantile) polycystic disease of the kidney and liver. Implications for genetic counseling. In: Bartsokas CS, editor. Genetics of kidney disorders. New York: Alan R Liss; 1989. p. 45–54.

11. Gang DL, Herrin JT. Infantile polycystic disease of liver and kidneys. Clin Nephrol 1986;25:28–36.

12. Worthington JL, Shackelford GD, Cole BR, et al. Sonographically detectable cysts in polycystic disease in newborn and young infants. Pediatr Radiol 1988;18:287–93.

13. Beaunover M, Snehal M, Li L, et al. Optimizing outcomes for neonatal ARPKD. Pediatr Transplant 2007; 11:267–71.

Part 5: Bladder Exstrophy

Alan B. Retik, MD, and
John T. Herrin, MBBS, FRACP

Bladder exstrophy is a condition in which lack of bladder closure results in the urinary bladder remaining open anteriorly.

Embryology

- Development of the pronephros, mesonephros, ureteric bud, and metanephros are more fully described in "Part 1: Obstruction of the Urinary Tract, including Hydronephrosis." Lack of development of the pronephros leads to absence of the mesonephros and subsequently lack of metanephric development, resulting in renal agenesis or marked renal dysplasia and absence of gonadal development in male.
- The ureteric bud arises from the mesonephric duct in close proximity to the cloaca and migrates into the trigone of the bladder and in the same period (4 to 6 weeks) induces mesenchymal development. Simultaneous cloacal subdivision is taking place; hence, combined defects in urinary, genital, and rectal elements are common.
- ΔNp63 80 homolog of the *PE53* tumor suppressor gene has an anti-apoptotic role in the central bladder development
- The ventral midline defect follows exaggerated growth of the cloacal membrane, which prevents normal lateral to medial ingrowth of outer ectodermal and inner endodermal layers. Inadequate mesenchymal ingrowth between these layers results in deficient development of the abdominal wall musculature and the pubic bones. This maldevelopment leads to premature rupture of the cloacal membrane, with exstrophy of the bladder, toward displacement of the anus and cleft genitalia. The extent of the defect is determined by the time at which the cloacal membrane ruptures. Diastasis of the symphysis pubis results from outward rotation of the innominate bones.
- Bladder exstrophy is part of the spectrum of omphalocele-cloacal exstrophy-imperforate anus-spinal dystrophy and of other syndromes. Tethered cord is common.

Incidence

- 1 in 30,000 (range 1 in 10,000 to 1 in 50,000) live births
- male 2 to 3:female 1

Prenatal Diagnosis/Treatment

There is often a family history of abdominal wall abnormalities.

A prenatal sonogram may demonstrate the defect in the abdominal wall. This is often associated with nonvisualization of the bladder, a lower abnormal bulge, small penis, anterior placed scrotum, a low-set umbilical cord insertion, and abnormal widening of the iliac crests.

Diagnosis allows contact with a team experienced in management of bladder exstrophy and arrangement for delivery at a site near such a center to facilitate early transfer for postnatal care.

Postnatal Presentation

Physical examination confirms the abdominal wall defect and open bladder and defines its nature and extent.

Postnatal Diagnosis

- Physical examination provides an evaluation of associated anomalies and definition of the genital and alimentary system integrity.
- Abdominal and pelvic ultrasonography is necessary to exclude renal anomalies (hydronephrosis and renal agenesis) and assess genital anatomy.

Differential Diagnosis

- Cloacal exstrophy is distinguished from bladder exstrophy by involvement of bowel and genital abnormalities.
- Covered or occult exstrophy may result from mesodermal invasion of the abnormally persisting infraumbilical membrane.

Preoperative Management

- Plan for delivery or early transfer to a tertiary center.
- Protect the exposed bladder mucosa by covering with clear plastic wrap to minimize abrasive contact.
- Assess for renal anomalies with physical examination and renal ultrasonography.
- Assess for associated anomalies of other organ systems: gastrointestinal, genital, and urinary.
- Maintain hydration: anticipate increased insensible losses, avoid fluid restriction, and provide intravenous fluid when NPO preoperatively.
- Assess renal function: measure blood urea nitrogen (BUN), creatinine, electrolytes, and CO_2 or bicarbonate levels.
- Initiate prophylactic antibiotics for surgery with a dose and an agent appropriate for the level of renal function.

ANESTHESIA

- Avoid overhydration or underhydration intraoperatively.
- Replace urinary losses.

Surgical Management

- Total early reconstruction should be performed as early as possible, preferably within the first 48 hours, when soft and pliable bones and joints allow closure of the symphysis pubis without the need for osteotomy.
- Later-staged repairs:
  - Antireflux surgery may be indicated at a later date.
  - Epispadias repair
- Augmentation and clean catheterization may be necessary in patients with a small, noncompliant bladder.

POSTOPERATIVE MANAGEMENT

- Careful fluid balance: monitor and replace losses. Renal function is usually normal.
- Monitor electrolytes, BUN, and creatinine.
- Continue prophylactic antibiotic coverage.

- Buck's traction: Adhesive skin traction is used with the patient in a position in which the hips have 90° of flexion with the knees slightly bent to protect the arterial tree.
- Clean intermittent catheterization is instituted early after removal of the indwelling catheter after reconstructive surgery. Education and supportive group therapy around the staged repairs and outcomes is arranged.

COMPLICATIONS/OUTCOME

- Overall survival is excellent for isolated bladder exstrophy. Exstrophy in association with other syndromes has a survival dependent on associated anomalies.
  Renal function is usually normal, and normal sexual function and fertility are possible.
- Early complications may include surgical wound dehiscence and infection of osteotomy sites.
- Late complications include urinary incontinence and a small, noncompliant bladder, which may require bladder augmentation and clean intermittent catheterization.

Recommended Readings

Avery LB. Developmental anatomy. 6th ed. Philadelphia (PA): WB Saunders; 1974.

Cheng W, Jacobs WB, Zhang JJ, et al. Delta Np63 plays an apoptotic role in ventral bladder development. Development 2006;133:4783–92.

Gearhart JP, Jeffs RD. Exstrophy complex and bladder anomalies. In: Walsh PC, Retik AB, Vaughan ED Jr, Wein AJ, editors. Campbell's urology. 7th ed. Philadelphia (PA): WB Saunders; 1997. p. 1939–90.

Kaplan GW. Embryology of the genitourinary tract. In: Retik AB, Cukier J, editors. Pediatric urology. Vol. 14. p. 96–113.

Stephens FD, Cook WA. Congenital urologic anomalies. In: Schrier RW, Gotschalk C, editors. Diseases of the kidney. 4th ed. Boston (MA): Little, Brown and Co; 1988. p. 691–714.

Silva RI. Evaluation and initial management of infants with bladder extrophy. www.UptoDate. 2007

Silva RI. Surgical management and postoperative care of children with bladder extrophy. www.Uptodate. 2007

Woolf AS. Embrology. In: Barratt TM, Avner ED, Harmon WE, editors. Pediatric nephrology. 4th ed. Baltimore (MD): Lippincott Williams and Wilkins; 1998. p. 1–20.

Part 6: Cloacal Exstrophy

John T. Herrin, MBBS, FRACP, and
Alan B. Retik, MD

Embryology

- Development of the pronephros, mesonephros, and ureteric bud and metanephros are more fully described in "Part 1: Obstruction of the Urinary Tract, including Hydronephrosis." Lack of development of the pronephros leads to absence of the mesonephros and subsequently to lack of metanephric development, resulting in renal agenesis or marked renal dysplasia and absence of gonadal development in the male.

- Parallel development of the lower urinary tract occurs with opening of the mesonephric duct to the allantois. The mesonephric duct opens into the allantois and cloaca at 5 weeks. Approximately 1 week later, the urorectal fold forms as a septum dividing the gastrointestinal tract (posterior compartment) from the anterior genitourinary compartment (the urogenital sinus).

- By 7 weeks, separate vesicoureteral openings form, and the allantois degenerates to a cord that becomes the urachus and the upper bladder, whereas the trigone develops from the wolffian duct remnant. The müllerian system development produces a ureterovaginal cord that opens into the urogenital sinus caudal to the development of the mesonephric duct. In the female, the müllerian duct forms the vaginal vestibule and lower vagina; the median septum becomes the vagina and uterine cervix. In the male, müllerian system regression leads to the prostatic urethra.

- At 6 months, there is further development of the mesonephric (Wolffian) and Müllerian systems directed by the presence or absence of a Y chromosome. Under the influence of the Y chromosome, testes form and produce Müllerian-inhibiting substance, which leads to Müllerian system regression while stimulated Wolffian development occurs. In the absence of a Y chromosome, ovarian development occurs. In the female, the

Müllerian duct forms the vaginal vestibule and lower vagina; the median septum becomes the vagina and uterine cervix. In the male, Müllerian system regression leads to the prostatic urethra.

- A defect occurs if the large cloacal membrane ruptures prematurely before the urorectal septum has partitioned the cloacal pouch.
- Two laterally placed hemibladders with exstrophy are formed with an open everted cecum between. The colon is rudimentary and hangs down to end blindly in the pelvis.
- The penis is small and paired in 50%; however, penis and scrotum are absent in 10% of patients.
- Female genitalia are also paired: septate in 50% but absent in 25%.
- In all, 50% of patients have an associated myelomeningocele.
- Associated anomalies are common, particularly imperforate anus and omphalocele.
- Covered or occult exstrophy may result from mesodermal invasion of the abnormally persisting infraumbilical membrane.

Incidence

The incidence is 1 in 250,000 live births.

Prenatal Diagnosis

Prenatal ultrasonography may demonstrate the defect in the abdominal wall and a myelomeningocele. Diagnosis allows contact with a team experienced in management of cloacal and bladder abnormalities and allows arrangements for delivery at a site near such a center to facilitate early transfer for postnatal care.

Postnatal Presentation

- Physical examination confirms the abdominal wall defect and open bladder and defines its nature and extent. The lateral hemibladders and open everted cecum are hallmarks of cloacal rather than simple bladder exstrophy. Other bowel anomalies,

associated spinal abnormalities–abnormal curvature, dysraphism, and menigomyelocele are common and should be defined.
- Imperforate anus and omphalocele are common.

Postnatal Diagnosis

- Physical examination provides an evaluation of associated anomalies and definition of the genital and alimentary system integrity.
- Abdominal and pelvic ultrasonography are necessary to exclude renal anomalies (hydronephrosis, renal agenesis).
- Genital anatomy must be assessed because bifid and even absent genitalia are possible.

Differential Diagnosis

- Bladder exstrophy differs in the lack of bowel and genital abnormalities. The defect is midline with a single open bladder and open bowel or visible colon not present.
- Covered exstrophy: Persisting infra-abdominal membrane may confuse diagnosis, and ultrasonography will be helpful in defining anatomy.

Preoperative Management

- Arrange for delivery at a tertiary center or a site where a specialized urological team experienced in the care of patients with cloacal abnormalities is available.
- Protect the exposed bladder mucosa by covering with a clear plastic wrap to minimize abrasive contact. Periodically irrigate the bladder with sterile saline.
- Assess for renal anomalies by physical examination and renal ultrasonography.
- Assess for associated anomalies of other organ systems including gastrointestinal, genital, and urinary systems.
- Maintain hydration. Insensible losses are increased and renal anomalies may have concentrating defects. Avoid fluid restriction. Provide intravenous fluid or an oral or PG water load of 10 mL/Kg at the time when made non per os preoperatively.

- Assess renal function: Send blood urea nitrogen (BUN), creatinine, electrolytes, and CO_2 or bicarbonate levels.
- Initiate prophylactic antibiotic coverage for surgery (ampicillin and gentamicin versus cephalosporin, depending on renal function).
- Discuss with parents the genital abnormalities and the issues regarding gender assignment. Because the phallus in large proportion of these patient is so inadequate, routine assignment of female gender has been the recommendation. The data pertaining to routine sexual assignment of patients with phallic inadequacy has become controversial[1,2,3] with suggestions that assignment be made on the basis of potential for functional phallic reconstruction,[1] that assignment of female gender is not necessarily resulting in childhood psychological, emotional, or behavioral distress[2] and of unpredictable sexual identification requiring re-examination.[3] In this time, it is clearly a matter of considering longer term studies. In the interim, cooperative multidisciplinary discussion among urologist, surgeon, endocrinologist, neonatologist, parents, and counselors is the best course.

Anesthesia

- Avoid fluid overload intraoperatively.
- Replace urinary losses.

Surgical Management

Surgical management focuses on separating the gastrointestinal from the genitourinary tract.

- The hemibladders are mobilized and sewn together, and the bladder is closed.
- The bowel is usually exteriorized as a colostomy, and the omphalocele is closed.
- Delayed urologic reconstruction often involves constructing a bladder pouch by augmenting the small bladder with intestine or stomach. This is usually a secondary procedure when bowel length has been defined.
- Intermittent catheterization is usually required to empty. Construction of a lower abdominal stoma from a tapered

bowel conduit may be required. A perineum may be constructed if sufficient tissue persists to construct a continent bladder neck.
- Genital reconstruction is considered controversial with further follow-up and assessment ongoing.[1,2,3]

Postoperative Management

- Careful fluid balance: Monitor and replace losses. Renal function is usually normal.
- Monitor electrolytes, BUN, and creatinine.
- Continue prophylactic antibiotic coverage.
- Intermittent catheterization to empty via a lower abdominal stoma (tapered bowel conduit).

Complications

- Early complications include the following:
  1. Surgical wound dehiscence
  2. Tension from large wound and open area of pelvic bone diastasis
  3. Infection of osteotomy sites
  4. Urinary incontinence
  5. Bladder diversion to bowel reservoir or augmented reconstructed bladder has the potential for metabolic and electrolyte abnormalities. Monitoring of electrolytes and renal function will allow appropriate supplementation.
- Abnormalities in bowel function: Short-bowel syndrome with need for special feeding and parenteral nutrition. There is potential for electrolyte losses, and the need for a supplemental regimen is high.
- Stoma complications (see chapter on stoma management) Rectal prolapse is common.
- Late complications include urinary infections, calculi, bladder mucosal metaplasia, and carcinoma.

Outcomes

- Overall survival depends on associated anomalies.
- Sex assignment and genital reconstruction are controversial issues and should be addressed individually.

References

GENERAL

Stephenson CD, MacKenzie AP, Lockwood CJ. Obstetrical and neonatal management of body stalk anomalies and cloacal exstrophy. Up-to-Date online 2007.

Hendren WH. Cloaca, the most severe degree of imperforate anus: experience with 195 cases. Ann Surg 1998;228:331–46.

SPECIFIC

1. Lund DP, Hendren WH. Cloacal exstrophy: a 25 year experience with 50 cases. J Pediatr Surg 2001;36:68–75.
2. Baker Towell DM, Towell AD. A preliminary investigation into the quality of life, psychological distress and social competence in children with cloacal exstrophy. J Urol 2003;169:1850–3.
3. Reiner WG, Gearhart JP. Discordant sexual identity in some genetic males with cloacal extrophy assigned to female sex at birth. N Engl J Med 2004;350:333–41.

Part 7: Urolithiasis in Neonates

*Bartley G. Cilento Jr, MD, FAAP, FACS, and
John T. Herrin, MBBS, FRACP*

Renal stone formation in the neonate is rare but can occur as a result of inherited metabolic changes such as inherited hypercalciuria, primary hyperoxaluria, and cystinuria. Stone formation can also result from iatrogenic causes such hyperalimentation or diuretic therapy. The conditions favoring stone formation may be exacerbated by obstructive conditions as with ureteropelvic junction obstruction (UPJ), ureterovesical junction obstruction (UVJ), congenital megaureter, or infection, or the use of certain medications such as furosemide, Diamox, and Topamax. Later in life, other unusual structural renal anomalies that may lead to urolithiasis include medullary sponge kidney, horseshoe kidney, and dominant polycystic kidney disease.

Classification of Neonatal Urolithiasis

METABOLIC

Hyperoxaluria is defined as spot urinary oxalate/creatinine rate > 360 mmol/mol creatinine or > 0.12 mg/mg creatinine or 24-hour > 0.5 mmol/1.73 m2 or 52 mg/1.73 m2. These values apply to patients under 6 months of age.

1. Primary: Type I is autosomal recessive and the most severe form caused by a defect in alanine-glycolate aminotransferase, causing hyperglycolaturia. It results in whewellite stones and nephrocalcinosis. Type II (rarer) is caused by a defect in glyoxylate reductase, causing excess urinary excretion of L-glyceric acid. The presence of glycolate is pathognomonic for type I and glyceric acid for type II. Both etiologies can be confirmed by liver biopsy.

2. Secondary: This type is the result of intestinal malabsorption of fats and bile acids, which preferentially now bind with calcium in the gut, resulting in unbound oxalate, which is absorbed and subsequently excreted in the urine. Such conditions include cystic fibrosis, ileal resection, and inflammatory

bowel disease. Stones are rare in the newborn but develop later in childhood.

Hypercalciuria is defined as a random urinary calcium/creatinine rate > 0.7 mmol/mmol (> 0.8 mg/mg and decreasing to 0.4 mg/mg by 6 months of age) or 24-hour excretion > 0.1 mmol/kg (> 4 mg/kg). In the first 5 days of life, preterm infants have a high calcium excretion of approximately 6.6 mg/24 hours associated with a high concurrent sodium excretion, which increases the calcium excretion.

1. Primary: This was formerly classified as absorptive or renal but likely represents a continuum of disease with suggested etiologies such as genetic variation in vitamin D receptors.
2. Secondary: This type induces hypercalciuria from autosomal recessive distal renal tubular acidosis, Wilson's disease, type 1 glycogenosis, Bartter's syndrome, primary hyperparathyroidism, steroid therapy, vitamin D excess, and, most commonly, furosemide therapy. All of these conditions most often result in nephrocalcinosis as well as nephrolithiasis.

Distal Renal Tubular Acidosis (Type I)

These stones are rare in younger patients

1. Form of secondary hypercalciuria
2. Autosomal recessive disorder of urine acidification resulting in an inability to acidify the urine. Urine pH always greater that 5.5. Serum acidosis results with hypokalemia and hyperchloremia. Low urinary levels of citrate are characteristic along with elevated levels of urinary phosphate, sodium, potassium, and calcium.

Urate Abnormalities

Urate abnormalities are defined as 24-hour > 0.6 mg/dL glomerular filtration rate or > 4 mmol/1.73 m2. These stones are rare in younger patients.

1. Primary: Hyperuricosuria owing to inherited purine metabolism disorders such hypoxanthine guanine phosphoribosyltransferase deficiency, also known as Lesch-Nyhan syndrome. There are at least three other unusual disorders; refer to "Recommended Reading"

2. Secondary: Hyperuricosuria owing to inflammatory bowel disease, dehydration, myeloproliferative diseases, and lympho-proliferative diseases. Except for dehydration, these are rare in neonates.

Cystinuria

Cystinuria is defined as spot urinary cystine/creatinine rate > 0.03 mmol/mmol or 24-hour > 0.13 mmol/1.73 m2 (31 mg/day). Qualitatively defined as the presence of increased dibasic amino acids in the urine. Autosomal recessive disorder resulting in abnormal transport of dibasic amino acids: cystine, ornithine, lysine, and arginine (COLA) through renal proximal tubule and intestinal epithelium. Cystine has a very low solubility coefficient in the urine, thereby resulting in stone formation. There appears to be three subtypes of enzymatic deficiency, with the homozygotes at greatest risk for early and recurrent stone disease. Calculi may occur in early life in association with chronic diarrhea such as seen in glucose-galactose malabsorption, although stones are more common in later life than in the neonate.

ACQUIRED

- Furosemide: Patients with bronchopulmonary dysplasia or congestive heart failure who are treated with furosemide (Lasix) may form stones because it causes calciuresis and stimulates parathyroid activity, resulting in secondary hyperparathyroidism.
- Parenteral nutrition: Premature infants are particularly susceptible to nephrocalcinosis and stone formation owing to vitamin D and calcium imbalance.
- Obstruction: Obstruction with infection or metabolic disease will increase the risk of stone formation. Concurrent obstructive lesions (UPJ or UVJ) enhance metabolic stone formation.
- Infection: In the nursery, infection is a rare cause of stone formation. Certain bacteria produce urease, which converts urea into ammonia. This causes a rapid rise in the urinary pH, resulting in a marked decrease in solubility of most urinary solutes, particularly magnesium, phosphate, and calcium. The most common urease-producing bacteria are *Proteus*, *Pseudomonas, Klebsiella, Providencia*, and some *Staphyloccus* species.

Incidence

Stones are rare in the neonatal population. The incidence depends on the etiology. The most common etiology of stone formation in the neonate is iatrogenic hypercalciuria resulting from furosemide therapy for bronchopulmonary dysplasia with or without parenteral nutrition. Cystinuria is rare: 1 in 7,000 to 1 in 120,000, and stones rarely occur in the neonate in the absence of obstructive abnormalities or vesicoureteric reflux. Other less common etiologies include inherited hypercalciuria and hyperoxaluria.

Prenatal Diagnosis and Treatment

- In general, ultrasonography is the only prenatal imaging modality necessary for evaluation. The prenatal detection of renal stones is rare. If detected, early postnatal evaluation is necessary to exclude obstructive lesions. Early therapy includes maintaining adequate hydration.
- If stones are prenatally detected, arrangements should be made for transfer to a center after birth where appropriate solute:creatinine ratios and 24-hour urine collections can be made so that early diagnosis and specific therapy can be instituted.

Postnatal Presentation

- Irritability
- Blood-stained diaper due to hematuria
- Renal sonogram demonstrating nephrocalcinosis and/or renal stones in the collecting system
- Nephrocalcinosis
- Hydronephrosis and rarely urinoma may follow obstruction from renal calculi

Postnatal Diagnosis

- Renal ultrasonography to demonstrate or exclude stones, nephrocalcinosis, or other renal anomalies such as obstruction
- Urine studies: Spot solute ratios and others:
  1. Calcium/creatinine
  2. Cystine/creatinine
  3. Oxalate/creatinine
  4. Urate/creatinine

  5. Amino acids
  6. Urinary pH
  7. Specific gravity
  8. Urinalysis and urine culture

- Urine chemical profile from 24-hour urine collection (used to confirm above solute:creatinine ratios):
  1. Calcium
  2. Oxalate
  3. Urate
  4. Cystine
  5. Citrate
  6. Others: Sodium, potassium, phosphate, urea, magnesium, creatinine, total volume
- Serum chemical profile:
  1. Electrolytes
  2. Calcium
  3. Phosphate
  4. Blood urea nitrogen and creatinine
  5. Uric acid
  6. Bicarbonate or CO_2

   Spiral computed tomography or intravenous pyelography may be necessary if ultrasonography is equivocal or to better determine the presence of obstruction requiring surgical intervention.

- If a stone is available or recovered, compositional stone analysis may provide valuable clues regarding the metabolic etiology. For example, the "whewellite" form of calcium oxalate strongly implies hyperoxaluria, whereas the "weddellite" form of calcium oxalate suggests hypercalciuria. The urinary calcium excretion may also assist in differentiation because hyperoxaluria most often occurs with mild or no increase in calcium:creatinine ratio.

Differential Diagnosis

- Urinary tract infection
- Hematuria secondary to the following:
  1. Coagulation abnormalities
  2. Renal vein thrombosis

3. Recent catheterization: urethral or traumatic umbilical artery catheterization (rare)

Preoperative Management

- Avoid dehydration
- Conservative therapy by increasing fluid intake (dilute feedings or supplemental intravenous fluids) and decrease sodium intake using low-sodium formulas
- Review solute:creatinine ratios:
  1. Elevated urinary calcium:creatinine ratio:
     a. Increase water intake (dilute feedings) to maintain hydration.
     b. Check blood vitamin D metabolites, calcium, phosphate, CO_2, parathyroid hormone levels.
     c. Check urine calcium, sodium, phosphate, and magnesium.
     d. Thiazide therapy and magnesium supplementation may be helpful in preventing further stone formation and may dissolve present stones.
     e. If there are multiple stones, a trial of potassium citrate should be undertaken.
     f. If 1,25-hydroxyvitamin D is elevated and urine phosphate is low, a trial of phosphorous supplementation is reasonable. This is designed to decrease hydroxylation of vitamin D and to decrease calcium absorption and excretion, thereby decreasing stone risk.
  2. Normal urinary calcium:creatinine ratio and stone present:
     a. Check urine ratios for cystine:creatinine and oxalate:creatinine.
     b. If elevated oxalate excretion, confirm with a 24-hour urine collection for creatinine, oxalate, and calcium. Also, obtain a random urine sample for creatinine, glycolate, and glycerate.
     c. While awaiting these studies, begin a trial of pyridoxine (250 to 300 mg/m2). After 1 week of therapy, obtain a repeated 24-hour urine collection as before and random urine for creatinine, glycolate, and glycerate.
     d. Continue therapy until the results have confirmed or excluded hyperoxaluria.

     e. If oxalate excretion is elevated and there is no response to therapy, consider liver biopsy to elucidate the type of hyperoxaluria.

     f. If oxalate excretion is elevated and there are normal levels of glycolate and glycerate, consider liver biopsy to elucidate the type of hyperoxaluria (ie, type III).

- Surgery (extracorporeal shockwave lithotripsy [ESWL] or endoscopic removal) is rarely needed in the neonate.
- Surgery is performed to relieve obstruction if present.

Anesthesia

Intravenous fluids should be given from the time the patient is made non per os and continued until oral intake is resumed.

Surgical Management

- Rarely needed in the neonate
- Indicated in the presence of obstruction
- Indicated if conservative therapy is not successful or stones do not pass
- ESWL is becoming the first treatment of choice in most cases, but this generally involves older children.

Postoperative Management

CONTINUATION OF CONSERVATIVE THERAPY TO PREVENT RECURRENCES

Complications/Outcome

- Primary risk is morbidity, not mortality.
- Specific complications are
  1. Recurrent stone formation
  2. Growth or enlargement of current stone(s), which can ultimately lead to obstruction, acute or chronic pyelonephritis, and loss of renal function
  3. Infection: Acute pyelonephritis, chronic pyelonephritis, or, ultimately, xanthogranulomatous pyelonephritis (rare in the neonate and a long-term complication)

4. Surgical complications: Hematoma, perforation of renal pelvis or ureter during endoscopic intervention, ureteral stricture after endoscopic intervention

Recommended Readings

Bert S, Gouyon JB, Semama DS. Calcium, sodium and potassium excretion during the first five days of life in very preterm infants. Biol Neonate 2004;85:37–41.

Nicoletta JA, Lande MB. Medical valuation and treatment of urolithiasis. Pediatr Clin North Am 2006;53:479–91.

Lottmann H, Gagnadoux MF, Daudon M. Urolithiasis in children. In: Gearhart JP, Rink RC, Mouriquand PDE, editors. Pediatric urology. Philadelphia: WB Saunders; 2001. p. 828–59.

Thomas SE, Stapleton FB. Urolithiasis in children. In:Gonzales ET, Bauer SB, editors. Pediatric urologic practice. Philadelphia: Lippincott Williams & Wilkins; 1999. p. 607–19.

Part 8: Dialysis/Catheters

*John T. Herrin, MBBS, FRACP, and
Craig Lillehei, MD*

Need for dialysis in the neonate is uncommon. Renal failure is usually nonoliguric and as such is manageable without dialysis. Furthermore, nonoliguric and acute oliguric renal failure has a shorter time course when compared with older children and adults. Chronic oliguric renal failure in the very small infant has a poor prognosis. It is most often associated with other anomalies. Supportive therapy, such as nutrition, electrolyte, and drug therapy, is limited by the need for fluid restriction. Catheters may need to be placed to provide access for calorie maintenance, intermittent hemodialysis, continuous dialysis modes (continuous venoatrial hemodialysis, continuous venovenous hemodialysis), or peritoneal dialysis.

Classification/Etiology of Renal Failure

* Prerenal
  1. Reduced effective circulating volume from hemorrhage, shock, dehydration, sepsis, congenital heart disease, necrotizing enterocolitis, large intracranial bleed
  2. Hypoxia/asphyxia
  3. Increased renal vascular resistance: Polycythemia, indomethacin (as treatment for patent ductus arteriosus)
* Intrinsic or parenchymal causes: Acute tubular necrosis, congenital renal anomalies, dysplasia, renal venous thrombosis, nephrotoxins such as aminoglycosides or radiocontrast agents, cystic disease of the kidney
* Obstructive lesions: Posterior urethral valves, ureteropelvic junction or ureterovesicle junction obstruction, neurogenic bladder (myelodysplasia), spinal lesions

Postnatal Diagnosis

* Laboratory testing: Electrolytes, blood urea nitrogen (BUN), creatinine, and blood gases

- History, physical examination: Assess renal size, blood pressure, signs/symptoms of sepsis
- Renal ultrasonography to demonstrate or exclude anomaly, cystic disease, or changes consistent with medical renal disease
- Renal scan

Differential Diagnosis

- Renal failure: Congenital or acquired
- Electrolyte abnormalities:
  1. Adrenal etiology: Electrolyte abnormality, hemorrhage, congenital adrenal hyperplasia
  2. Functional lesions: Renal tubular acidosis, hyperkalemia secondary to low sodium output

Preoperative Management

- Correct volume deficit. Slow rather than rapid (bolus) correction is necessary to avoid solute diuresis and further dehydration. Rapid delivery results in increased solute output and obligate fluid loss, preventing reabsorption.
- Check electrolyte and blood gas profile, BUN, creatinine, electrolytes, calcium, phosphorous, and CO_2.
- Correct electrolyte and acid-base abnormalities. Priority is determined by a change in the electrocardiogram, blood gases, calcium, and potassium.
  1. In hypercalcemia and hyperkalemia, initial therapy includes removal of calcium or potassium from parenteral solution and modification of feedings. For hypercalcemia, saline (0.9% NaCl) expansion and administration of a loop diuretic (furosemide) may be necessary. For hyperkalemia, acidosis should be corrected. Sodium polystyrene sulfonate (Kayexalate) (1 g/kg per rectum) may be needed for control. Kayexalate is carried in hypertonic sorbitol or glucose, posing a risk of necrotizing enterocolitis. If potassium control is difficult,
     a. search for significant tissue damage (sequestered hemorrhage [cephalohematoma, intraventricular hemorrhage]) or bowel necrosis, consider hypoadrenal syndromes, and provide dialysis as definitive therapy.

2. If serum potassium and/or calcium are normal or low in the presence of acidosis, potassium and/or calcium should be corrected before or concurrently with correction of the acidosis. This will prevent the risk of arrhythmia or respiratory paralysis from hypokalemia with intracellular translocation or painful tetany or seizures from a decrease in ionized calcium.

- Transfusion, if necessary, is likely to require volume correction with furosemide (Lasix) or dialysis if the patient is oliguric. Dialysis or exchange transfusion may be necessary to avoid fluid overload and pulmonary edema.
- Check BUN and creatinine to provide a rough guide to renal function. Measure urine specific gravity or osmolality and urine volume output to provide an estimate of fluid replacement requirements. If there is a high urine output of hypotonic urine, extra care with replacement fluid will be necessary to avoid solute diuresis and dehydration.
- Control hypertension at the time of surgery. Patients with oliguric renal failure, acute or chronic, are extremely sensitive to fluid volume (hypervolemia or hypovolemia) and electrolyte replacement.
- Specific problems in renal failure:
  1. Hypertension
  2. Anemia
  3. Risks of acidosis and hyperkalemia
- Monitor and treat for infection, for which these patients are at increased risk.

Anesthesia

- Drug choices may be limited owing to decreased renal function.
  1. Opiates are the preferred choice for pain control. Demerol metabolites are excreted by the kidney and hence accumulate and can cause seizures and respiratory depression.
  2. Muscle relaxants have a significantly decreased excretion that may lead to prolonged paralysis; hence, care in the choice of these agents is required. Aminoglycosides, kanamycin, and hypocalcemia potentiate the muscle-blocking effects. Succinylcholine is often associated with muscle damage and hence significant risk of hyperkalemia.

- Potassium-free fluid should be used intraoperatively unless there is a known potassium-losing state from a renal tubular disorder (Fanconi's syndrome, renal tubular acidosis) or continuing bowel losses.
- If chronic acidosis is present preoperatively, hyperventilation may be necessary to prevent hyperkalemia from relative underventilation (when ventilated at normal rates).

Replacement of Dialysis Catheters

HEMODIALYSIS

- Preoperative imaging, such as ultrasonography, may be useful to clarify available vessels.
- Hemodialysis is most often accomplished via a relatively large-bore catheter (8 to 10F) entering either a subclavian or internal jugular vein and terminating at the right atrial entry. Access via femoral veins may be used but may poses additional difficulties with infection, thrombosis, and stabilization of the catheter. Extracorporeal membrane oxygenation circuits may be modified for ultrafiltration and/or hemodialysis.
- Intraoperative fluoroscopy is useful to facilitate central passage of the guidewire and dialysis catheter. It may also allow early recognition of such complications as pneumothorax or hemothorax.

Peritoneal Dialysis

- Peritoneal dialysis is not as efficient as hemodialysis. However, it is preferable for long-term dialysis in infants.
- It is best accomplished using a multiholed Silastic catheter with a subfascial grommet for tissue ingrowth. A second subcutaneous grommet is not used in infants owing to erosion of the overlying soft tissue.
- Partial omentectomy may be performed at the time of placement to reduce catheter occlusion by the omentum.
- Allowing the surrounding tissue to heal before using the catheter is optimal to reduce any leakage of dialysate.

Postoperative Management

- Dressing technique: Sterile dressing is changed with dialysis.
- The catheter should be heparinized (the catheter is filled with heparinized saline) and used exclusively for dialysis.

Complications/Outcome

- Common complications of dialysis:
  1. Volume imbalance
  2. Bleeding from heparinization
  3. Potential for seizure or disequilibrium (a state in which a rapid change in extracellular fluid osmolarity leads to cerebral swelling) with intracellular hemorrhage, changes in conscious state, coma, intracellular hemorrhage, or death
  4. Infection
- Catheter complications:
  1. Infection at the catheter insertion site. If it spreads proximally, it can cause catheter infection, bacteremia/sepsis, or endocarditis.
  2. Bleeding may occur around the catheter at the insertion site.
  3. Thrombosis of catheter or large vessels around the catheter.
  4. Late complication includes stenosis of vessel.
- Complications of peritoneal dialysis:
  1. Acute leakage around the catheter
  2. Respiratory distress from volume overload
  3. Lack of ultrafiltration with or without absorption, which may lead to fluid overload
  4. The fluid volume may produce fullness during dwell time, causing feeding difficulties, including vomiting. This effect often requires nasogastric continuous feedings or parenteral feedings.
- The outcome of renal failure depends on underlying etiology.

Part 9: Neurogenic Bladder Dysfunction in the Newborn

Stuart B. Bauer, MD

Embryology and Anatomy

- Neurogenic bladder dysfunction occurs when a lesion affects the peripheral and/or central nervous system sensory and/or motor pathways that control lower urinary tract function. The most common cause of neurogenic bladder dysfunction in the neonate is attributable to a spinal dysraphic state produced by faulty closure of the spinal canal. The spinal canal closes in a caudad direction from its most cephalad extent beginning at 14 days of fetal development and is completed by day 21. Incomplete fusion of the neuroectoderm and the adjacent lateral mesodermal components results in a defect in the posterior portion of the canal, creating the possibility of neural elements protruding outwardly (open myelodysplasia). The specific lumbar and sacral elements that actually herniate determine the type of neurologic lesion affecting the lower urinary tract. In some cases, there is no defect in the closure of the spinal canal, but abnormal ectodermal structures become incorporated within it, leading to tethering of the cord as the child grows (occult dysraphism).
- The various types of neurospinal dysraphisms are classified as follows:
  1. Open myelodysplasia (85%)
     a. Meningocele (10%): a protruding dural sac with no neural elements
     b. Myelomeningocele (75%): a protruding sac with neural elements
     c. Lipomyelomeningocele (15%): the protrusion of fatty elements with the sac
  2. Closed (occult) neurospinal dysraphism (15%)
     a. Lipoma (75%): an intradural fatty mass attached to the spinal cord

    b. Split cord malformation (10%): a bony spur or fibrous band causing a split in the lumbar portion of the developing spinal cord.

    c. Tethered cord (15%): a thickened filum terminale that prevents the conus from ascending up the canal as the fetus develops.

Incidence

The incidence is directly related to the incidence of myelodysplasia. In the early 1990s, this was 1 in 1,000 live births, but the current incidence is much less owing to the widespread advocacy of folic acid for women of childbearing age to prevent spinal dysraphic states.

Postnatal Clinical Presentation

There are no outward signs of neurogenic bladder dysfunction; rather, it is the abnormal spinal condition that signifies its presence.

- For myelomeningocele, an open spinal defect covered by a thin transparent membrane is obvious at the time of delivery.
- For lipomyelomeningocele, a large mass protruding from the midline lower spinal area is evident at birth.
- For occult dysraphic states, a subtle cutaneous lesion of the back is manifested in over 85% of the cases consisting of a small fatty mass, a hair patch, a dermal vascular malformation, a dimple in the L3–4 area (as distinguishable from a pilonidal dimple caudad in the gluteal cleft), or an abnormal or asymmetric gluteal cleft.
- For sacral agenesis, flattened buttocks and a shortened gluteal cleft are characteristic findings of the lower spinal area.

Diagnosis

There are no outward signs of neurogenic bladder dysfunction in the neonate; only the abnormal appearance of the skin overlying the middle lumbar and/or sacral areas of the spinal canal signify its presence. Therefore, diagnosis begins when the lower midline area of the spine is inspected.

- For open spinal defects, the diagnosis is obvious at birth; with occult dysraphisms and sacral agenesis, visual inspection of the back and lower spine is required, specifically looking for any cutaneous manifestation of the underlying disease process. With sacral agenesis, it is important to palpate the lower spine to denote the absence of sacral vertebrae.
- For open spinal defects, the lower limbs may be deformed with inversion of the feet, loss of muscle mass, and/or absence of spontaneous movements, especially when the neurologic defect involves the lumbar level. Often with an occult spinal lesion or sacral agenesis, the lower extremities are normal in appearance and on neurologic assessment.
- If a lesion is suspected, spinal ultrasonography performed within the first 2 to 3 months of life can delineate the position of the conus medullaris, the presence of an intraspinal lipoma, and the thickness and extent of the filum terminale.
- Magnetic resonance imaging of the spinal cord is needed to more specifically outline the intraspinal pathology.

Preoperative Management

- Ten percent or less of newborns with myelodysplasia have an abnormal renal sonogram owing primarily to bladder outlet obstruction from dyssynergy between the detrusor and external urethral sphincter muscles during a voiding contraction. It is important to identify these children early in postnatal life for this dictates intervention with clean intermittent catheterization (CIC). Consequently, renal and bladder ultrasonography are mandatory either before spinal canal closure or as soon as feasible after surgery.
- For children with occult lesions of the spine, ultrasonography of the kidneys is not required in the immediate postnatal period because the incidence of deterioration of the urinary tract in utero is rare; however, imaging is still mandated within 2 to 3 months of age.
- Measurement of urine residuals after spontaneous voiding is needed in all these children to test the ability of the child to empty his/her bladder. If high (> 5 mL),

1. Crede voidings are instituted to ensure complete bladder emptying.
2. If this maneuver is not feasible/effective, then CIC is begun.

- Urodynamic studies measure the function of the bladder and external urethral sphincter by monitoring the intravesical pressure and the electromyographic activity of the sphincter during the phases of bladder filling and emptying. These studies are necessary to determine bladder compliance and contractility, as well as innervation of the external urethral sphincter and its responsiveness to bladder filling and emptying. This identifies babies at risk for bladder and upper urinary tract deterioration owing to the potential deleterious effects of bladder sphincter dyssynergy. These infants require CIC with or without anticholinergic medication to maintain a compliant bladder with good storage capability and to prevent reflux and hydronephrosis from occurring.
- For children undergoing spinal cord untethering secondary to an occult lesion, preoperative urodynamic studies provide a baseline for comparison with postoperative assessments to denote new onset or progressive changes with subsequent tethering.
- Sacral agenesis is a relatively stable lesion, but urodynamic studies are indicated soon after the diagnosis is made to determine the presence of bladder sphincter dyssynergy (for the reasons stated above) and to plan appropriate treatment of the lower urinary tract.

Complications

- Complications from CIC rarely occur in infancy but are seen more commonly in the older pediatric and adult population (eg, false passage, stricture, meatitis, epididymitis).
- Urinary tract infection in children who require CIC is not more common than that seen in children followed expectantly and it is readily treated. The incidence of urinary tract infection is inversely related to the frequency of the CIC and the completeness of bladder emptying with each catheterization.
- Prenatal closure of the open spinal canal defect has been performed at some institutions but findings on postnatal observations have been mixed. The need for postnatal ventricular

shunting has been reduced considerably but postnatal urody-namic assessment has revealed extensive loss of urethral sphincter function with poor detrusor compliance in some.

Outcomes

- Early intervention in babies at risk for urinary tract deterioration has lowered the incidence from 40% to < 5% when prophylactic treatment is initiated.
- Children who begin CIC early in life tend to accept the program and to become independent at an earlier age compared with those who start CIC at a later age.
- Early initiation of CIC also improves achievement of continence. Improved compliance and larger storage capacity of the bladder markedly reduce the need for augmentation cystoplasty at a later age.

Recommended Readings

Bauer SB. Neuropathology of the lower urinary tract. In: Belman AB, King LR, Kramer SA, editors. Clinical pediatric urology. 4th ed. London: Martin Dunitz; 2001. p. 371–408.

Edelstein RA, Bauer SB, Kelly MD, et al. Long-term urologic response of neonates with myelodysplasia treated proactively with intermittent catheterization and anticholinergic therapy. J Urol 1995;150:1500–4.

Part 10: Testicular Torsion

Neil R. Feins, MD, FAAP, FACS, and
Konstantinos Papadakis, MD FAAP, FACS

Etiology

Torsion of the testicle in neonates is almost always different than that seen in older children and adults. Normally, the tunica will invest the epididymis and posterior surface of the testicle, fixing it to the scrotum and making unable to twist. The older child is more likely to develop an intravaginal torsion due to failure of the tunica vaginalis to invest the cord and testicle and thus, creating a "bell clapper deformity" that is allowing the testis to twist freely within the tunica.

The fetus and neonate are more likely to experience an extravaginal type of torsion, involving all the elements of the cord. The torsion occurs due to poor fixation of the tunica vaginalis to the adjacent dartos muscle. This allows the cord to twist resulting in severe ischemia, necrosis, and loss of the gonad. These events invariably occur prenatally and always lead to loss of the affected testis. Depending on when the torsion occurs in pregnancy, the presentation can range from edematous and fixed scrotal skin with an indurated, intrascrotal mass (closer to the time of delivery), to a marble-like testis without any associated scrotal skin changes, and to a vanished testis (early in pregnancy).

Incidence

Five percent of all torsions occur before or soon after birth. Of these, 72% occur prenatally and 28% postnatally. Twenty-one percent are bilateral, and 3% are asynchronous bilateral.

Prenatal Diagnosis

This is not technically possible at this time. Some mothers describe a sudden increase in fetal activity that could possibly, in hindsight, represent a prenatal torsion event.

Postnatal Diagnosis

If the testicle was in torsion in utero, the neonate is generally asymptomatic, afebrile, and comfortable. The only finding is an enlarged scrotum associated with a nontender, swollen, and firm scrotal mass. There may be a red to blue discoloration. The scrotal skin is frequently fixed to the infarcted gonad. The cremasteric reflex is absent. Transillumination is negative. If the torsion is acute, it will be extremely tender to palpation.

Doppler ultrasonography can be helpful in difficult cases. However, verifying arterial flow to the testicle is not a reliable finding in neonates due to extremely small testicular vessels and can be operator dependent. Demonstration of diminished arterial flow in the symptomatic testis as compared with normal flow in the asymptomatic testis is strongly suggestive of torsion.

A high level of suspicion is a satisfactory indication for surgical intervention and exploration.

Differential Diagnosis

This includes torsion of the testicular appendage, inflammatory and neoplastic processes affecting the testicle, and the intrascrotal processes. (the testicular appendages are Mullerian duct remnants on the superior pole of the testis, and the epididymal appendages are Wolfian duct remnants.) On certain occasions, a hydrocele and/or an inguinal hernia may be mistaken for neonatal torsion. An abnormal scrotal appearance may be the result of testicular trauma during a difficult vaginal delivery.

Preoperative Management

Neonatal torsion is commonly diagnosed at birth or soon after. If the baby is well hydrated and if no life-threatening problems exist, all child needs a routine physical examination, nasogastric tube, and antibiotics.

Anesthesia

Experienced pediatric general anesthesia with a local field block.

Surgical Management

In the vast majority of cases, the testicle is already necrotic and
rarely salvageable; therefore, emergent, neonatal surgery without
experienced pediatric anesthesia is not recommended. However,
exploration and orchiectomy are necessary because a tumor could
present with identical clinical and imaging findings. If there is any
possibility that the torsion could be acute and the patient is otherwise healthy, emergency exploration and detorsion should be
performed within 4 to 6 hours of presentation. The patient should
be explored with an inguinal incision on the affected side. The testicle should be brought up into the wound and examined. If there
is any chance it could be viable, the gonad should be detorsed and
pexed in the scrotum. Most testes that are torsed in the prenatal
and postnatal period are clearly necrotic, with no chance of salvage, should be removed.

Because of reported cases of bilateral testicular torsion, the
contralateral testis must be prophylactically secured, usually at the
time of the original surgery to prevent the future risk of torsion.
The most important step is to evert the tunica vaginalis and
expose the tunica albuginea of the testis to the dartos; this may be
done either through a transcrotal or inguinal approach.

Although asynchronous extravaginal torsion is rare, there are
reports of this unfortunate situation. There are many case reports
of bilateral simultaneous neonatal torsion. Each case must be evaluated by the clinical findings. The chance of salvage of either testis
is extremely small, but in bilateral cases, detorsion, fixation,
antibiotics, and treating expectantly are an option unless both
testes are clearly necrotic, liquefied, or abscessed, in which case,
bilateral orchiectomy must be carried out.

Postoperative Management

This is usually unremarkable unless the testis was detorsed and
secured; then antibiotics should be given for 3 to 5 days. If a scrotal incision was used, povidone-iodine ointment should be
applied to the scrotum every 6 hours. The testicle should be evaluated for viability over the ensuing months and again at puberty

for growth. Evaluation can be done by physical examination and ultrasonography.

Complications/Outcome

The torsed testicle that was detorsed and pexed could necrose and liquefy and ultimately be absorbed. Under some circumstances, it could form an abscess and require scrotal drainage.

Management of testicles of questionable viability is controversial; they may go on to be of cosmetic and even functional use. However, there are reports that the ischemically damaged testicle may have a propensity to cause an autoimmune-mediated injury to the contralateral testis, with resultant abnormality in semen analysis.

Absent testes can be cosmetically corrected with prostheses as a teenager. In cases of bilateral orchidectomy, hormonal replacement is mandatory.

Part 11: Circumcision

Neil R. Feins, MD, FAAP, FACS, and
Konstantinos Papadakis, MD, FAAP, FACS

Embryology

The distal urethra is formed from the endoderm of the urethral plate and the fossa terminalis from the endodermal ingrowth from the surface of the glans. By 10 to 11 weeks' gestation, the preputial fold is present.

The skin at the distal margin overgrows the glans leaving an epithelial plate of fusion between the glans and prepuce. The prepuce covers the glans by 10 to 11 weeks' gestation.

The preputial space forms by breakdown of the fused epithelial surfaces from the deepest portion outward. The prepuce is retractable in 4% of infants at birth, in 50% at 1 year of age, and in 92% by 5 years of age. Phimosis is physiologic during the first year of life. During the first 3 to 5 years of life, the natural process of intermittent erections and progressive accumulation of desquamated residue separate the inner epithelial surface of the prepuce from the glans. By 3 years of age, 90% of foreskins are easily retractable. Forcible retraction of the prepuce is painful and unnecessary.

Incidence

Circumcision is currently the most commonly performed surgical procedure in the United States.

The decision to have a boy circumcised is largely cultural/religious. The medical risk:benefit analysis is controversial as both are low. Benefits include improved hygiene, decreased rate of infection (urinary tract, venereal, balanitis), paraphimosis, and penile carcinoma. There appears to be decreased rates of infection and transmission of HIV and other sexually transmitted infections for circumcised adult males.

Evaluation

Prior to circumcision, it is important to identify a normal foreskin, meatus, and phallus.

Contraindications to Neonatal Circumcision

- Hypospadias and/or chordee: circumcision should be delayed as the foreskin may be needed for future reconstructive procedures.
- Abnormal foreskin: possible accompanying anomalies, that is, hypospadias
- Congenital concealed penis: nonfixation of the penile skin to the corpora should prompt further evaluation and delay circumcision with possible penoplasty at 6 to 9 months of age.
- Spinal cord anomalies that may lead to incontinence (eg, myelominingocele): external collecting devices can fit better if the prepuce is intact.

Preoperative Management

- Make sure that an informed consent has been signed.
- Obtain the appropriate circumcision restraint board and instruments.
- NPO for 2 hours prior to the procedure.
- In premature infants, delay the procedure until 48 hours prior to discharge.
- Investigate any bleeding diathesis.

Surgical Management

- Place the patient on the circumcision board and secure extremities.
- Penile block 1 mL 1/2% lidocaine.
- Prepare the area with povidone-iodine or other antibacterial solution.

- Free the foreskin from the underlying glans, accurately place the appropriate mechanical instrument, and amputate the excess foreskin. There are 3 commonly used types of circumcision instruments: the Gomco clamp, the Mogan clamp, and the Plastibell. All are adequate if used properly.

CAUTION

IF using the Gomco or Mogan devices: never use cautery to excise the redundant foreskin. The transmission of the electrical current can destroy the underlying corpora, resulting in complete loss of the penis.

1. Check for bleeding.
2. Sutures are rarely needed in the routine newborn circumcision.
3. Outside of the immediate newborn period (2 to 6 weeks of age), after circumcision, place 6-0 chromic sutures in each quadrant to prevent separation of the shaft skin from the mucosal collar.

Postoperative Management

- Dress the site with vaseline and gauze.
- Apply povidone-iodine or other antibacterial ointment to the penis every 6 hours for 10 days to avoid infection, fungal overgrowth, and adherence of the raw penile tip to the diaper.
- Prescribe acetaminophen for pain.
- The infant should not be bathed for 48 hours.

Complications

- Infection is very rare: treat with intravenous antibiotics and topical antibiotic ointment.
- Penile adhesions can be prevented by having the parents stretch the skin if adhesions are noted to be developing.
- Removal of an excessive amount of shaft skin can be corrected immediately if identified by replacing a portion of the foreskin and suturing it in place. If found late, a formal penoplasty and rotation of flaps or grafting may be necessary.

1. Amputation of a portion of the glans or shaft.
2. Hypospadias and epispadias may result if the glans penis is slit on the dorsal or ventral aspect in preparation for the actual excision of the prepuce.

- Redundant foreskin following circumcision can be corrected by circumcision revision, usually after 6 months of age. Contraction of the excess foreskin can result in phimosis.
- Bleeding may be controlled by pressure, topical clotting agents, suture ligature, and possible repair in the operating room using optimal visual aids.
- Meatal stenosis occurs only in circumcised males, probably owing to scar formation secondary to the diaper rubbing on the delicate, previously protected meatus with a resultant cicatrix formation. The scarred narrow opening does not enlarge with the growing penis.
- Inclusion cysts secondary to implanting smegma or rolling in epidermis at the time of circumcision.
- Skin bridge formation between the penile shaft and the glans. Treatment is simple division.
- Concealed penis when excessive skin has been removed but an inadequate amount of inner preputial epithelium is removed, and a stenotic preputial ring results in pushing of the shaft beneath the pubis.
- Keloid at the anastomotic site can be treated with triamcinolone injections.
- Retained devices, a Plastibell circumcision relies on the device to release with sloughing of the redundant prepuce occurring. Incomplete sloughing may not allow the device to separate and may lead to ascending infections.

NINE

Neurological Disorders

Part 1: Neonatal Hydrocephalus

Janet S. Soul, MDCM, FRCPC, and
Joseph R. Madsen, MD, FACS, FAAP

Embryology

- Communicating hydrocephalus may have its origin as early as 6 weeks of gestation in relation to the formation of the subarachnoid spaces, where cerebrospinal fluid (CSF) is absorbed.[1]
- Hydrocephalus associated with aqueductal stenosis and the Arnold-Chiari malformation likely has its origin around 15 to 17 weeks' gestation in relation to the elongation of the mesencephalon and evolution of the constriction of the aqueduct.[1]
- Posthemorrhagic hydrocephalus (PHH) occurs as a complication of intraventricular hemorrhage (IVH) originating from blood vessels in the subependymal germinal matrix. These vessels are immature in preterm infants, consisting of simple endothelium-lined channels located in the caudothalamic groove. The fragility of the vessels renders them susceptible to rupture and consequent hemorrhage into the germinal matrix (GMH, also called a grade I IVH). If the hemorrhage is large, the bleeding extends into the lateral ventricles (IVH). A grade II IVH is one where the hemorrhage generally occupies less than 50% of the normal ventricular volume on a parasagittal view by cranial ultrasonographic scan (CUS), whereas a grade III IVH occupies greater than 50% of the ventricular volume and is associated with acute ventricular distension.[2] IVH may also result from hemorrhage originating in the vessels of the choroid plexus; this origin contributes more significantly to IVH in the term infant than in the preterm infant.

Incidence

- The incidence of hydrocephalus (all types) in newborns is about 1 in 1,000 live births.
- PHH occurs much more commonly in premature than in term infants. The incidence of PHH increases markedly with the severity of IVH; thus, it occurs in less than 15% of infants with grade II IVH but occurs in up to 75% of infants with grade III IVH with or without periventricular hemorrhagic infarction (sometimes called grade IV IVH).[3]

Prenatal Diagnosis

- Prenatal ventriculomegaly may be diagnosed by routine prenatal ultrasonography. A detailed sonogram should be performed to rule out brain malformations and/or other anomalies suggestive of a syndrome or in utero infection. Fetal magnetic resonance imaging (MRI) is more sensitive than ultrasound for the detection of parenchymal abnormalities that may be associated with hydrocephalus and therefore is preferred, when available.
- Amniocentesis should be considered, particularly if other anomalies are detected (cytogenetic abnormalities occur in 20 to 30% of cases of overt fetal hydrocephalus).
- PHH is occasionally diagnosed prenatally, although the incidence of prenatal IVH is quite low. A large in utero IVH resulting in PHH may occur, for example, in the setting of hypercoagulable disorders or bleeding disorders, significant acute maternal illness, trauma, or demise of a twin fetus, particularly when there is a shared placental circulation.
- In utero surgical treatment of fetal hydrocephalus is not recommended owing to minimal benefit and high risk of the procedure. This is largely attributable to the inability to identify a subgroup of fetuses with ventriculomegaly in whom early shunt placement would significantly improve outcome. Early delivery and delivery by cesarean section may be considered in some cases with marked hydrocephalus and macrocephaly.

Postnatal Presentation

- Idiopathic hydrocephalus and hydrocephalus caused by aqueductal stenosis, Dandy-Walker malformation, myelomeningocele, and other brain malformations will usually be clinically apparent in the first days after birth by physical examination.
  1. Clinical signs include macrocephaly, abnormally rapid head growth (crossing percentiles), large anterior and posterior fontanelle, and splitting of sutures.
  2. Lethargy, weakness, hypotonia, impaired upgaze (sunsetting sign), and/or poor feeding are often evident with careful examination but may be absent despite significant hydrocephalus.
- In premature infants, IVH occurs within the first 72 hours after birth in most cases and is diagnosed by routine CUS. PHH usually develops in the first few days or weeks after birth, following the occurrence of IVH.
  1. In premature infants, PHH may develop rapidly or slowly.
     a. Rapidly progressive ventricular dilation (over days) following IVH (1) often occurs in very low birth weight infants (< 1,000 g); (2) may be clinically apparent with excessive head growth, splitting of sutures, and bulging or full fontanelle and may be accompanied by nonspecific signs of lethargy, apnea/bradycardia, and worsening respiratory status or feeding difficulties (signs that can be thought to indicate sepsis); and (3) rarely resolves without medical and/or surgical therapy.
     b. Slowly progressive ventricular dilation (over weeks) after IVH (1) is often clinically silent with a gradual increase in head circumference and fontanelle size but without signs of increased intracranial pressure and (2) often resolves, with or without medical therapy.[3]
     c. Onset of PHH may rarely recur weeks or even months after the onset of IVH in preterm infants.[4] Therefore, this history and risk must be communicated to the outpatient primary care provider for careful follow-up of head growth, neurologic examination, and development.
  2. In term infants, PHH usually develops fairly rapidly following the onset of IVH. The infant may present because of clinical signs related to PHH rather than to the original IVH.

Postnatal Diagnosis

- The diagnosis of hydrocephalus is usually suspected by clinical signs of increased intracranial pressure and macrocephaly/increased head growth (see "Postnatal Presentation" above).
- CUS may confirm the presence of ventriculomegaly, but MRI (and, to a lesser extent, computed tomography [CT]) are better for the detection of any associated abnormalities such as parenchymal injury related to a TORCH infection, aqueductal stenosis, posterior fossa cyst, and vermal agenesis or hypoplasia that will shed light on the etiology and prognosis of the hydrocephalus.
- The diagnosis of PHH is usually made by CUS, although clinical signs (increasing head circumference, full fontanelle, split sutures, lethargy, apnea) may suggest the diagnosis prior to CUS.
  1. Follow-up CUS should be performed frequently in the weeks following IVH (particularly grade III IVH) diagnosed by routine CUS obtained in the first week after birth. Follow-up CUS scans should be performed at least every 1 to 2 weeks, and as often as every 2 to 3 days in preterm infants with very low birth weight (< 1000 g) and/or large IVH (grade III IVH).
  2. A CUS should also be obtained in a preterm infant who displays clinical signs of hydrocephalus (as outlined above).
  3. The CUS in infants with PHH typically shows enlarged and rounded ventricles, suggestive of excessive CSF accumulation and increased pressure.
  4. Serial CUS (eg, performed at 1–2 week intervals) may be required to make the diagnosis of PHH in infants in whom ventricular dilation progresses slowly.
  5. Serial measurement of the resistive index (RI) in the anterior cerebral artery can be determined by Doppler ultrasonography using the formula below, where "systolic" refers to systolic blood flow velocity and "diastolic" refers to diastolic blood flow velocity.

$$RI = \frac{(systolic - diastolic)}{systolic}$$

RI may increase from normal values of 0.5 to 0.6 up to 0.8 or even greater than 1 (RI > 1 means reversal of diastolic flow). A significant increase in RI with a gentle compression of the anterior fontanelle compared with baseline measurement (ΔRI) may indicate hemodynamic compromise and the eventual need for surgical intervention.[5]

6. If the diagnosis of PHH is in doubt, obtaining a CUS before and after a lumbar puncture (LP) in which 10 to 15 mL/kg of CSF is removed may be helpful in establishing the diagnosis (and the effectiveness of LP) by demonstrating a significant improvement in ventricle size ± reduction in RI.

Differential Diagnosis

The differential diagnosis of hydrocephalus in the newborn includes a number of associated brain malformations and syndromes, and atrophic ventriculomegaly attributable to a variety of causes. It is most important to determine whether the ventriculomegaly is caused by excess CSF accumulation (and therefore requires treatment) or is the result of cerebral malformation or tissue destruction accompanied by stable ventriculomegaly (which requires no treatment).

HYDROCEPHALUS REQUIRING TREATMENT

Exclusive of PHH, which is discussed in detail elsewhere in this chapter, other causes of hydrocephalus in the newborn include the following:

- Aqueductal stenosis (33% of congenital/neonatal hydrocephalus)
- Myelomeningocele with associated hydrocephalus (28%)
- Congenital "communicating" hydrocephalus (22%)
- Dandy-Walker malformation with associated hydrocephalus (7%)
- Other: associated with other genetic syndromes, or with congenital infection (eg, toxoplasmosis) (10%)

STABLE VENTRICULOMEGALY: CAUSED BY ATROPHY OR BRAIN MALFORMATION

- Brain malformations: holoprosencephaly, lissencephaly, agenesis of the corpus callosum

- Hydranencephaly caused by destruction of cerebrum
- Atrophy resulting from congenital infection, for example, cytomegalovirus, toxoplasmosis
- Periventricular leukomalacia (PVL)—most common in preterm infants. PVL often coexists with IVH; thus, the atrophic ventriculomegaly in a preterm infant with both IVH and PVL can be mistaken for PHH; however, in these cases, ventricular dilation does not progress.[6]

Preoperative Management

SUPPORTIVE MEASURES

Supportive measures are required prior to definitive surgical treatment in cases of hydrocephalus that require placement of a ventriculoperitoneal (VP) shunt in the newborn period (ie, hydrocephalus owing to aqueductal stenosis, myelomeningocele, Dandy-Walker malformation, and communicating hydrocephalus).

FURTHER DIAGNOSTIC STUDIES

Further diagnostic studies may be required to elucidate the etiology of the hydrocephalus.

- Appropriate neuroimaging should be obtained to establish a diagnosis of hydrocephalus (MRI or CT, serial CUS, see "Postnatal Diagnosis" above) and to determine the presence of any other parenchymal abnormalities (eg, brain malformation).
- Any infant with anomalies of other organs and/or dysmorphic features should have a karyotype and be evaluated by a geneticist.
- Any male infant with aqueductal stenosis and/or adducted thumbs and/or agenesis of the corpus callosum should undergo specific chromosomal analysis for mutations in the *L1CAM* gene on the X chromosome (Xq28) because the recurrence risk will be 50% for future male fetuses if the mother is carrying the mutation.
- Infants with hydrocephalus (or stable ventriculomegaly, particularly if ventricular margins are irregular) and any evidence of in utero infection (eg, calcifications in the brain parenchyma,

chorioretinitis, hepatitis, purpura) should undergo diagnostic testing for such infections because prompt treatment of the underlying infection can improve both short- and long-term outcome.

PRETERM INFANTS

The preoperative management of PHH in preterm infants may be prolonged because definitive treatment with a VP shunt may not be technically feasible until the infant has reached a weight of 1,500 to 2,000 g.

- In slowly progressive ventricular dilation (progressive dilation over weeks), close clinical observation and serial CUS may be sufficient until the dilation spontaneously resolves, which occurs in up to two-thirds of cases. However, infants with persistent ventricular dilation by CUS (with or without clinical signs of hydrocephalus) that does not resolve will require medical therapy with serial LPs and/or medication to reduce CSF production. Medical therapy may also be used as a temporizing measure to treat ventriculomegaly until an infant is large enough and/or sufficiently stable to undergo surgical treatment. Medical therapy may reduce parenchymal injury secondary to ventricular dilation, whether or not the infants eventually require a shunt.
  1. LPs: LPs may be performed every 1 to 3 days to remove excess CSF. Ideally, opening pressure should be measured, and 10 to 15 mL/kg of CSF should be removed. Direct ventricular tap may be performed by specially trained personnel but is less favored because of the risk of infection, particularly with repeated taps. A CUS performed before and after CSF drainage will determine whether the procedure was effective in reducing ventricle size and ΔRI or baseline RI.
  2. Medications to decrease CSF production: The use of acetazolamide and furosemide together to treat PHH is controversial, as one study suggests that the two medications used together resulted in a worse neurologic outcome.[7,8] Acetazolamide therapy may be effective in addition to taps if taps alone are ineffective or if adequate amounts of CSF cannot be removed by LP (usually owing to obstruction of

the egress of the fourth ventricle by particulate matter from IVH). There have been no large studies of the use of acetazolamide alone in the treatment of PHH (with or without LPs); thus, its safety and efficacy are unknown. One study showed short-term benefit of acetazolamide alone in the management of 3 of 5 infants with PHH; the medication was discontinued in the other 2 infants because of metabolic acidosis.[9] A dose of 25 to 100 mg/kg/d of acetazolamide divided twice or thrice daily may be used, starting with a low dose and increasing over subsequent days, depending on the response to therapy (measured by serial CUS). Electrolytes must be monitored frequently. Additional sodium citrate/citric acid, potassium, or other electrolyte supplements may be required to treat resultant electrolyte abnormalities. Furosemide may also be added to acetazolamide therapy, but this combination showed no significant benefit over "standard therapy" and possibly a worse neurologic outcome.[7,8] There is also a high incidence of nephrocalcinosis and electrolyte abnormalities in infants in whom these two medications are used together.[10] Thus, these risks should be considered carefully before initiating therapy with both acetazolamide and furosemide.

3. Fibrinolytics: Five trials of intraventricular administration of various fibrinolytics showed no clear efficacy in reducing shunt placement or improving long-term outcome in preterm infants with established PHH.[11] A pilot trial of drainage, irrigation, and fibrinolysis (DRIFT) to treat PHH in premature newborns yielded promising results.[12] However, the subsequent multicenter randomized trial of DRIFT therapy showed no benefit over standard therapy in terms of shunt placement or neonatal death.[13] This lack of efficacy was due in large part to the high incidence of secondary IVH in the DRIFT group (35%) compared with the standard therapy group (8%).

- Rapidly progressive ventricular dilation (over days to less than a few weeks) usually requires eventual placement of a VP shunt. If the infant is too small for placement of a VP shunt, serial LPs may be attempted. If LPs are ineffective in removing an adequate volume of CSF (eg, because of a lack of communication between the ventricles and lumbar subarachnoid space), consideration should be given to placement of a subgaleal shunt, ventricular access device, or external drain (see "Choice of Neurosurgical Procedure for Assistance with CSF Diversion" below).

- The effect of medical therapy should be monitored by clinical response and serial CUS for the measurement of ventricular size, RI, and ΔRI. The CUS studies should be performed every 2 to 7 days, depending on the rate of ventricular dilation and the frequency of taps.

Indications for Surgical Intervention for Hydrocephalus Management

- Progressive hydrocephalus as evidenced by increasing head circumference over expected growth, full fontanelle, apnea and bradycardia, and limitation of eye movements.
- RIs may further quantify changes in CSF hydrodynamics, with reversal of flow during compression, raising specific concern about the hemodynamic consequences of intracranial pressure.
- Failure of attempts at nonsurgical therapy for progressive ventricular dilation (see "Preterm Infants" above).

Goals of Surgical Intervention

- Control of intracranial pressure and relief of neurologic compromise
- Decreasing volume of ventricles to minimize white matter damage
- Temporization for patients who may "outgrow" resistance to CSF flow and the need for CSF diversion

Choice of Neurosurgical Procedure for Assistance with CSF Diversion

- Ventricular access device, with intermittent or continuous (rarely practiced locally) drainage
  1. Advantages: Requires only one incision and allows removal of CSF without lumbar punctures.
  2. Disadvantages: Risk of infection, difficult to manage as an outpatient if the infant is otherwise ready for discharge.
- Ventriculosubgaleal (VSG) shunt[14]
  1. Technically similar to ventricular access device but drains fluid directly into the subgaleal pocket.

   2. Advantages: Can be placed in infants of less than 1,500 g, diminishes the need for taps, may be left in as the patient is discharged if the CSF dynamics are unbalanced.
   3. Disadvantages: Relatively high rate of failure to drain CSF (see "Surgical Complications" below); protruding fluid collection can be cosmetically concerning.
- VP shunt
   1. Placement of a VP shunt requires a reasonable body mass, generally between 1,500 and 2,000 g. Consequently, very low birth weight, premature infants typically require a temporizing procedure before receiving a shunt.
   2. Valve choices now include adjustable settings, protection against overdrainage with antisiphon devices, and other technical modifications.

Surgical Management

- Careful preparation and draping from the scalp to the abdomen is mandatory.
- A small incision is made to allow access to the region where the ventricular catheter is to be placed. In infants, this is typically just above the Landolt suture, 2 to 2.5 cm off midline, with the direction of the catheter toward the foramen of Monro, generally aiming for a point in the middle of the forehead. The length of the catheter can be judged from the distance to the coronal suture, which would deliver the tip into the frontal horn, just lateral to the foramen of Monro.
- Abdominal opening is in a subcostal or midline exposure. Typically, a small incision, about 1 cm long, is adequate for entering the peritoneum. We typically do not use a trocar in these infants. A tunneling catheter is used to connect the two incisions to bring the shunt system from above to below.

Postoperative Management

- Initial avoidance of overdrainage is accomplished by keeping the patient flat for approximately 24 hours to minimize the risk of subdural hematomas.

- Gradually elevate the head of the bed to diminish the likelihood of overdrainage and monitor by palpating the anterior fontanelle. Monitoring with CUS, possibly combined with RI, can be helpful in assessing the functioning of the shunt.

Complications

SURGICAL COMPLICATIONS

- Infection occurs in ~ 5% of infants with ventricular access devices but can also occur in infants with internalized shunts.
- Infants with VSG shunts commonly show a recrudescence of progressive ventricular dilation, necessitating placement of a VP shunt. This occurs at an average of 9 weeks following VSG shunt placement (range 2.5 to 27 weeks).[14]
- A trapped fourth ventricle may occasionally occur in PHH owing to obstruction by particulate matter of the aqueduct of Sylvius and foramina of the fourth ventricle. This may become evident after lateral ventricles have been decompressed by placement of a VP shunt.

MEDICAL COMPLICATIONS

- Electrolyte abnormalities and acidosis may occur as a consequence of treatment with acetazolamide and/or furosemide.
- Meningitis may occur at a higher rate than expected, even in infants who do not undergo LPs.

Outcome

Outcome relates primarily to the etiology of the hydrocephalus (ie, associated syndrome, chromosomal abnormality, brain malformation, or parenchymal brain injury). Secondary factors in outcome include shunt infections and malfunctions, which may have a negative effect on neurologic outcome.

- Aqueductal stenosis—spectrum of clinical phenotypes; depends on the presence of other anomalies, congenital infection, chromosomal abnormality, etc; very wide range of outcomes reported in the literature.[15,16]

1. Overall prognosis—up to two-thirds will be able to work and live independently, although one-third of those will have neurologic abnormalities (including cognitive and visual impairments, spasticity/cerebral palsy, epilepsy), one-quarter will have moderate disability, and 8% will have severe disability; up to 15% will have epilepsy.[16]

2. X-linked hydrocephalus (with aqueductal stenosis) due to a mutation of the *L1CAM* gene on chromosome Xq28—is associated with mental retardation, spastic paraparesis, adducted thumbs, and/or agenesis of the corpus callosum. There is some correlation between phenotype and genotype.[17]

- Myelomeningocele with Arnold-Chiari malformation—about 75% will have an intelligence quotient greater than 80 and be ambulatory with aggressive (early) treatment of hydrocephalus and myelomeningocele.

- Congenital communicating hydrocephalus—at least two-thirds will have a normal neurologic outcome.

- Dandy-Walker malformation

  1. Outcome determined by associated anomalies in most children (incidence of 86%), chromosomal abnormalities (eg, trisomy 13, trisomy 18, translocations, etc; incidence of 32 to 46%)[18]

  2. Isolated Dandy-Walker malformation—up to 75% with normal intelligence and development

  3. Isolated Dandy-Walker "variant", that is, hypoplasia of the inferior vermis—several small series have shown that outcome is generally favorable although there can be mild motor, cognitive, language, and behavioral abnormalities.[18-20]

- PHH—outcome largely related to the size of the initial IVH, the presence of any parenchymal lesions (PVL or periventricular hemorrhagic infarction), and gestational age at birth. Overall mortality is 15 to 20% (related to the severity of the IVH, gestational age, and other significant illness), and major neurologic morbidity is up to 55% (significant motor and/or sensory handicap and/or mental retardation).[7,21] Children with a small IVH, for example, grade I or II IVH, do not appear to have an increased risk of neurologic sequelae compared with infants of the same gestational age and severity of illness without an IVH.[22] However, as many as 50% of children born at less than 32 weeks' gestational age have school difficulties whether or not they had IVH± PHH, even though the risk is clearly higher among children and adolescents with a history of IVH and lower birth gestational age/weight.[23,24] There are no data that demonstrate definitively the separate contributions of IVH and cerebral white matter injury in infants with PHH, especially because the latter is often missed by CUS. Children with grade III or IV IVH with PHH are often grouped together in outcome studies. However, children with a definitive periventricular hemorrhagic infarction in addition to a large IVH (ie, what is typically called a grade IV IVH) usually have significant neurologic sequelae related largely to the parenchymal injury.[25-27] One recent study showed that for children with IVH and periventricular hemorrhagic infarction, about two-thirds will have a motor deficit (hemiplegia with/without diplegia, or quadriplegia) and up to one-half had significant cognitive, language, and visual impairments, with relative sparing of adaptive skills.[27]

References

1. Volpe JJ. Neural tube formation and prosencephalic development. In: Neurology of the Newborn. 4th ed. Philadelphia: W.B. Saunders Co.; 2001. p. 1–44.

2. Volpe JJ. Intracranial hemorrhage: subdural, primary subarachnoid, intracerebellar, intraventricular (term infant), and miscellaneous. In: Neurology of the Newborn. 4th ed. Philadelphia: W.B. Saunders Co.; 2001. p. 397–427.

3. Murphy BP, Inder TE, Rooks V, et al. Posthaemorrhagic ventricular dilatation in the premature infant: natural history and predictors of outcome. Arch Dis Child Fetal Neonatal Ed 2002;87:F37–41.

4. Perlman JM, Lynch B, Volpe JJ. Late hydrocephalus after arrest and resolution of neonatal post- hemorrhagic hydrocephalus. Dev Med Child Neurol 1990;32:725–9.

5. Taylor GA, Madsen JR. Neonatal hydrocephalus: hemodynamic response to fontanelle compression—correlation with intracranial pressure and need for shunt placement. Radiology 1996;201:685–9.

6. du Plessis AJ. Posthemorrhagic hydrocephalus and brain injury in the preterm infant: dilemmas in diagnosis and management. Semin Pediatr Neurol 1998;5:161–79.

7. International PHVD Drug Trial Group. International randomised controlled trial of acetazolamide and furosemide in posthaemorrhagic ventricular dilatation in infancy. Lancet 1998;352:433–40.

8. Kennedy CR, Ayers S, Campbell MJ, et al. Randomized, controlled trial of acetazolamide and furosemide in posthemorrhagic ventricular dilation in infancy: follow-up at 1 year. Pediatrics 2001;108:597–607.

9. Mercuri E, Faundez JC, Cowan F, Dubowitz L. Acetazolamide without frusemide in the treatment of posthaemorrhagic hydrocephalus. Acta Paediatr 1994;83: 1319–21.

10. Libenson MH, Kaye EM, Rosman NP, Gilmore HE. Acetazolamide and furosemide for posthemorrhagic hydrocephalus of the newborn. Pediatr Neurol 1999;20:185–91.

11. Haines SJ, Lapointe M. Fibrinolytic agents in the management of posthemorrhagic hydrocephalus in preterm infants: the evidence. Childs Nerv Syst 1999;15:226–34.

12. Whitelaw A, Pople I, Cherian S, et al. Phase 1 trial of prevention of hydrocephalus after intraventricular hemorrhage in newborn infants by drainage, irrigation, and fibrinolytic therapy. Pediatrics 2003;111(4 Pt 1):759–65.

13. Whitelaw A, Evans D, Carter M, et al. Randomized clinical trial of prevention of hydrocephalus after intraventricular hemorrhage in preterm infants: brain-washing versus tapping fluid. Pediatrics 2007;119:e1071–8.

14. Rahman S, Teo C, Morris W, et al. Ventriculosubgaleal shunt: a treatment option for progressive posthemorrhagic hydrocephalus [see comments]. Childs Nerv Syst 1995;11:650–4.

15. Hanigan WC, Morgan A, Shaaban A, Bradle P. Surgical treatment and long-term neurodevelopmental outcome for infants with idiopathic aqueductal stenosis. Childs Nerv Syst 1991; 7:386–90.

16. Villani R, Tomei G, Gaini SM, et al. Long-term outcome in aqueductal stenosis. Childs Nerv Syst 1995;11:180–5.

17. Finckh U, Schroder J, Ressler B, et al. Spectrum and detection rate of L1CAM mutations in isolated and familial cases

with clinically suspected L1-disease. Am J Med Genet 2000; 92:40–6.

18. Ecker JL, Shipp TD, Bromley B, Benacerraf B. The sonographic diagnosis of Dandy-Walker and Dandy-Walker variant: associated findings and outcomes. Prenat Diagn 2000; 20:328–32.

19. Estroff JA, Scott MR, Benacerraf BR. Dandy-Walker variant: prenatal sonographic features and clinical outcome. Radiology 1992;185:755–8.

20. Limperopoulos C, Robertson RL, Estroff JA, et al. Diagnosis of inferior vermian hypoplasia by fetal magnetic resonance imaging: potential pitfalls and neurodevelopmental outcome. Am J Obstet Gynecol 2006;194:1070–6.

21. Dykes FD, Dunbar B, Lazarra A, Ahmann PA. Posthemorrhagic hydrocephalus in high-risk preterm infants: natural history, management, and long-term outcome. J Pediatr 1989;114(4 Pt 1):611–8.

22. Krishnamoorthy KS, Kuehnle KJ, Todres ID, DeLong GR. Neurodevelopmental outcome of survivors with posthemorrhagic hydrocephalus following Grade II neonatal intraventricular hemorrhage. Ann Neurol 1984;15:201–4.

23. Bowen JR, Gibson FL, Hand PJ. Educational outcome at 8 years for children who were born extremely prematurely: a controlled study. J Paediatr Child Health 2002; 38:438–44.

24. van de Bor M, den Ouden L. School performance in adolescents with and without periventricular-intraventricular hemorrhage in the neonatal period. Semin Perinatol 2004; 28:295–303.

25. Guzzetta F, Shackelford GD, Volpe S, et al. Periventricular intraparenchymal echodensities in the premature newborn: critical determinant of neurologic outcome. Pediatrics 1986;78:995–1006.

26. Bassan H, Benson CB, Limperopoulos C, et al. Ultrasonographic features and severity scoring of periventricular hemorrhagic infarction in relation to risk factors and outcome. Pediatrics 2006;117:2111–8.

27. Bassan H, Limperopoulos C, Visconti K, et al. Neurodevelopmental outcome in survivors of periventricular hemorrhagic infarction. Pediatrics 2007;120:785–792.

Part 2: Myelodysplasia

Laurie J. Glader, MD, FAAP, Ellen R. Elias, MD, FAAP, and Joseph R. Madsen, MD, FACS, FAAP

Failure of the neural tube to close in early embryonic development can give rise to a range of neural tube defects, both open and closed. Myelomeningocele is the most common open form of spinal dysraphism.

Embryology/Definition

A. The neural tube closes by the fourth week of gestation in normal spinal cord and brain development. This closure probably occurs in zipper-like fashion, rostral to caudal, resulting in a cylindrical structure with anterior and posterior apertures. Most recent studies suggest that this closure involves at least five zippers located between the rostral and caudal ends, each mediated by different genes and affected by different teratogens.[1] Interruption of this closure results in a variety of defects, depending on the timing and location of the interruption.

B. Types of neural tube defects:
   1. Anencephaly is a lethal condition resulting from interrupted closure of the anterior aperture at 26 days. The cranial vault and cerebral hemisphere are absent, generally resulting in stillbirth or death in the immediate neonatal period.
   2. Encephalocele is a defect of the skull that allows for herniation of meninges and brain tissue. In all, 70 to 80% of cases occur in the occipital region but encephaloceles also occur in the fronto-facial area.
   3. Spina bifida results when there is failed closure of the posterior aperture and can be further subcategorized:

   A myelomeningocele is a complex anomaly involving failure of the posterior vertebral elements to fuse. A cyst or "cele" results that contains cerebrospinal fluid and neural elements, including spinal cord and nerves. In all, 80% of myelomeningoceles occur in the lumbar (thoracolumbar, lumbar and lumbosacral) regions. The spinal cord itself ends in an abnormally low and flattened

structure called the *placode*. The placode is usually visible
through the skin defect and resembles an open book with
a raphe down the middle, sometimes with nerve roots
exiting ventrally.

A meningocele contains no neural elements.

Spina bifida occulta results when there is normal formation of spinal cord and soft tissues, but when there is
failure of vertebral arch fusion.

A lipomeningocele is a skin-covered lesion consisting of
a lipoma attached to the spinal cord that is often tethered
in the spinal canal. It may be marked superficially by a
hemangioma or hairy patch.

Incidence and Survival

A. Between 3.6 and 10 per 10,000 live births, depending on ethnic background. This incidence is decreasing secondary to folic
   acid supplementation and pregnancy termination after prenatal diagnosis.[2]
B. The risk for a second affected child from the same parent is 2
   to 3%. Adults with neural tube defects have a 5% chance of
   having an affected child. Siblings of a child with a neural tube
   defect, as well as siblings of the parent, have a 1 to 2% risk of
   having an affected child.
C. The 1-year survival is 87%; approximately 78% of all individuals with spina bifida survive to age 17, although there
   are a number of factors affecting morbidity throughout
   adulthood.[3]
D. Long-term survival and quality of life after closure of the primary defect have improved for a number of reasons:
   1. Aggressive neurosurgical intervention
   Shunting for hydrocephalus
   Treatment of symptomatic Chiari II malformations
   Spinal cord detethering
   2. Clean intermittent catheterization for treatment of neuro-
      genic bladder, resulting in reduced incidence of recurrent
      urinary tract infection, vesicoureteral reflux, and chronic
      renal failure
   3. Orthopedic management of spinal and lower extremity
      deformities

Prenatal Diagnosis and Preventive Treatment

A. Screening for neural tube defects via maternal serum α-fetoprotein (AFP) levels at the sixteenth week of gestation is now standard. Elevated AFP for gestational age (> 2 multiples of the mean [MOM]) should prompt further investigation via high resolution ultrasound to look for fetal anomalies. Elevated amniotic fluid AFP and acetylcholine esterase provide further support for the diagnosis.[4]

B. Radiographic signs of open neural tube defects specifically include signs of the associated Chiari malformation (ibanana signî or a flattened cerebellum) and a transient frontal bone anomaly called a "lemon sign." Ultrasound can also demonstrate level of termination of the normal cord and placode. Fetal magnetic resonance imaging (MRI) can further define anatomy, though the effect on patient management is still evolving.

C. Folate supplementation has been demonstrated to reduce the incidence of neural tube defects by 50 to 70% in women who take it for at least 3 months prior to conception and during the first month of pregnancy.[5]

D. Prenatal surgery may offer improved outcomes[6] and is currently being evaluated as part of a randomized, prospective trial funded by the National Institutes of Health (<http://www.spinabifidamoms.com>). This study is still accruing patients in an attempt to determine the benefits of prenatal neural tube repair. Because the surgery is associated with an increased risk of premature birth, the potential benefits require close quantitative analysis, which will hopefully be forthcoming from this study.

E. Prenatal diagnosis makes possible a planned cesarean section prior to the onset of labor, which is the preferred mode of delivery because it decreases the likelihood of rupturing the meningeal sac[7] and is associated with improved neurological outcome.

Postnatal Clinical Presentation

A. There is uniformly a defect in the axial skeleton with a variable amount of dermal covering, depending on the specific lesion. Neural tissue may appear plate-like.

B. The fontanelles and sutures must be assessed for indication of increased intracranial pressure. Macrocephaly may be present.

C. Visible abnormalities of the lower extremities often include clubfeet and limited range of motion.

D. The neurological exam reveals variable abnormalities, depending on the lesion. Reflexes may be absent, including (with the highest lesions) knee, ankle, and anal wink. Voluntary motor control is also variably limited from hip to toe flexion. Sensory impairment reflects the level of the lesion.

E. There may be visible associated congenital anomalies, including cleft lip and palate, imperforate anus, and cryptorchidism.

Differential Diagnosis

A. In all, 85% of all neural tube defects occur in isolation and inheritance is multifactorial.

B. Possible etiologies include as follows:
1. Chromosomal abnormalities (especially trisomy 13 and 18)
2. Mutant genes (Meckel syndrome)
3. Teratogen exposure (alcohol, valproate, thalidomide)

Preoperative Management

A. The infant should be placed in a prone position and wet sterile dressings applied to the lesion, covered by plastic wrap. Moisture prevents adherence of the dressing to the sac. This combination results in negligible insensible losses; thus, standard intravenous fluid management is generally used. It is important to emphasize to the care team that the point of any plastic wrap is to keep the lesion clean and moist, not to be somehow occlusive. Placing the baby into a large plastic bag, which keeps meconium and other contaminants in close proximity to the cele, is counterproductive. Though most open neural defects leak cerebrospinal fluid, it is useful to protect the lesion because a widely open sac increases the risk of central nervous system bacterial infection. Intravenous antibiotics (generally ampicillin and gentamicin in meningitic dosages) are indicated in the preoperative and perioperative period.[8]

B. Early repair significantly reduces infection risk. Transfer in prone position to tertiary care setting for surgical repair of the defect within 24 to 48 hours.

C. Clean intermittent catheterization is indicated to check postvoid residuals until urologic and renal function are clearly understood.

D. Latex allergy was a common problem in the past in children with spina bifida who underwent repeated surgical procedures because of frequent and repeated exposure to latex in the medical environment. To minimize this problem, use nonlatex gloves and equipment.

E. A cranial ultrasound should generally be obtained soon after birth. Arnold Chiari type II malformations result from premature fusion of the posterior fossa leaving insufficient space for the cerebrum, cerebellum, and brainstem. Brainstem and portions of the cerebellum may herniate through the foramen magnum into the upper cervical spinal canal. Obstructed flow of cerebrospinal fluid (CSF) results in hydrocephalus the majority of the time.

1. It has been believed that 85% of children with myelomeningocele will require shunting for hydrocephalus, though recent reappraisal, prompted by the success of some prenatal surgical centers in decreasing this number, have led many neurosurgeons to be in less of a hurry to shunt these babies. The presumption that the vast majority need shunts has perhaps elevated the percentage of patients shunted in the past. Approximately 25% of children with myelomeningocele are born with hydrocephalus significant enough to warrant shunting at birth. An additional 25 to 60% are at risk for developing hydrocephalus subsequent to back closure, although the number receiving shunts at any particular age varies from center to center.

2. The most common type of shunt is the ventriculoperitoneal shunt. Rarely, if the peritoneal surface is scarred following infection, a ventriculoatrial or ventriculopleural shunt may be placed, though these alternative sites for CSF drainage rarely work well in infants. If significant hydrocephalus is present at birth, a shunt may be placed at the same time as the back closure. Otherwise, the infant is

closely monitored after back closure for signs of rapidly enlarging head circumference and symptoms of increased intracranial pressure.

3. A head MRI is frequently obtained electively during the first year of life in children with myelomeningocele to assess the severity of the Chiari malformation. An MRI of the lower back may be necessary preoperatively to define anatomy in skin-covered lesions. Plain spine films can be useful if there is a significant kyphus (ventral angulation) deformity that may have to be reduced prior to skin closure.

F. Careful neurological assessment to detect motor and sensory levels of the lesion is critical. Children with myelomeningocele present with neurological deficits corresponding to the level of their lesion. Serial neurological examinations should include assessment of anal wink in addition to lower and upper extremity motor and sensory function. Degree of impairment depends on location of the myelomeningocele, with lower lesions causing less disability.

1. Higher levels are more commonly associated with hydrocephalus.

2. Lumbar lesions result in paralysis and decreased sensation from the proximal lower extremities down.

3. Lesions in S1-S2 region are associated with decreased innervation to the distal lower extremities.

4. Lesions below S2 generally have no orthopedic sequelae, allow for independent ambulation, and are not usually associated with scoliosis.

5. All lesions above S1 are associated with neurogenic bowel and bladder issues.

G. Monitor for seizures. There is a 20 to 25% incidence of seizures in this population.[9] Brain anomalies in addition to Chiari malformation are found in association with myelomeningocele, especially in children with higher level lesions.

H. Assess for other congenital malformations, including other central nervous system and vertebral anomalies, cardiac defects (particularly ventriculoseptal defects), cleft lip and palate, tracheoesophageal fistulas, renal anomalies, imperforate anus, and cryptorchidism.

I. Consideration should be given to certain syndromes (including trisomy 13 and 18 and cri du chat) if dysmorphic features and other anomalies are present.

J. Neural tube defects may be associated with common teratogens, including ethanol, and the anticonvulsant valproate.

Anesthesia

A. General anesthesia is used for closure of the myelomeningoceles. A bladder catheter is placed to decompress the bladder pending urodynamic workup.

B. Minimization of trauma to the neural placode may require intubating the baby in the lateral position or building up the area around the defect to avoid any pressure on it in the supine position.

C. All infants with spina bifida are assumed to be at risk for developing latex allergy, and every effort is made to avoid latex exposure.

Surgical Management

A. Sterile preparation of the defect with toxic solutions (such as alcohol) should be avoided.

B. The placode is dissected free of any possible adherent dermal tissue (which could form late postoperative dermoid tumors).

C. Thin, translucent tissue and skin too thin to use are trimmed away around the circumference of the defect.

D. The placode is frequently rolled into a more normal shape and gently held in this configuration with fine sutures to the pial edge.

E. Exploration around the placode and within the spinal canal above the lesion is performed to rule out another tethering lesion, such as diastematomyelia (a bone or soft-tissue band passing through the neural elements, tethering them at a different level).

F. The dural edge is identified, usually as it thins out and blends with skin around the perimeter of the defect. The dural edge is undermined (generally separating it from the lumbar fascia), and it is rolled up around the dura and closed in a watertight fashion.

G. Some surgeons prepare a flap of lumbar fascia to bring over the placode, but this is associated with risk of compression and should usually be avoided.

H. Subcutaneous and cutaneous levels are closed, with goal of attaining a well-vascularized, watertight closure.

I. A ventriculoperitoneal shunt may be placed at the time of the first operation, but in most cases, this can be postponed with close postoperative monitoring.

Postoperative Management

A. Typical hospital course is 1 to 2 weeks, allowing time for pre-operative assessment, postoperative recovery, and evaluation of possible associated conditions.

B. The infant must remain prone or on the side until the wound heals.

C. Head circumference needs to be plotted daily, particularly in the child who has not had shunt placement.

D. Feeding difficulties are commonly associated with the Chiari II malformation. Growth and nutritional status, as well as a child's ability to suck and swallow, must be watched closely. Acute deterioration of feeding skills may signal a shunt mal-function.
   1. Plot daily weights and closely monitor input and output.
   2. Observe for spitting, gagging, choking, and hypoxia.

E. Urologic and renal evaluation
   1. A urologic consult should be obtained.
   2. Ultrasound will detect associated renal anomalies and pos-sible hydronephrosis from vesiculoureteral reflux.
   3. Voiding cystourethrogram will help identify VU reflux.
   4. Postvoid residuals and urodynamic studies must be obtained.
   5. Urine culture, urinalysis, and serum creatinine are obtained as a baseline, if not already done preoperatively.
   6. Clean intermittent catherization (CIC) is recommended for those infants who have large postvoid residuals, evi-dence of significant hydronephrosis, and/or increased blad-der pressure on UDS studies. Those infants who do not manifest these problems can safely be allowed to void into

diapers. CIC is started in the hospital and continued at discharge.

F. Hip dysplasia and clubfeet may be present at birth.
    1. An orthopedic consult should be obtained.

G. Sensory impairment can be associated with myelomeningocele.
    1. Strabismus is commonly associated with Chiari malformation.
    2. Hearing and vision screens may be performed prior to discharge

H. Psychological and social strain associated with myelomeningocele cannot be underestimated.
    1. From the beginning, a social worker should be available for the family.
    2. An excellent information and support resource is the Spina Bifida Association of America (phone number (202) 944-3285 or available online at <www.sbaa.org>).

Complications/Outcomes

A. Neonatal period
    1. Increased intracranial pressure from evolving hydrocephalus in the unshunted child, or shunt malfunction or infection in the shunted child requires urgent assessment as symptoms may progress rapidly and death may ensue.[10]

    Signs include irritability, bulging fontanelle, stridor, apnea, sixth nerve palsy, paralysis of upward gaze, worsening oromotor function, vomiting, and upper extremity weakness.[11]

    Shunt infection should be suspected if the above symptoms are accompanied by fever and increased white blood cell count.

    A shunt series and computed tomographic scan must be obtained in conjunction with neurosurgical evaluation.

    A shunt tap is necessary to rule out a shunt infection.

    2. Respiratory complications may occur secondary to the Chiari malformation, generally presenting with vocal cord paralysis and stridor. Central and obstructive apnea also occur. Mechanism for all of these abnormalities is secondary to lower brain stem dysfunction. Surgical decompression of the Chiari malformation should be considered

under such circumstances, but it is critically important to be sure the CSF drainage is adequate before going forward with this surgery. Tracheostomy is occasionally necessary.

3. Oromotor dysfunction can occur again secondary to the Chiari malformation.

A videofluoroscopic swallowing study may be indicated to assess risk of aspiration with oral feeds.

Some children require gastrostomy tube placement secondary to aspiration risk or inability to take in adequate calories by mouth.

4. Urinary tract infections are common. Frequently, children with myelomeningocele are colonized with multiple organisms secondary to routine catheterization.

A positive urine culture alone may be inadequate to address need for treatment.

Positive urine cultures are generally treated with antibiotics when the child has fever, increased white blood cell count, and/or there is a single organism with a high colony count on a catheterized urine specimen.

Prophylactic antibiotics may be indicated, especially if vesicoureteral reflux is present. Amoxicillin is a common antibiotic used for prophylaxis in newborns and young infants. Other antibiotics, such as Bactrim and Nitrofuradantoin are used in older children.[12]

5. Intensive rehabilitation therapies are critical in optimizing the health and general development of a child with myelomeningocele.

Therapies may include physical, occupational, and speech/language services.

Initially, services should be established through state Early Intervention (EI) programs, which are mandated under the Individuals with Disabilities Education Act. EI referral should be made early during an infant's initial hospitalization as there can be waiting lists.

After age three, services are provided through the public school system.

B. On-going issues in childhood
1. There are a wide variety of medical and developmental issues associated with myelomeningocele. As a result, children with myelomeningocele require a comprehensive

multidisciplinary team of providers including combinations of neurosurgery, orthopedic surgery, urology, physiatry, gastroenterology, endocrinology, pulmonary medicine, and physical, occupational, and speech therapists.

2. Increased ICP continues to be a risk. In addition to symptoms described above, signs may include as follows:

Headache or visual changes

New onset of respiratory complications, particularly stridor from vocal cord paralysis

New onset of difficulty in swallowing or change in oromotor function

Change in cognitive function

3. Growth and nutrition continue to be an important area of concern. Failure to thrive is a common problem in infants and young children.

Arm span may more accurately reflect growth because growth below the waistline is usually disproportionately slow or distorted by lower extremity or spinal deformities.

Skinfold thickness is another valuable measure of nutrition.

Some children may need gastrostomy tube placement.

Bowel incontinence and constipation are prominent problems. An aggressive, consistent bowel program is often required and may include laxatives, suppositories, enemas, or even antegrade colonic enemas.[13]

4. Certain endocrinopathies are common.

The most common type of endocrinopathy is precocious puberty.[14] Leuprolide acetate (Lupron) may reverse the development of early sexual characteristics.

Growth hormone deficiency should be suspected in the child who is receiving adequate nutrition but is growing poorly. Wrist x-ray for bone age, serum insulin-like growth factor-I (IGF-I), and IGF-binding protein-3 (IGBP-3) can help to define a deficiency.[15]

5. Orthopedic complications

Worsening scoliosis or kyphosis may cause restrictive lung disease.

Osteopenia, particularly in the nonambulatory patient, increases the risk for pathological fractures.

Contractures of hips, knees and ankles, and hip dislocation are common. Treatments include physical therapy,
orthotics, neuromuscular blockades, and surgeries.

6. Decubitus ulcers are common secondary to limited movement
   and diminished peripheral sensation and occur commonly on
   the feet.

   Risk of infection exists.

   Wheelchairs and other seating systems, which the child
   uses, must be reviewed regularly for appropriate fit, padding,
   and positioning.

7. Latex allergy

   Ongoing avoidance of latex-containing products.

   Some foods are cross-reactive with latex and should be
   avoided, such as avocado, banana, and water chestnuts.

8. Cognition

   Approximately 75% of children with myelomeningocele
   have intelligence quotient scores greater than 80. Verbal
   scores tend to be higher than performance. Of those with
   normal cognition, 60% have specific learning disabilities.
   Although most children demonstrate adequate language skills
   in terms of grammar and lexicon, most experience challenges
   in language processing.[16] Many children with myelomeningocele require some sort of special education.

   A formal neurodevelopmental assessment should be
   obtained if any questions arise about a child's social and
   cognitive abilities.

9. Hearing and vision status must be formally reassessed to
   rule out any exacerbation of learning difficulties. Hearing
   loss has historically been a problem associated with antibiotic use in the setting of urinary tract infections but has
   been dramatically reduced with the advent of clean intermittent catheterization.

10. Seizures remain a risk, and families should be familiar with
    signs and symptoms for which to monitor as well as an ini-
    tial treatment approach.

11. The primary care physician plays a critical role in coordi-
    nating the care of a child with myelodysplasia.[17] The role
    includes general pediatric care and surveillance for compli-
    cations, communication with multiple subspecialists, and
    advocacy in school programs and the community.

References

1. Van Allen MI, Kalousek DK, Chernoff GF, et al. Evidence for multi-site closure of the neural tube in humans. Am J Med Genet 1993;47:723.

2. Kaufman B. Neural tube defects. Pediatr Clin North Am. 2004;51:389–419.

3. Mitchell LE, Adzick NS, et al. Spina bifida. Lancet 2004; 364:1885–95.

4. Milunsky A. Maternal serum screening for neural tube and other defects. In: Milunsky A, editor. Genetic disorders and the fetus: diagnosis, prevention, and treatment. 3rd ed. Baltimore: The Johns Hopkins University Press; 1992. p. 324–662.

5. Padmanabhan R. Etiology, pathogenesis and prevention of neural tube defects. Congenit Anom (Kyoto) 2006;46:55–67.

6. Sutton LN, et al Improvement in hindbrain herniation demonstrated on serial fetal magnetic resonance imaging following fetal surgery for myelmeningocele. JAMA 1999; 282:1826–31.

7. Luthy DA, Wardinsky T, Shurtleff DB, et al. Cesarean section before the onset of labor and subsequent motor function in infants with myelomeningocele diagnosed antenatally. N Engl J Med 1991;324:662.

8. Neural Tube Defects in the Neonatal Period. Available at: www.emedicine.com/ped

9. Talwar D, Baldwin M, Horbatt C. Epilepsy in children with meningomyelocele. Pediatr Neurol 1995;13:29.

10. Madikians A, Conway E. Cerebrospinal fluid shunt problems in pediatric patients. Pediatr Ann 1997;26:613.

11. Charney E, Rorke L, Sutton L, et al. Management of Chiari II complications in infants with myelomeningocele. J Pediatr 1987;111:364.

12. Bauer SB. The management of the myelodysplastic child: a paradigm shift. Br J of Urol 2003;92(suppl 1):23–28.

13. Leibold S, Ekmark E, Adams R. Decision making for a successful bowel continence program. Eur J Pediatr Surg 2000; 10:26–30.

14. Elias ER, Sadeghi-Nejad A. Precocious puberty in girls with myelodysplasia. Pediatrics 1994;92:521.

15. Lopponen T, Saukkonen A, Serlo W, et al. Reduced levels of growth hormone, insulin-like growth factor-1, and binding protein-3 in patients with shunted hydrocephalus. Arch Dis Child 1997;77:32.

16. Fletcher J, Barnes M, Dennis M. Language development in children with spina bifida. Semin Pediatr Neurol 2002;9:201–8.

17. Elias ER, Hobbs N. Spina bifida: sorting out the complexities of care. Contemp Pediatr 1998;15:156.

TEN

Retinopathy of Prematurity

Jane E. Stewart, MD, and
Deborah K. VanderVeen, MD

Embryology

Normal retinal blood vessel development begins at about the fourteenth week of gestation and is complete at approximately term. Blood vessels grow from the optic nerve outward toward the ora serrata. Thus, infants who are born prematurely have incompletely vascularized retinas, and factors such as the relative hyperoxia of the extrauterine environment in some infants leads to abnormal fibrovascular proliferation of the retina called retinopathy of prematurity (ROP).

Incidence

The risk of ROP is highest in the smallest, most premature infants. In the Cryotherapy for Retinopathy of Prematurity (CRYO-ROP) natural history study, 66% of all infants weighing less than 1,251 gm at birth developed ROP, and 90% of infants weighing less than 750 gm at birth developed ROP. Similarly, in the Early Treatment for Retinopathy of Prematurity (ETROP) study, 68% of infants ≤ 1,251 gm at birth developed ROP and 93% of those less than 750 g developed ROP. The rate of moderately severe (prethreshold) ROP in the ETROP study was 37%, and there was an increased incidence of zone 1 disease at 9%, compared with 2% in the CRYO-ROP study. Approximately 8% of the premature infant population of birth weight less than 1,251 gm is expected to meet criteria for treatment.

Postnatal Presentation

There are no signs or symptoms of ROP. Therefore, screening eye examinations are critical for diagnosis. Examinations are performed by indirect ophthalmoscopy or in some centers by using Retcam digital images.

Postnatal Diagnosis

All infants born at $\leq$ 30 weeks or with a birth weight $\leq$ 1,500 g should be examined by an ophthalmologist experienced in the diagnosis of ROP in preterm infants. Infants weighing over 1,500 g with an unstable clinical course (eg, those who have had severe respiratory distress syndrome, hypotension requiring pressor support, or surgery in the first several weeks of life) should also be considered for screening.

Screening examinations to detect ROP are performed in the beginning 3 to 6 weeks after birth and are continued every 2 to 3 weeks until the retina shows complete vascularization. If ROP is detected, more frequent examinations are indicated, based on the severity and progression of the ROP. Our schedule for screening is 6 weeks after birth for infants born at $\leq$ 26 weeks, 5 weeks after birth for those born at 27 to 28 weeks, 4 weeks after birth for those born at 29 to 30 weeks, and 3 weeks after birth for all others.

Most ROP is mild and regresses without treatment. However, ROP that becomes more severe may warrant treatment. Treatment may be considered when type 1 prethreshold ROP is diagnosed. Type 1 prethreshold ROP includes in zone 1, eyes with any ROP and plus disease (Figure 1) or stage 3 (Figure 2) with or without plus disease, and in zone 2, stage 2 or 3 with plus disease. Observation is recommended for type 2 prethreshold ROP. Type 2 prethreshold includes zone 1, stage 1 or 2 ROP without plus disease, or zone 2, stage 3 ROP without plus disease. Treatment should be considered for an eye with type 2 ROP when progression to type 1 status or threshold ROP occurs.

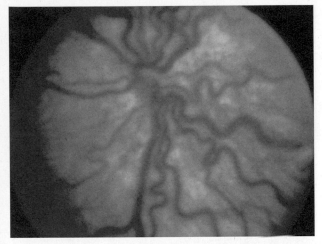

Figure 1 Plus disease (abnormal dilation and tortuosity of retinal vessels)

Differential Diagnosis

There are no other ophthalmologic conditions with similar clinical presentation in the premature infant population.

Preoperative Management/Anesthesia

- The pupils should be dilated prior to the procedure. We use cyclopentolate 1% and cyclomydril (see "Complications/ Outcomes" below).
- Laser treatment should be performed in a separate room or area within the nursery (Figure 3) to avoid possible laser damage to the eyes of others. Often laser treatment is performed with sedation and topical anesthesia but occasionally is performed in the operating room. We prefer to use fentanyl ± versed for sedation, with

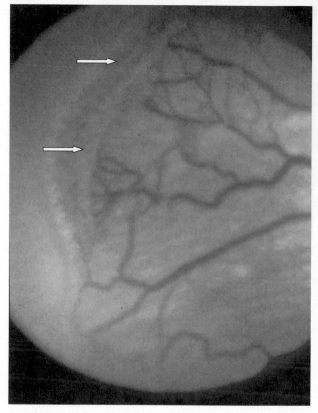

Figure 2 Stage 3 ROP (arrows: areas of abnormal pre-retinal fibrovascular proliferation)

oral sucrose and topical ophthalmic proparacaine. Cryotherapy and retinal reattachment surgeries are usually performed in the operating room under general anesthesia. Protective eyewear specific to the laser wavelength should be provided to personnel involved in the care of the infant during the procedure.

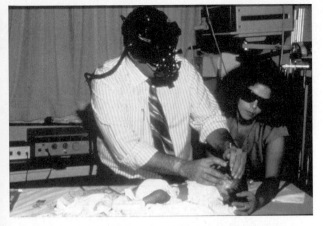

Figure 3 Laser treatment at bedside in NICU

- The patient's overall medical status, extent of treatment required, and preference of the clinician performing the procedure all contribute to the choice of anesthesia, which may range from topical plus restraint, with or without sedation to general anesthesia with intubation and muscle relaxation. Infants who have severe chronic lung disease are at risk for pulmonary exacerbation related to the intubation and sedation. Infants who have received steroid therapy for their lungs in the past may have adrenal suppression, and stress steroid replacement treatment during the perioperative period may be warranted.

Surgical Management

Treatment for ROP consists of ablation of the peripheral avascular retina by either laser therapy or cryotherapy.

- Laser treatment is generally the first-line treatment for ROP unless there are factors limiting the delivery of the laser or visualization of the retina via an indirect ophthalmoscope (ie, small pupils or vitreous hemorrhage).

- Cryotherapy is equally effective but generally causes more inflammation and discomfort. It is needed when laser cannot be adequately delivered and may be useful for cases with early retinal detachment.
- If the ROP does not improve with the initial treatment, retreatment may be considered after 10 to 14 days.
- If the ROP progresses to cause a retinal detachment, then surgery to reattach the retina will be required and may include placement of a scleral buckle (encircling band around the eye) or vitrectomy (removal of the vitreous gel), with or without removal of the lens.

Postoperative Management

- Most ophthalmologists will prescribe a cycloplegic agent and topical steroid (with or without antibiotic) to reduce inflammation after the laser treatment or cryotherapy.
- After treatment, the eyelids and conjunctiva may appear red and edematous from manipulation; cryotherapy often produces more inflammation than laser therapy.
- Topical antibiotics and anti-inflammatory medications are similarly prescribed after eye surgery for retinal detachment.

Complications/Outcomes

Most ROP regresses without treatment. Treatment is performed for eyes with moderately severe ROP to help the ROP regress before retinal detachment occurs, because eyes that develop a retinal detachment involving the macula are usually blind.

Treatment at type 1 prethreshold reduces the incidence at one year of age for poor visual outcomes to 14.5% and poor structural outcomes to 9.1%. Even with treatment, however, the incidence of poor vision remains significant for eyes treated for zone 1 ROP (33.3%).

Eyes that develop a retinal detachment have extremely poor visual outcomes even if vitrectomy is performed and the retina is successfully reattached. In a case series of 42 eyes treated surgically for stage 4 and 5 ROP, only 15% achieved a visual acuity of 20/300 or better (legal blindness is defined as worse than 20/200).

Although outcomes were poor, intervention did result in some useful vision, with 48% achieving ambulatory vision and 72% achieving light perception or better.

Short-term complications of laser therapy or cryotherapy include transient inflammation or hemorrhage in the eye. One long-term effect is a minor loss of peripheral vision. Rare complications include cataract formation, glaucoma, infection, bleeding inside the eye, and inadvertent laser treatment to other parts of the eye. Infants with more severe ROP are more likely to develop other ocular problems such as myopia, strabismus, and nystagmus, whether they required laser treatment or not.

Side effects of mydriatic eye drops (phenylephrine, cyclopentolate, and atropine) have been noted in premature infants including hypertension, feeding intolerance, and reactive airway disease in infants with chronic lung disease. Infants should be given the lowest dose of these drugs possible to achieve optimal mydriasis and should be monitored closely for side effects.

Close follow up of all extremely premature infants by an ophthalmologist is important after discharge from the NICU until the retinal vessels are mature and then again at 8 to 12 months to evaluate for possible ocular or visual functional problems.

References

1. An International Committee for the Classification of Retinopathy of Prematurity. The International Classification of Retinopathy of Prematurity Revisited. Arch Ophthalmol 2005;123:991–9.
2. American Academy of Pediatrics, Section on Ophthalmology. Screening examination of premature infants for retinopathy of prematurity [published erratum appears in Pediatrics 2006;117:572–6]. Pediatrics 2006;117:572–6.
3. Palmer EA, Flynn JT, Hardy RJ, et al. Incidence of early course of retinopathy of prematurity. Ophthalmology 1991;98: 1628–40.
4. Early Treatment for Retinopathy of Prematurity Cooperative Group. The incidence and course of retinopathy of prematurity: findings from the early treatment for retinopathy of prematurity study. Pediatrics 2005;116:15–23.

5. Early Treatment for Retinopathy of Prematurity Cooperative Group. Revised indications for the treatment of retinopathy of prematurity. Arch Ophthalmol 2003;121:1684–96.

6. Quinn GE, Dobson V, Barr CC, et al. Visual acuity of eyes after vitrectomy for retinopathy of prematurity. Follow-up at 5 1/2 years. Ophthalmology 1996;103:595–600.

7. Trese MT, Droste PJ. Long-term postoperative results of a consecutive series of stages 4 and 5 retinopathy of prematurity. Ophthalmology 1998;105:992–7.

8. Quinn GE, Dobson V, Repka MX, et al. Development of myopia in infants with birth weights less than 1251 grams. Ophthalmology 1992;99:329–40.

9. Page JM, Schneeweiss S, Whyte HE, Harvey P. Ocular sequelae in premature infants. Pediatrics 1993;92:787–90.

10. VanderVeen DK, Coats D, Dobson V, et al. The prevalence and course of strabismus in the first year of life for infants with prethreshold ROP: findings from the Early Treatment for Retinopathy of Prematurity study. Arch Ophthalmol 2006;124:766–73.

11. Phelps DL. Retinopathy of prematurity. Pediatr Clin North Am 1993;40:705–14.

12. Mirmanesh SJ, Abbasi S, Bhutani VK. Alpha-adrenergic bronchoprovocation in neonates with bronchopulmonary dysplasia. J Pediatr 1992;121:622–5.

13. Hermansen MC, Sullivan LS. Feeding intolerance following ophthalmologic examination. Am J Dis Child 1985;139:367–8.

ELEVEN

Intravenous Extravasation Injuries

Arin K. Greene, MD, MMSc, and
Charles A. Hergrueter, MD

- Although extravasation or infiltration is used to describe the leakage of intravenous (IV) fluid out of a vein and into the interstitial tissue, extravasation (Latin extra + vas vessel) is a more accurate term. Extravasation is the escape of fluid from a vessel or channel. Infiltration describes the permeation of tissues by fluid and can occur without extravasation (ie, subcutaneous injection). In the context of a catheter delivering IV fluid, infiltration cannot happen without extravasation.

- Approximately 11% of IV catheters in children cause extravasation. In the pediatric intensive care unit, the rate of extravasation is as high as 28%. Infants are at greater risk than children older than 12 months because of the fragility and small caliber of their peripheral veins, as well as their inability to verbalize discomfort. The risk of extravasation is dependent on the substance being delivered. For example, the extravasation rate for chemotherapeutic agents is 6.5%, whereas only 0.23% of patients have extravasation of IV contrast.

- Most IV extravasations involve small volumes of benign fluids (normal saline, lactated ringers, 5% dextrose) that do not cause morbidity. In one series of 1,800 IV extravasations, only 2.2% of extravasations resulted in skin injury, and no child had a compartment syndrome or required a skin graft.

- IV catheters are located in the superficial venous system, above the level of the muscle fascia. Thus, extravasations occur in the suprafascial space, and the risk of injury to deep structures, such as muscle, is low. However, depending on the type of the infiltrated substance, location of the injury, and volume of extravasated material, limb viability can be threatened. For example, deep catheters or extravasation of toxic substances (chemotherapeutic agents) can cause subfascial damage and compartment syndrome.

- Almost all IV extravasations are managed conservatively by removing the catheter, elevating the extremity, and then implementing local wound care if skin injury occurs. Currently, there are no randomized prospective studies in humans regarding the optimal management of IV extravasation injuries.
- Signs of an infiltrated catheter
  1. Cannot be flushed
  2. No return of blood
  3. Surrounding edema
- Complications of IV infiltration
  1. Minor: erythema, pain, swelling
  2. Moderate: partial or full-thickness skin injury
  3. Severe: compartment syndrome, muscle compromise, neurovascular damage

Mechanism of Damage

- Osmotic
  1. Urea, hypertonic fluids, cation solutions (calcium, potassium), hyperalimentation
  2. Osmolarity greater than serum can alter the osmotic gradient across the cell membrane leading to intracellular dehydration and cell death.
  3. Injury from computed tomography or magnetic resonance imaging contrast extravasation is dependent on the osmolarity of the contrast. In general, commonly used types of IV contrast have a favorable osmolarity, similar to serum. In one study, none of the 56 patients who suffered an IV contrast extravasation had tissue injury requiring intervention.
- Ischemia
  1. Vasopressors (dopamine and epinephrine)
  2. Cause local vasoconstriction leading to necrosis of the overlying skin and deep tissues

3. Long duration of extravasation is more problematic than the concentration of the drug.
4. Certain cation solutions (calcium and potassium) can cause ischemia by prolonged depolarization of capillary smooth muscle.

- Pressure necrosis
  1. Large volume extravasation, usually from an infusion pump, can lead to pressure-induced necrosis from the infiltrated fluid.
  2. Increased interstitial pressure leads to venous outflow obstruction followed by arterial insufficiency and local ischemia.

- Cellular toxicity
  1. Chemotherapeutic agents (adriamycin, methotrexate) cause the most severe extravasation injury because, in addition to pressure necrosis, they are directly cytotoxic to cells.
  2. Inhibition of DNA replication and the extent of injury are related to the drug concentration.
  3. Cation solutions (calcium and potassium) can cause protein precipitation, leading to cell death.

Prevention

- Most institutions require central venous access or peripheral venous shunts for the administration of caustic agents such as total parenteral nutrition, electrolyte solutions, or chemotherapeutic drugs.
- The risk and severity of extravasation is dependent on the location of the peripheral catheter.
  1. The dorsum of the hand and foot are prone to tissue damage from extravasation because of minimal subcutaneous tissue in these areas.
  2. The scalp is a common site for IV catheter placement in the neonate, and extravasation can cause alopecia.
  3. Areas near joints, such as the antecubital fossa, should be avoided in young children because the catheters are prone to malposition with motion.
- Mechanical pumps should not be used for the administration of IV therapies if possible.

    1. A delivery of no more than 20 pounds per square inch should be set to limit continued infusion in the event when the IV catheter becomes dislodged.

    2. Pressure alarms have not been shown to be effective.

- Frequent monitoring of the catheter site
    1. The IV site must be visible, not hidden under dressings or tape.
    2. Hourly assessment by primary nurse for signs of swelling, blanching, firmness, or leakage around the catheter. Decreased flow rates or difficulty flushing an IV catheter must be investigated.
    3. Daily assessments by the IV team

Physical Examination

- An assessment of skin injury should be made.
    1. Stage 1: erythema of the skin
    2. Stage 2: partial-thickness injury to the dermis (blistering)
    3. Stage 3: full-thickness skin injury into the subcutaneous tissue
    4. Stage 4: injury through all soft tissue with visible bone
- Investigation for deeper injury
    1. Palpate pulses and assess warmth and capillary refill of the extremity.
    2. Examine muscle compartments and evaluate active and passive range of motion.
    3. Signs of compartment syndrome: tenderness on palpation of fascial compartments, pain on passive flexion or extension, decreased range of motion, a fixed posture of the extremity, decreased sensation, reduced pulses (only a late finding).
    4. If physical exam findings suggest a compartment syndrome, then fascial compartment pressures can be measured. Fascial release is indicated for pressures greater than 30 mm Hg.

Initial Management

- Conservative management is the mainstay of treatment and is successful in 98% of extravasation injuries.

1. The catheter is aspirated and removed.
2. New IV catheters should not be inserted anywhere in the affected extremity.
3. Limb elevation above the level of the heart using pillows or an IV pole.
4. Splinting the extremity in a position of function will enhance venous return and promote edema reduction.
5. Serial examinations over the first 48 hours after injury

- The use of ice and heat is controversial. Ice is believed to limit the inflammatory reaction as well as the diffusion of the infiltrated substance by causing vasoconstriction. Heat is felt to stimulate the evacuation of the infiltrate through vasodilatation and increased blood flow. However, we do not advocate ice or heat because they may exacerbate the injury. For example, both ice and heat have been shown to worsen tissue damage after the extravasation of chemotherapeutic agents, depending on the type of drug. Heat can cause thermal injury and ice can cause an ischemia from vasoconstriction. Sensation in the extravasated area may be impaired and thus the patient may not be able to appreciate pain from the application of heat or ice. In addition, young children or intubated patients are unable to verbalize discomfort from hot or cold packs. Thus, heat or ice may cause a "second hit", converting a partial-thickness skin injury into a full-thickness wound, for example. *The most important maneuver to eliminate the extravasated fluid is elevation of the extremity.*

- Debridement after IV extravasation also is controversial. In general, we do not advocate debridement; *elevation and observation* is the best course of action. If skin injury is going to occur, conservative management will allow the area to demarcate, and the resulting wound then can be managed secondarily. Initial debridement may create a wound that would not have ever formed.

- The use of antidotes after IV extravasation also is controversial, and we generally do not recommend their use. Hyaluronidase, phentolamine, and nitroglycerin are the most commonly described antidotes for IV extravasations, but randomized prospective studies on their efficacy are not available. These can be injected through the infiltrated catheter before it is removed, administered subcutaneously, or applied topically. The antidotes such as isoproterenol, propranolol, dimethyl sulfoxide, sodium bicarbonate, and corticosteroids have not been proven effective in animal studies. If an antidote is to be effective, it must be administered *early*. Unfortunately, most extravasations are not appreciated immediately and by the time plastic surgical consultation arrives and the antidote is ordered and available for administration, the substance has already diffused or its effects have worn-off. For example, phentolamine, an alpha-adrenergic antagonist, has been used to treat epinephrine extravasation, but the effects of epinephrine wear off in 60 to 90 minutes, and the added volume of phentolamine has been shown to *worsen* tissue injury. Injection of an antidote increases the volume of fluid in the interstitial space and worsens pressure necrosis. In contrast to injectable antidotes, topical nitroglycerin for the treatment of extravasated vasopressors should not be harmful because it does not add volume to the infiltrate. Saline flushout, using stab incisions through which saline is flushed, also should not be harmful for the dilution and removal of harmful infiltrations because the stab incisions cause minimal morbidity and the added volume of saline escapes through the stab wounds.

Treatment of Wound Complications

- The true extent of tissue damage often is not appreciated initially. If skin damage is to occur, it will become evident by 72 hours after the initial insult.
- Partial-thickness skin injuries
  1. Managed by topical antibiotic ointments or dressings
  2. Typically heal without scarring by epitheliazation in 7 to 14 days.
- Full-thickness skin injuries
  1. Dry eschars are managed with topical antibiotic ointments and dressings.
  2. Debridement is indicated for necrotic tissue to reduce the risk of infection and to facilitate healing by secondary intention. Following debridement, damp-to-dry saline dressing changes twice daily are used.

3. Small full-thickness skin injuries are allowed to heal secondarily. Large wounds may require skin grafting or flap closure to expedite healing or to prevent functional limitations due to contractures or hypertrophic scarring.

More Aggressive Interventions

- The most serious complication of an IV extravasation is compartment syndrome. This occurs when injury to tissues beneath the muscle fascia cause swelling. Because the subfascial compartments are tight spaces, swelling can first occlude deep venous outflow and ultimately arterial inflow leading to myonecrosis. Muscle is extremely sensitive to ischemia, and irreversible damage occurs after 6 hours of hypoperfusion.
- If physical examination findings of compartment syndrome exist, then emergent operative release of the involved compartments is indicated. By incising the fascia during the compartment release, the underlying tissues may swell without constriction thus preserving adequate venous and arterial flow.

Recommended Readings

Brown AS, Hoelzer DJ, Piercy SA. Skin necrosis from extravasation of intravenous fluid in children. Plast Reconstr Surg 1979;64:145–50.

Cohan RH, Bullard MA, Ellis JH, et al. Local reactions after injection of iodinated contrast material: detection, management, and outcome. Acad Radiol 1997;4:711–8.

Ener RA, Meglathery SB, Styler M. Extravasation of systemic hemato-oncological therapies. Ann Oncol 2004;15:858–62.

Friedman J. Plastic surgical problems in the neonatal intensive care unit. Clin Plast Surg 1998;25:599–17.

Garland JS, Dunne WM, Havens P, et al. Peripheral intravenous catheter complications in critically ill children: a prospective study. Pediatrics 1992;89:1145–50.

Gault DT. Extravasation injuries. Br J Plast Surg 1993;46:91–6.

Greene AK. Management of epinephrine injection injury to the digit. Plast Reconstr Surg 2005;115:1800–1.

Harris PA, Bradley S, Moss ALH. Limiting the damage of iatrogenic extravasation injury in neonates. Plast Reconstr Surg 2001;107:893–4.

Mathes SJ, Hentz VR. Plastic Surgery. St. Louis (MO): Elsevier; 2006.

Upton J, Mulliken JB, Murray JE. Major intravenous extravasation injuries. Am J Surg 1979;137:497–506.

Yilmaz M, Demirdover C, Mola F. Treatment options in extravasation injury: an experimental study in rats. Plast Reconstr Surg 2002;109:2418–23.

TWELVE

Orthopedic Considerations in the Surgical Neonate

Michael P. Glotzbecker, MD, and
John B. Emans, MD

General Considerations

Although rarely life- or limb-threatening, orthopedic abnormalities are commonly encountered in the neonatal setting. Some deformities will be purely postural, are a result of months of intrauterine positioning, and will correct without treatment with normal development. However, recognition of other abnormalities is critically important because when discovered these may be most easily treated in the newborn period. Knowledge of the appropriate care of orthopedic conditions can simplify the task of the neonatologist while reassuring the parents. Although some situations, such as the isolated clavicular fracture without associated brachial plexus or vascular injury, may not require orthopedic consultation, most musculoskeletal pathology encountered in the newborn nursery or neonatal intensive care unit (ICU) should be followed by an orthopedic surgeon to optimize the long-term result.

Neural tube defects, congenital scoliosis and kyphosis, positional or congenital foot abnormalities, limb deficiencies or abnormalities, and many skeletal dysplasias can be diagnosed prenatally by ultrasonography. Prenatal knowledge of such problems is helpful, facilitating prenatal parental education and postnatal specialist care. Prenatal consultation with the appropriate specialists helps families understand possible postnatal care and long-term disability and helps to lessen the surprises and disappointment associated with the discovery of a congenital musculoskeletal problem. Early diagnosis also allows for consideration of fetal surgery. Surgical intervention in utero to correct structural abnormalities holds promise in several fields, orthopedics notwithstanding. However, its role is controversial in nonfatal conditions, given the possible risk to the fetus and mother and early results of fetal surgery in myelodysplasia have been met with guarded enthusiasm.

The development of the musculoskeletal system begins at approximately 12 days of gestation, as cells migrate between endoderm and ectoderm to form mesoderm in a caudal to cephalad progression. Between days 5 and 20 of gestation, the ectoderm differentiates into the notochord at the cephalad end of the primitive streak. The paraxial mesoderm, located on both sides of the neural tube, subsequently undergoes segmentation in a cephalad to caudad progression, forming somites, transitional embryonic organs that eventually disintegrate, and give rise to both axial and appendicular connective, muscular, and skeletal structures. Development of the vertebral column and limbs occurs concurrently with the creation of many of the other major organ systems, including the renal, cardiac, gastrointestinal, and hematologic systems. Understanding this developmental timing is important to the neonatologist, as musculoskeletal abnormalities are often quite obvious, and disruption of musculoskeletal development may prompt evaluation for other systemic abnormalities.

Skeletal Birth Trauma–Fractures and Dislocations

GENERAL CONSIDERATIONS

Pseudoparalysis is the most common manifestation of underlying musculoskeletal birth trauma. Management of birth fractures, like all neonatal fractures, is almost always nonoperative. Diagnosing the cause of lack of voluntary motion of an arm or leg can be challenging and subtle. Nonmusculoskeletal causes of musculoskeletal malfunction such as cerebral hemorrhage and other intracranial processes or infection must also be considered in the differential diagnosis of pseudoparalysis. Physeal fractures may be difficult to recognize radiographically because there is no calcification of the epiphysis to show the displacement of epiphysis relative to metaphysis. The limb may appear deformed or the joint may appear dislocated or swollen, whereas the true pathology is a fracture through the physis. Clinical examination, ultrasonography, arthrography, and magnetic resonance imaging (MRI) can be useful in the diagnosis of physeal fractures. Furthermore, multiple fractures in the neonate should prompt investigation of a systemic condition such as osteogenesis imperfecta or should raise suspicion for possible nonaccidental trauma, especially if the baby has been discharged from the hospital. Neonatal joint sepsis may manifest as joint dislocation or epiphyseal separation, further confusing the apparent diagnosis of trauma.

Embryology

CLAVICLE

The clavicle is the first bone in the body to begin ossification, and the medial physis of the clavicle is the last to close during growth and development. Ossification begins by the fifth or sixth week of gestation, and by the eighth week of gestation its general "S"-shaped pattern has been established. Fusion of the epiphysis to the shaft may occur as late as 23 to 25 years of age.

HUMERUS

The proximal humeral epiphysis is not ossified to any appreciable extent until 6 months after birth. The diaphysis, however, has begun ossification and should be visible on plain radiographs in full-term infants.

FEMUR

Endochondral ossification begins around the eighth week of gestation from a single proximal femoral physis, with medial growth exceeding lateral growth, giving rise to the characteristic elongated femoral neck. The capital femoral epiphysis does not ossify until approximately 4 months of age in females and slightly later in males. The trochanteric apophysis does not ossify until almost 4 years of age.

SPINE

Developmental anatomy of the spine is complex, with each vertebra arising from multiple ossification centers. Ossification becomes evident in the vertebral arches during the eighth week. At birth, there is typically a radiographically visible centrum, or ossification center in the middle of the developing vertebral body, and a visible center in each of the neural arches. The three bony parts are connected by cartilage.

Incidence and Etiology

CLAVICLE

Clavicular fractures represent the most common musculoskeletal birth trauma, occurring in as many as 5% of all births. Clavicle fractures account for nearly 90% of all obstetrical fractures. Specific factors identified as predictive of clavicular fracture include vaginal delivery, prolonged gestation, epidural anesthesia, forceps delivery, shoulder dystocia, macrosomia, and the experience of the obstetrician. Despite this, efforts at predicting clavicular fractures based on predelivery factors have been largely unsuccessful.

HUMERUS

- Proximal humerus: Injuries to the proximal humeral physis, though not as common as clavicular fractures, can occur as the arm is placed in a variety of abnormal positions during a vaginal delivery. Hyperextension or forceful rotation of the affected arm is hypothesized to generate the forces necessary to fracture through the proximal humeral physis. Although seen in newborns of all obstetric presentations, breech positioning and macrosomia in particular are considered risk factors for proximal humeral fracture.
- Humeral diaphysis: Fractures of the humeral diaphysis are rare, with an incidence of between 0.035 and 0.34% of live births. This injury may occur with maneuvers to bring the arm down during version and extraction with the upper extremities in an overhead position, particularly with breech presentations.

FEMUR

Fractures of the femur are uncommon in the newborn period and should raise concerns regarding abuse or fragile bone. Twin pregnancies, breech presentation, and prematurity may be associated with this injury.

SPINE

With the exception of breech positioning, injury to the newborn's spine in the absence of abuse is decidedly uncommon. Breech deliveries can be associated with injury to the lower cervical or upper thoracic spine, with traction as the supposed mechanism. Cephalic deliveries, on the other hand, can produce upper cervical spine injury with rotation as the putative mechanism.

PRENATAL DIAGNOSIS AND TREATMENT

Efforts at predicting clavicular or proximal humeral fractures based on predelivery factors have been largely unsuccessful.

Postnatal Diagnosis

CLAVICLE

As with any fracture at any age, the standard signs of injury include swelling, deformity, and eventually warmth and bruising over the site of the fracture. Although it is normally easy to palpate the clavicular margins in the newborn, swelling associated with fracture can make this palpation difficult. Also, in the setting of generalized edema, palpation of the normal clavicular margins may be difficult. Pseudoparalysis, characterized by voluntary splinting or immobilization of the ipsilateral arm, may also be present as the infant attempts to limit movement on the affected side to minimize pain. This is frequently mistaken for a brachial plexus palsy. Infants may also turn their heads toward the affected side, thereby relaxing the ipsilateral sternocleidomastoid muscle (SCM) and reducing its pull on the fractured clavicle. A fractured clavicle in the acute setting can also generate an asymmetric Moro's reflex. Frequently, the presence of a mass (healing fracture callus) over the clavicle 7 to 10 days after the initial trauma confirms the diagnosis. After clinical evaluation, diagnosis is by plain radiographs (often as an incidental finding). Ultrasonography can also be useful in establishing this diagnosis, particularly when plain radiographs are normal yet a suspicion of clavicular fracture remains.

Differential diagnosis includes proximal humeral fracture, congenital pseudoarthrosis of the clavicle, brachial plexus injury, sternoclavicular joint dislocation, and septic arthritis. Concern about septic arthritis or neurovascular injury accompanying clavicular fracture or failure of standard imaging techniques to show the diagnosis should prompt orthopedic consultation.

HUMERUS

- Proximal humerus: Although presentation can be subtle, refusal to use the ipsilateral extremity and irritability when the ipsilateral extremity is manipulated suggest proximal humeral injury. Swelling and ecchymosis may be present, as well as tenderness in the region of the proximal humerus. A proximal humerus fracture may also present as a pseudoparalysis. An asymmetric Moro's reflex may be present. As the proximal humeral epiphysis does not appear on plain radiographs until approximately 6 months of age, ultrasonography (or MRI) can be invaluable in establishing the diagnosis of proximal humeral fracture in the neonate. A physeal fracture may appear to be and be mis-read on plain radiograph as dislocation (pseudo-dislocation). Physeal fracture is significantly more common than a true traumatic dislocation, as most dislocations in the neonatal period are only found in babies with underlying birth trauma to the brachial plexus or central nervous system.
- Humeral diaphysis: Swelling, erythema, and ecchymosis may be apparent over the diaphyseal region of the affected brachium. Presentation may also include a pseudoparalysis or an asymmetric Moro's reflex. A humeral diaphysis fracture is diagnosable by plain radiographs. Differential diagnosis includes septic arthritis, clavicular fracture, brachial plexus injury, and posterior dislocation of the glenohumeral joint.

FEMUR

Swelling may be present in the thigh and pseudoparalysis present in the affected extremity. Diagnosis is by plain radiographs.

Dislocation of the ipsilateral hip and septic arthritis should be considered.

SPINE

The newborn with injury to the spine may present with respiratory distress of unclear etiology (eg, in the case of cervical spine injury), abnormal motor response, hypotonia, or hypertonia. Plain radiographs, consisting of antero-posterior and lateral views, should be obtained. MRI may be useful in select cases when plain radiographs are unremarkable yet a suspicion remains. Of note, MRI has the advantage of showing spinal cord and other soft tissue anomalies. Brachial plexus injury and intracranial pathology should be considered.

Management

CLAVICLE

Treatment of the isolated clavicular fracture is nonoperative and does not generally require orthopedic consultation. Regardless of the degree of immobilization, the fracture typically stabilizes 7 to 10 days following injury. Using a safety pin to fasten the ipsilateral sleeve to the torso of the baby's garment provides adequate immobilization for comfort and healing to take place.

HUMERUS

Orthopedic consultation should be obtained.

- Proximal humerus: The potential for remodeling is tremendous in the newborn, and treatment typically consists of immobilization using a safety pin to attach the sleeve of the affected extremity to the torso of the baby's garment. In rare cases of severe epiphyseal displacement reported by ultrasonographic studies, gentle bedside reduction with minimal anesthesia, followed by ultrasonographic confirmation of reduction may be necessary. These fractures should be stable within 7 to 10 days and completely healed in 2 to 3 weeks.
- Humeral diaphysis: Treatment consists of immobilization as neonatal fractures of the diaphysis have remarkable remodeling capacity. Up to 70 degrees of angulation and total displacement

can be accepted and expected to remodel. Reported treatments include a sling and swathe or a traction device using a von Rosen splint. However, to prevent the loss of external rotation that can result from healing in an internally rotated position, the extremity should be splinted in a position of extension along the patient's torso. The affected extremity can be secured to the neonate's torso with a loose wrap if needed.

FEMUR

Orthopedic consultation should be obtained. Fractures of the femoral diaphysis have tremendous potential for remodeling and are stabilized to some degree by a thick periosteal sleeve and the adjacent thigh musculature. If the fracture is minimally angulated, then splinting will most likely suffice and should be continued for 2 to 3 weeks. For a stable fracture, this is likely to be sufficient, and will allow access to the feet if needed. To prevent worsening of fracture angulation, care must be taken to avoid ending the splint near the fracture site. For more severely angulated fractures, particularly those of the proximal and midshaft femoral diaphysis, application of a Pavlik harness can be a successful mode of treatment. The harness keeps the hip in flexion and abduction and usually produces acceptable alignment. One disadvantage of the Pavlik harness is that it may make venous access to the baby's feet difficult. Acceptable amounts of angulation include 30 to 40 degrees of anteroposterior angulation, 10 to 15 degrees of varus angulation, up to 30 degrees of valgus angulation, and no more than 10 degrees of rotational malalignment.

Although rare, fractures that shorten excessively (more than 1 to 2 cm) and those with excessive residual angulation after treatment in a Pavlik harness may demand more complex modes of treatment such as spica cast application or skeletal traction, both of which place a demand on the nursery or ICU staff. Overhead traction, or so called "Bryant's" traction consists of gentle longitudinal overhead traction applied to both legs. This permits easy nursing care for the infant, but arranging a traction apparatus may be difficult around incubators and other equipment. It is also associated with some risk of skin injury and compartment syndrome, as it requires circumferential wrapping of the legs.

SPINE

Urgent orthopedic consultation should be obtained. The head should be supported in such a manner to maintain appropriate spinal alignment. The occiput should rest on a surface inferior to the surface of the back to prevent inadvertent flexion of the cervical spine because of the proportionately large head of the infant. Treatment is typically nonoperative, consisting of proper alignment and relative immobilization of the infant. If the spinal injury is unstable or associated with neurologic injury, operative intervention may be needed.

Complications and Outcomes

CLAVICLE

Nonunion of fractures in this age group is extremely rare. Caretakers and parents should be cautioned to avoid unnecessary movement of the affected extremity to prevent causing pain to the patient. Parents should be informed that the infant would develop a mass, which is healing callus, over the fracture site that will typically resolve within 6 months.

HUMERUS

Caretakers and parents should be cautioned to avoid unnecessary movement of the affected extremity to prevent causing pain to the patient.

- Proximal humerus: Fractures of the proximal humeral epiphysis heal rapidly and typically do not leave functional or cosmetic defects. A rare, late complication of a proximal humerus fracture in the newborn is that of humerus varus, in which there is a significant reduction in the humeral neck-shaft angle, producing shortening of the extremity and mild limitation in shoulder abduction. Fortunately, the mild functional deficits resulting from this deformity do not generally need later surgical correction. Osteonecrosis of the humeral head is an extremely rare complication of proximal humerus fractures in this age group.

- Humeral diaphysis: Humeral shaft fractures in the neonate almost always heal and remodel, with up to 40 to 50% remodeling within 2 years. Loss of external rotation resulting from mal-union in an internally rotated position is the most common potential complication. This can be avoided by splinting the extremity with the elbow in extension. Up to a 15 degree loss of external rotation can easily be tolerated without functional compromise.

FEMUR

The vast majority of femoral fractures heals and remodel, resulting in restoration of normal anatomy regardless of treatment method.

Short-term complications of the treatment of femoral shaft fractures derive from the treatment modalities employed. Hip spica casts can cause respiratory embarrassment, lead to skin breakdown beneath the cast, make hygiene problematic, and access to an ill neonate difficult. Skeletal traction requires meticulous care to ensure that traction is applied along the correct vector and that pin sites are kept clean. The usual circumferential wrapping of the legs for traction in Bryant's overhead traction carries a risk of compartment syndrome, requiring careful monitoring, as well as intermittent wrapping and unwrapping of the legs.

Although a femur fracture often shortens and may lead to a limb that is shorter than the contralateral side, healing at the site of a femoral diaphyseal fracture may result in growth acceleration of the affected limb that can cause a leg length discrepancy. The average amount of overgrowth of the injured limb is 0.9 cm, with a range from 0.4 to 2.5 cm. This may or may not produce relative lengthening of the injured side, depending on the amount of shortening that was accepted during treatment. Growth acceleration is uncommon after infant femur fractures, but is expected after femur fractures occurring from age 18 months to 10 years.

Excessive residual varus angulation of the femur can lead to a hypoplastic lateral femoral condyle and a valgus deformity at the knee. Particularly severe cases may need to be corrected with osteotomy later in life.

SPINE

Paresis or paralysis can be short-term complications. Recovery is variable. Post-traumatic syringomyelia may occur late after spinal cord injury. Progressive scoliosis with growth is a nearly universal complication if paralysis persists.

Brachial Plexus Injury

EMBRYOLOGY

Motor nerve fibers arising from the spinal cord appear near the end of the fourth week of gestation. Nerve fibers arise from the developing spinal cord from cells in the basal plates, emerging as a continuous series of rootlets along its ventrolateral surface. The fibers for a developing muscle group become arranged in a bundle (ventral nerve root). Neural crest cells migrate to the dorsolateral aspect of the spinal cord where they differentiate into cells of the spinal ganglion. The distal processes of these cells join the ventral nerve root to create a spinal nerve. The ventral primary ramus contributes to the innervation of the limbs and ventrolateral parts of the body wall. The nerves from the spinal cord segments opposite each limb bud elongate and grow into the limb. Nerve fibers are distributed to muscles and the skin in a segmental manner. Early in development, successive ventral primary rami are joined by connecting loops of nerve fibers to form plexuses that supply the limbs (such as the brachial plexus). The dorsal divisions of these plexuses supply the extensor surface of the limbs, whereas the ventral divisions of the trunks supply the flexor muscles. Although typically the brachial plexus is composed of the nerve roots of C5-T1, 22% of cases have a prefixed cord in which there is a contribution of C4, and 1% of cases have a postfixed cord in which there is a contribution from T2.

Incidence and Etiology

Brachial plexus injury is estimated to occur in 0.1 to 0.4% of live births. The incidence increases to between 8 and 23% of live births complicated by shoulder dystocia. Perinatal risk factors include large size for gestational age, multiparous pregnancy, prolonged labor, and difficult delivery.

Shoulder dystocia in the setting of vertex presentation can occur if the shoulders retain a strict antero-posterior orientation in relation to the maternal pelvis instead of a more physiologic obliquity. The anterior shoulder is then compressed against the symphysis pubis, and downward traction during delivery is translated into traction on the anterior brachial plexus. It is also possible for the posteriorly oriented brachial plexus to be injured via compression against the sacral promontory. Difficult arm or head extraction in breech deliveries also increases the risk of neural injury.

Almost 80% of brachial plexus injuries involve the C5–C6 roots, known as "Erb-Duchenne palsy." These injuries are typically postganglionic and have a relatively good prognosis for full recovery. Upper trunk injuries following breech delivery, however, can be preganglionic and have a more guarded prognosis. Similarly, the less commonly seen injuries to the lower C8–T1 roots, known as "Klumpke's" palsy, are typically preganglionic and have a lower rate of full recovery. Preganglionic lesions are avulsions from the spinal cord, which will not spontaneously recover. It is uncommon to see involvement of the entire brachial plexus.

Prenatal Diagnosis and Treatment

Risk factors associated with birth brachial plexopathy include shoulder dystocia, macrosomia, prolonged second stage of labor, and method of delivery (increased incidence with midforceps and vacuum extraction). Nevertheless, brachial plexus injury has been observed in the absence of all of these risk factors.

Postnatal Diagnosis

Diminished spontaneous movement of the affected extremity will be present from the time of birth. Flaccid paralysis is highly suggestive of brachial plexus injury. Presentation can be bilateral.

The level of neurologic involvement should be determined by physical examination. Spontaneous movement of specific muscle groups should be documented including shoulder abduction, internal and external rotation, elbow flexion/extension, wrist flexion/extension, and finger motion. The newborn may have asymmetric primitive reflexes (Moro and tonic neck). Provocative testing by stimulating these neonatal reflexes to induce elbow flexion and wrist and digital extension is useful in establishing a diagnosis. The presence of a Horner's syndrome (ptosis, miosis, anhidrosis, and enophthalmos) should be documented as this indicative of a preganglionic injury and therefore predicts a worse natural history. The presence of an elevated hemidiaphragm (phrenic nerve) or a winged scapula (long thoracic nerve) may also suggest that there has been a preganglionic injury to the plexus. Several classification systems have been developed to assess the severity of brachial plexus injury and help predict the need for microsurgical intervention.

Diagnosis can be confirmed through serial examinations and elimination of other possible etiologies. It is imperative to rule out common causes of pseudoparalysis such as a clavicle fracture, proximal humeral fracture, or septic arthritis (particularly when spontaneous upper extremity movement is present at birth and later diminishes), cervical spine injury, and intracranial pathology such as an ischemic insult to the brain. Electromyography and nerve conduction velocity testing most likely do not have a place in the immediate neonatal setting.

Management

If brachial plexus injury is suspected based on birth history and presentation, orthopedic consultation should be obtained. Conditions requiring emergent surgical intervention such as septic arthritis should be ruled out.

In the United States, microsurgical or other invasive intervention in the immediate newborn period is uncommon because the majority of brachial plexus injuries resolve during the first few months of life. Current recommendations include observation and serial examinations until age 3 months. This is because longitudinal studies have reported that if normal biceps function fails to return by 3 months of age, the outcome at 2 years is generally abnormal. During this time, a physical therapist should be consulted to assist with passive range of motion of all affected joints. Perhaps, most important among these joints is the glenohumeral joint, which one should move passively while taking care to stabilize the scapulotho-racic articulation. The infant affected by a brachial plexus injury is at risk for the development of glenohumeral capsular contraction, which is more difficult to treat than to prevent.

For the infant who fails to show adequate recovery, potential surgical interventions include microsurgery (typically performed around 3 months of age), tendon releases and transfers (for children ages 2 to 7 years), and osteotomies (for older children).

Complications and Outcomes

Joint stiffness of the affected extremity can develop if passive range of motion is not instituted in a timely fashion.

Prognosis varies with the level of the lesion (preganglionic versus postganglionic), degree of involvement (ie, number of nerve roots involved), presence or absence of Horner's syndrome, and amount of recovery observed at 2 to 3 months of age. There is consensus that several factors consistently predict poor outcome: total plexus involvement, C5–C7 involvement, and/or the presence of Horner's syndrome. The majority of patients affected will show significant recovery by age 2 months and will subsequently enjoy normal function through childhood and adulthood.

In patients who fail to recover complete function, there will frequently be an internal rotation contracture of the shoulder, which may lead to subsequent posterior dislocation of the gleno-humeral joint. Muscle transfers used to augment external rotation can be used successfully in children aged 2 to 7 and result in functional improvements. An external rotation osteotomy of the humerus in older children also successfully restores global shoulder function in patients with an internal rotation contracture at the shoulder.

Musculoskeletal Infection

GENERAL CONSIDERATIONS

Compared with other children, neonates have an immature host defense mechanism. Those admitted to the neonatal ICU are at even heightened risk of infection, and therefore osteomyelitis, both because of the underlying disease process prompting admission and the increased exposure to invasive procedures, diagnosis is challenging, as the neonate will often present with nonspecific signs. The usual markers of musculoskeletal infection such as fever, reluctance to move an extremity or joint swelling are commonly absent in the neonate requiring ICU care owing to the compromised status of the child, sedation for ventilatory control, etc. More common sources of infection (pneumonia, line sepsis) may both seed and obscure the musculoskeletal infection. The microbiology of offending organisms is also different in the neonatal population, resulting in different first line treatment choices.

Embryology

The synovial membrane is a distinct anatomic structure separate from the joint capsule. The main arterial supply travels through the fibrous capsule into the synovium where rapid division forms an intercommunicating network, allowing rapid transfer of both antibiotics and bacteria from the arterial vessels into the joint. The metaphyses of long bones are areas of relative venous stasis in the skeletal system that can potentially harbor bacteria. Furthermore, until approximately age 8 to 18 months, there is continuity of metaphyseal sinusoids through the developing physis into the epiphysis, ending in epiphyseal venous lakes and giving pathogens access to the joint via a pre-epiphyseal osteomyelitic focus. An estimated 70% of cases of osteomyelitis involve concomitant seeding of the adjacent joint in the neonate.

Incidence and Etiology

SEPTIC ARTHRITIS

Incidence is 0.12 per 1,000 live births and 0.67 per 1,000 admissions to the neonatal ICU. Risk factors include presence of an indwelling intravenous catheter or umbilical catheter, prematurity, ventilator dependence, and concomitant systemic sepsis as reported through positive blood culture. Maternal gonococcal infection may be an additional risk factor.

Septic arthritis occurs as a result of hematogenous seeding, local spread form contiguous infection, or primary seeding of a joint secondary to trauma or surgery. Metaphyses of long bones in four joints (hip, shoulder, ankle, and elbow) have an intrarticular component, and therefore allow for seeding of the joint from a metaphyseal osteomyclitis. Bacterial infection of the joint space leads to an inflammatory effusion that leads to articular destruction through the release of proteolytic enzymes.

The most common organism in pediatric septic arthritis is *Staphylococcus aureus* (56%) followed by group A strep (22%), *S. pneumoniae* (6%), other gram-negative organisms and *Neisseria gonorrheae*. In the neonate, group B β-hemolytic streptococcus and gram-negative bacilli are common infecting agents in addition to *S. aureus*.

OSTEOMYELITIS

The reported incidence of neonatal osteomyelitis is 1 to 3 per 1,000 neonatal hospital admissions. Both trauma and bacteremia contribute to the development of osteomyelitis. Risk factors are similar to those listed for septic arthritis, although an additional consideration is repeated heel sticks in the neonate. There are several reported cases of osteomyelitis of the os calcis secondary to repeated heel sticks.

Infection begins at the metaphyseal venous sinusoid, where there is a change from high-flow arterioles to low-flow sinusoids. This occurs in a region with few reticuloendothelial cells available for phagocytosis. Thrombosis of vessels suppresses the delivery of immune cells, and subsequently an exudate is created. This may result in a periosteal abscess or seeding of an adjacent joint. The most common sites for acute hemolytic osteomyelitis are the growing ends of long bones such as the distal femur, proximal tibia, distal humerus, and distal radius.

It is important to note that the most common organisms that affect neonates are different than those that affect other children with osteomyelitis. Though *Staphylococcus aureus* remains the most common offending organism in neonates, Group B β-hemolytic streptococcus, gram-negative enterics, and *Candida* have a much higher incidence in neonates when compared with older children.

VERTEBRAL OSTEOMYELITIS

Intervertebral disk infection and vertebral osteomyelitis are exceedingly uncommon in the neonate. When infection does occur, younger children are more susceptible to diskitis because their disks have a rich arterial blood supply that is derived from the vertebral body. In older children and adults, this blood supply is limited.

Prenatal Diagnosis and Treatment

Prolonged rupture of membranes, maternal colonization/infection, and premature labor may put a newborn at increased risk for osteomyelitis. The presence of these risk factors in a newborn should increase the index of suspicion when considering the diagnosis of osteomyelitis.

Postnatal Presentation and Diagnosis

- Unlike childhood or adult musculoskeletal sepsis, the typical signs of fever, bony tenderness, limp, and diminished voluntary motion may not be apparent in the infant in an ICU setting. Sedated infants on respirators may not show asymmetric motion of extremities. Fever may be reported as temperature instability or be completely absent. Nevertheless, fever, pseudoparalysis of the affected limb, irritability with passive motion, tenderness to palpation, and swelling over the involved site remain valuable clues to the possibility of osteomyelitis or joint sepsis. Poor feeding may be another nonspecific clue to the diagnosis. Although rare, patients with vertebral osteomyelitis may present with relatively unimpeded spontaneous movement of the upper extremities, although flexion and extension of the hip joints may produce irritability given the pull that this motion exerts on the iliopsoas muscle. Infants with vertebral osteomyelitis may become irritable when placed on their backs or simply repositioned. Advanced studies such as MRI are often necessary to show such infections.
- An orthopedic surgeon should be consulted on an urgent basis to confirm the diagnosis of septic arthritis and to perform aspiration of suspicious joints or subperiosteal fluid

collections to obtain cultures to direct antibiotic treatment. Musculoskeletal infection is commonly multifocal in the newborn in the neonatal ICU. All suspicious joints should be aspirated. In the case of osteomyelitis, reported yields from subperiosteal aspiration approach 90%. Depending on the center, aspiration of the hip may be facilitated by an interventional radiologist. A joint fluid white blood cell count greater than 50,000 or a positive gram stain suggests the diagnosis of septic arthritis.

- A generalized evaluation for sepsis should be obtained, including blood, urine, and sputum cultures; complete blood count with differential; baseline erythrocyte sedimentation rate; and C-reactive protein. Of note, the infant may be too ill to generate a leukocytosis. Blood cultures are positive in up to 50% of patients.

Imaging may include ultrasound, plain radiographs, or MRI.

1. Ultrasonography of suspicious areas may accurately diagnose periosteal elevation or abscess formation and can show effusions present in the hip, shoulder, and other joints. It can be a useful modality for guiding aspiration of joints or subperiosteal collections. It is the first line imaging study for the diagnosis of septic arthritis of the hip.

2. Early findings with plain radiography include blurring of soft tissue planes surrounding the affected site. Plain radiographs may also show subluxation or dislocation of an affected joint secondary to increased intracapsular pressure and distention from a fluid collection. Bony resorption (relative osteopenia) and periosteal elevation develop after 7 to 10 days. Visualization of bony resorption on plain radiographs requires a 30 to 50% loss of bone mineralization.

3. Bone scan can be misleading in the newborn. The normal physes of infants are extremely active on bone scan and may obscure an adjacent bone reaction. Also, bone scan may be cold if bony destruction has already taken place in patients with osteomyelitis of sufficient duration. However, bone scintigraphy using technetium 99m methylene diphosphonate can be useful in identifying multiple foci and will typically show pathology at 24 to 48 hours after onset.

4. MRI may be the earliest and most sensitive diagnostic tool. It will show early marrow edema, subperiosteal fluid, or bony destruction. Its requirement for transport from the neonatal intensive care setting, however, limits its feasibility for unstable infants.

- The differential diagnosis should include neoplasm, vascular malformation, fracture, and purulent myositis.

Management

GENERAL CONSIDERATIONS

Awareness of musculoskeletal infection as a possible diagnosis and appreciation for the risk of irrevocable harm to growth plates and joints is pivotal. Emergent orthopedic consultation is mandatory. Delay in diagnosis and institution of appropriate antibiotic therapy and/or surgical drainage and debridement carries with it a higher long-term morbidity for the infant. An infectious disease consultation should also be obtained. Clinical management guidelines are available for both osteomyelitis and septic arthritis. Aspiration of the affected part and blood cultures before initiation or change in treatment will increase the specificity and likelihood of success of antibiotic treatment.

SEPTIC ARTHRITIS

Once appropriate cultures have been obtained, antibiotics should be started. If the neonate is suffering from generalized sepsis, then administration of potentially life-saving antibiotic therapy should not be delayed in anticipation of aspiration or open biopsy. In lieu of culture and sensitivity results, general recommendations are to treat the neonate with appropriate coverage against *Staphylococcus*, Group B *Streptococcus,* and possible gram-negative bacilli (ie, cefazolin or oxacillin plus an aminoglycoside).

Urgent, open surgical drainage is often mandatory for the hip and shoulder and possibly elbow to minimize the risk of secondary avascular necrosis of the secondary centers of ossification of these joints, which reside wholly within the joint. Open drainage may be preferred in other joints, or repeated aspiration may suffice along with parenteral antibiotics, provided there is appropriate response, typically within approximately 48 hours.

OSTEOMYELITIS

Palpable subperiosteal fluid collections and those identified by ultrasonography or MRI should be aspirated. Soft metaphyseal areas of affected long bones can usually be aspirated directly with an 18-gauge needle, as one is readily able to penetrate the cortex. Antibiotics should be instituted, and in the absence of an adequate response to antibiotic therapy, open debridement of affected bone should take place. If the periosteal sleeve remains intact, even relatively large areas of bone may be able to reconstitute themselves following debridement. Because neonates have a poor absorption of oral antibiotics, they require a full 4 to 6 weeks of parenteral antibiotics.

VERTEBRAL OSTEOMYELITIS/DISKITIS

Isolated vertebral osteomyelitis is uncommon in infants and often not recognized until associated with psoas abscess or epidural abscess, which require drainage. Diskitis is more commonly encountered in childhood and most patients with diskitis can be successfully treated with antibiotics. A biopsy is indicated in atypical patients or when there is a poor response to antibiotics.

Complications and Outcomes

Osteomyelitis or septic arthritis in the neonate can be devastating in the long term. Neonates have substantially thinner cortex and more loosely adherent periosteum, which easily allows infection to track into adjacent joints. Recurrent and/or multifocal septic arthritis and osteomyelitis may occur and serve as a source for generalized sepsis. Chronic osteomyelitis, sequestrum, and involucrum formation is uncommon in the neonate. Poor outcome is associated with delay in diagnosis and a subsequent delay in treatment and principally relates to the long-term problem of growth disturbance and joint cartilage destruction.

Damage from musculoskeletal sepsis in infancy may profoundly alter subsequent growth and development of the musculoskeletal system. Prolonged sepsis in diarthrodial joints will frequently cause degenerative changes and may lead to premature stiffness and degenerative arthritis. Of equal significance is the potential for damage to growth plates or growing epiphyses. Established sepsis may destroy the sensitive, growing portion of the physis leading to retarded physeal growth and severe discrepancy in extremity length or asymmetric growth with angular deformity.

Orthopedic Congenital Deformities

"CONGENITAL" MUSCULAR TORTICOLLIS (WRYNECK)

Incidence and Etiology

Congenital muscular torticollis, also known as "wryneck," is a relatively common finding in the newborn period with a reported incidence ranging from 0.3 to 2%. The right hand side is more commonly affected. The condition is seen more commonly in the first born and carries with it a 20% association with developmental dysplasia of the hip and a 15% association with metatarsus adductus (both also thought to be intrauterine deformations). There is a strong correlation between torticollis and breech/assisted delivery as well as birth trauma.

The term "congenital" is a misnomer because the etiology of congenital muscular torticollis is unknown and may come from prenatal or postnatal causes. The etiology may include a component of intrauterine compartment syndrome involving one of the SCMs, more commonly on the right side. This intrauterine compartment syndrome gives rise to a fibrotic and contracted SCM, which, in turn, exerts an abnormal pull on the infant's head. Histologic and MRI studies have reported muscle atrophy and interstitial fibrosis in this condition. Other theories regarding its etiology include intrauterine crowding or a vascular phenomenon, a primary myopathy of the SCM, or fibrosis from peripartum bleeds associated with tearing of the muscle during childbirth. Paroxysmal torticollis of infancy has been linked to a calcium channel mutation.

PRENATAL DIAGNOSIS AND TREATMENT

Prenatal detection has little role in this disorder.

Postnatal Diagnosis

Congenital muscular torticollis typically first appears several weeks after delivery. The SCM is effectively shortened on the involved side leading to ipsilateral tilt and contralateral rotation of the face and chin. The affected baby presents with its head laterally flexed toward and rotated away from the affected side.

There are three main ways a child may present with congenital torticollis. Some may have a palpable fibrotic mass within the involved SCM (43 to 55% incidence, pseudotumor or fibromatosis colli). Others will have muscular torticollis with a tight SCM but no palpable tumor (30 to 34% incidence). The last group will have postural torticollis without a mass or tightness in the SCM (11 to 22% incidence).

The diagnosis is made by physical examination and by exclusion of more serious congenital conditions. Range of motion of the neck should be checked and the SCM should be palpated for the presence of a tumor. Visual field tracking and response to sound should be evaluated. A complete neurological examination should be performed. Plain radiographs of the cervical spine, including anteroposterior and lateral, should be considered to rule out congenital abnormalities of the cervical spine. Ultrasound is the imaging modality of choice for radiographic evaluation of congenital muscular torticollis, though it may be unreliable in early or mild cases. It is used to describe the extent of fibrosis in the muscle. US of the hips should be obtained to assess for developmental dysplasia of the hips.

When considering the differential diagnosis, it should be noted that as many as 18% of patients may have a neuromuscular condition that is contributing to the diagnosis. Idiopathic 'congenital' muscular torticollis typically is not present at birth. However, congenital vertebral anomalies such as hemiatlas, congenital cervical scoliosis, or Klippel–Feil syndrome may present at birth with head tilt or "wryneck." Atlantoaxial rotary displacement, cervical infection or inflammation, tumors or other conditions that affect the cerebellum and/or spinal cord, Arnold-Chiari malformations or syringomyleia, and ocular or hearing abnormalities should be considered as well in the differential diagnosis of torticollis in the infant.

Management

The diagnosis of torticollis should prompt an orthopedic consultation. Nearly all patients with congenital muscular torticollis can be treated successfully with stretching exercises and observation. Manual stretches are performed in flexion, extension, lateral bending, and rotation and can be learned by parents. Placing objects of interest away from the side of the tight SCM may encourage stretching. Improvement typically occurs by age 6 to 18 months.

BoTox and a tubular orthosis for torticollis ('T.O.T.') collar have been reported to be useful in persistent cases. Some cases persisting beyond 6 months to 1 year of age with persistent head tilt, deficits of passive rotation or lateral bending of more than 15 degrees, or a tight band palpable in muscle may require surgical release and lengthening to improve function and prevent permanent plagiocephaly. Custom-molded cranial helmets may help with early treatment of severe plagiocephaly and should be applied early enough to permit cranial remodeling.

Complications and Outcomes

The vast majority of these cases resolve with stretching and observation. If therapy is initiated within the first 4 months of life, the need for surgical intervention is highly unlikely. Larger SCM 'tumors', hip dysplasia, the presence of craniofacial asymmetry, and older age at presentation have all been shown to correlate with the need for surgical treatment. The presence of a pseudotumor as opposed to simple muscular torticollis or postural torticollis decreases the likelihood that a stretching program will be effective.

Care must be taken to prevent the development of plagiocephaly, as the affected patient will tend to lie exclusively on one side of their head. With time, secondary bony changes may occur to the base of the skull and the face. Plagiocephaly may have become more prevalent in patients with torticollis recently, as parents are discouraged from allowing the baby to sleep prone for risk of sudden infant death syndrome. Though this secondary skull and facial deformity frequently resolves without treatment by

2 years of age, it can be permanent if not treated appropriately before closure of the fontanelles.

Congenital Spine Problems

EMBRYOLOGY

The spinal cord and supporting column evolve from highly differentiated cells both ectodermal and mesodermal in origin. The notochordal process forms from a ventral invagination of midline ectoderm during the third week of fetal development. Notochordal cells complete separation from the parent ectoderm, forming the distinct structure known as the notochord. Midline ectoderm then undergoes further structural differentiation, folding in on itself to form the neural tube, which separates from remaining ectoderm. Neurulation, the process of neural tube formation, then proceeds as the tube closes first in the midline, then cranially, and, finally, caudally.

These early neural structures induce surrounding mesoderm to form somites, paired entities that give rise to dermatomal, myotomal, and sclerotomal structures. Somites undergo segmentation around week 6 of development, and the ventral, medial corner of the somite disintegrates as sclerotomal cells migrate medially to surround the notochord and developing neural tube. The process of resegmentation follows this as each sclerotome divides into cranial and caudal halves. The cranial portion of each sclerotome induces spinal nerve formation from adjacent neural tube ectoderm and eventually forms the inferior portion of the vertebral body. The caudal portion of each sclerotome gives rise to the intervertebral disk, as well as the superior portion of the vertebral body, the transverse processes, and the posterior elements. The notochord, completely surrounded by sclerotomal cells, gives rise to the nucleus pulposus, a gelatinous, central component of the mature annulus fibrosis. Finally, the adjacent myotome does not undergo resegmentation, resulting in muscular bridging across the intervertebral disks, a distinct mechanical advantage toward motion in the vertebral column. Myotomes then form beneath the still competent dorsolateral wall of the somite, giving rise to paraspinal musculature. Overlying dermatomes generate the well-known dermatomal pattern of cutaneous sensory innervation and form subcutaneous tissue beneath an epithelial layer of ectodermal origin.

At birth, the conus medullaris, or distal-most extent of the spinal cord, extends to the third lumbar vertebra. After birth, however, the disproportionate growth between the skeletal and central nervous systems continues, and by 2 months of age, the conus medullaris has taken up position at its adult level, the L1–L2 intervertebral space.

Other organ systems, in particular the genitourinary and cardiovascular systems, undergo key developmental changes around the same time as the spinal cord and column, and malformations affecting the latter should prompt serious investigations into possible malformations of the former. Up to 25% of patients with congenital scoliosis (entailing vertebral malformation) can be expected to have a concomitant genitourinary anomaly.

Spinal dysraphism is a general term describing failure of the mesoderm (sclerotomal, myotomal, and dermatomal cells) and/or ectoderm to fuse over the dorsal aspect of the neural tube. The mildest form of spinal dysraphism is known as spina bifida occulta and denotes a failure of sclerotomal fusion, resulting in absence of the normal bony posterior arch over the dorsal aspect of the spinal cord. In more severe forms of spinal dysraphism, such as myelomeningocele, both mesoderm and ectoderm have failed to fuse over the dorsal aspect of the neural tube, leaving neural elements exposed to the outside world with or without dural coverage.

Congenital scoliosis (spinal column deformity in coronal plane) entails one of two (or at times both) developmental defects: failures of somite formation and/or failures of somite segmentation (or resegmentation). Failures of formation lead to defects that range from mild wedging of the vertebral body to absence of half of the vertebral body, producing a hemivertebra. Hemivertebrae are further classified as fully segmented, semisegmented, or unsegmented, depending on whether both, one, or no growth plates are present. Additionally, a hemivertebrae can be either incarcerated or nonincarcerated, depending on the degree to which surrounding somites have incorporated it into the vertebral column. Failures in segmentation may be unilateral, leading to bar formation, or bilateral, resulting in block vertebra formation.

Congenital kyphosis (spinal column deformity in sagittal plane), similar to congenital scoliosis (the two often coexist), can be produced by either a failure of segmentation, failure of formation, or a mixture of the two.

Occipitocervical synostosis involves fusion (failure of segmentation) between the occiput and C1.

Klippel–Feil syndrome entails fusions (failure of segmentation) between one or more cervical levels, excluding the occipitocervical junction.

Incidence and Etiology

SPINAL DYSRAPHISM

The exact incidence of spina bifida is difficult to judge, given the likelihood that many cases go unnoticed during the lifetime of the patient. However, 5% of lumbar spine films performed in the United States show isolated lumbar defects. Myelomeningocele occurs in the United States with an incidence of 1 to 2 per 1,000 live births. Incidence can vary with geographic locale, and proposed etiologic factors include nutritional (lack of folic acid in the diet), pharmacologic (maternal exposure to valproic acid or carbamazepine), and maternal diabetes. Spinal dysraphism occurs most commonly in the lumbosacral region of the spine but can occur at any level. Associated neurologic conditions include hydrocephalus (present in and requiring ventriculoperitoneal shunting in 90% of cases), Arnold-Chiari malformation, hydromyelia, and tethered cord. Additionally, patients with sacral dysraphism have a greater than 50% coincidence of hip dislocation or subluxation. The vast majority (higher incidence with higher affected levels) will have progressive scoliosis, and up to 30% will have clubfoot.

CONGENITAL SCOLIOSIS, KYPHOSIS

The true incidence of congenital scoliosis is unknown, as many cases may be undetected. Estimates of the incidence range from 1 to 4% in the general population.

Anomalies in formation and segmentation of the spine lead to asymmetric growth of the spine and progressive deformity. Vertebral defects may arise from the disruption of genes involved in development, environmental insults during gestation, or a combination of both factors. Congenital spinal problems are frequently associated with other organ system abnormalities, most notably in the cardiovascular and genitourinary systems.

KLIPPEL–FEIL SYNDROME

The segmentation defects found in Klippel–Feil syndrome (fusion of cervical spinal elements) are reported to occur in approximately 0.7% of the population; however, this number may underestimate the true incidence as many cases may remain undetected or subclinical. There may be other congenital cervical spinal abnormalities. Abnormalities of other organ systems, such as the cardiac and/or genitourinary systems, is common.

Prenatal Diagnosis and Treatment

GENERAL CONSIDERATIONS

The spine can be seen at 7 to 8 weeks gestation and its calcification is well defined at 10 to 12 weeks. Ultrasound can detect hemivertebra, fused vertebrae, absence of vertebrae, widening of the spinal canal, or kyphoscoliosis. In addition, neural tube defects and isolated skin defects can be diagnosed.

α-fetoprotein levels are commonly used as a screening tool for prenatal detection of myelomeningocele.

Advances in fetal ultrasonography have made prenatal diagnosis of major spinal dysraphism more likely. As mentioned elsewhere, there is active interest in prenatal diagnosis and early fetal surgery for closure of myelomeningocele. Intrauterine repair of myelomeningocele has not been associated with improvement of lower extremity neurologic function, but has been associated with a reduction of the Chiari type 2 malformation and a decrease in the need of a cerebral spinal fluid shunt. If anticipated, babies with spina bifida may be better delivered by cesarean section than vaginally, and preparations can be made for early postnatal sac closure.

Postnatal Diagnosis

GENERAL CONSIDERATIONS

Congenital vertebral anomalies are easily missed in the neonatal period, barring gross malformation, and typically are noted on radiographs. Ultrasonography in infants up to 6 weeks of age can effectively detect major spinal cord malformation or low-lying conus medullaris. After 6 weeks of age, MRI is needed for assessment of the spinal cord, may be deferred until an older age depending upon the urgency of the situation.

Detection of vertebral anomalies may prompt further imaging by computed tomography or MRI to rule out hydrocephalus or intraspinal pathology such as low conus medullaris, intraspinal lipoma, diastematomyelia, syringomyelia, or tethered cord. A careful neurologic examination is important, as 20 to 40% of patients with congenital spinal deformities may have a congenital abnormality of the spinal axis. Spinal ultrasonography before age 6 weeks may also suffice to rule out major intraspinal anomalies. Intraspinal pathology should be called to the attention of a neurosurgeon with pediatric expertise.

A careful evaluation of pulmonary function is important, as congenital spinal deformities are associated with the inability of the thorax to support normal respiration or lung growth.

Associated genitourinary and/or cardiovascular anomalies are often present. Up to 55% of patients with congenital spine deformities may have associated organ defects. Cardiac (ventricular and atrial septal defects and patent ductus arteriosus) and genitourinary (renal hypoplasia, horseshoe kidney, and single kidney) conditions are common. Patients diagnosed with a congenital spinal deformity should have a screening renal ultrasound and cardiac evaluation. The differential diagnosis in a child with a spinal disorder includes VATER or VACTERL, Goldenhar syndrome (oculo-auriculo-vertebral defects), Jarcho Levin syndrome, and neurofibromatosis.

SPINAL DYSRAPHISM

Cutaneous abnormalities, hairy patches, fatty swellings, very asymmetric sacral creases, and deep clefts or 1dimpling may be present at birth. Absent abdominal reflexes may also suggest a spinal deformity. Although such findings are most often not associated with an underlying spinal cord abnormality, their presence should prompt investigation of potential spinal dysraphism or spinal cord tethering with early spinal ultrasound.

Open cases of myelomeningocele present with neural elements uncovered.

Anteroposterior and lateral radiographs may show absence of posterior vertebral elements. The presence of skeletal anomalies may be difficult to discern, given the degree of vertebral ossification in the neonatal period.

Clinical signs of a tethered cord occur in approximately 15% of patients with spina bifida. Clinical sings include changes in urologic function, development of spasticity, foot deformity, or scoliosis.

CONGENITAL SCOLIOSIS/KYPHOSIS

Cutaneous abnormalities similar to those found in spinal dysraphism may suggest the diagnosis. In congenital scoliosis, anteroposterior radiographs of the thoracolumbar spine will show vertebral anomalies in the coronal plane. Anomalies are sometimes visible only as an absence of symmetry. That is, all pedicles should appear in pairs and all vertebrae should have a roughly rectangular outline that spans the entire coronal dimension of the column. The presence of skeletal anomalies may be difficult to discern, given the degree of vertebral ossification in the neonatal period.

With congenital kyphosis or lordosis lateral radiographs of the spine will show failures of segmentation or formation or vertebral wedging with or without a change in the normal kyphosis and lordosis. The presence of skeletal anomalies may be difficult to discern given the degree of vertebral ossification in the neonatal period.

KLIPPEL–FEIL SYNDROME

Physical findings characteristic of Klippel–Feil syndrome are a low posterior hairline, a short, broad neck, torticollis, scoliosis, high scapula, and jaw abnormalities. Patients may have marked limitation in range of motion, particularly rotation. Occipitocervical synostosis can present with a similar presentation and should be in the differential diagnosis. Klippel–Feil syndrome can entail fusion of multiple cervical levels and therefore produce more limitation in range of motion than occipitocervical synostosis.

Management

SPINAL DYSRAPHISM

For closed spinal dysraphism without neurologic deficit, documentation of neurologic status, observation for progressive defects, and assessment of spinal neuroanatomy by ultrasound are sufficient. Open myelomeningocele or closed dysraphism with neurologic deficit requires urgent neurosurgical consultation, as skin closure should take place soon after birth (often within 48 hours). Ventriculoperitoneal shunting may also be needed soon after birth as hydrocephalus accompanies over 90% of cases of lumbosacral spinal dysraphism. Neurosurgical detethering has been shown to benefit patients presenting with tethered cord syndrome.

Management of hip dislocation and/or clubfoot in the context of spinal dysraphism is more complicated than their management as isolated cases and may be deferred or treated with early casting and manipulation. Urologic consultation is also needed to assist with assessment of bladder and upper urinary tract function. Where available, coordinated team care including a developmental pediatrician, nurse, and case manager is helpful to educate families. Orthopedic management concerns focus on maximizing long-term function and independence. Typical issues include paralytic foot deformities, pressure sores, hip dislocation and stiffness, and spinal deformities.

CONGENITAL SCOLIOSIS/KYPHOSIS

The natural history of congenital scoliosis has been well documented and depends on the type and magnitude of malformation. Balanced deformities may remain stable with growth, whereas unbalanced growth potential, especially if opposite a bony tether such as a congenital rib fusion mass or bony bar, may progress rapidly during infancy and later during the preadolescent growth acceleration. In general, bracing is ineffective for congenital scoliosis. Progressive curves should be treated promptly, irrespective of age. Hemivertebrae that are fully segmented (ie, have both a cranial and caudal growth plate), particularly if they are opposite a unilateral bar, tend to produce a rapidly progressive curve, and may require relatively early operative intervention to prevent significant deformity. Traditional treatment of progressive congenital spine deformities has focused on early fusion with arrest of deformity. Newer techniques include excision of vertebral elements and correction. Complex vertebral anomalies spanning a larger section of spine may be treated with growth-oriented techniques such as growing rods or Vertical Expandable Prosthetic Titanium Rib (VEPTR) devices.

The natural history of congenital kyphosis is potentially worrisome, with nearly all untreated curves proceeding to worsened deformity and some type I congenital kyphosis producing a high rate of neural deficit, including complete paraplegia. Almost all cases of congenital kyphosis need spinal fusion to halt progressive deformity and reduce the risk of neural compromise. Early in-situ fusion to halt progression is preferred to later higher-risk reconstructive procedures.

KLIPPEL–FEIL SYNDROME

Typically asymptomatic, but radiographically and often visually apparent during the patient's childhood, congenital cervical fusion may not be troublesome until the patient's second or third decade. At this time, neurologic symptoms secondary to instability or pain from early arthritis may develop. Three subpopulations of Klippel–Feil syndrome at particularly high risk for neurologic problems and early arthritis are those with C2–C3 fusion and concomitant occipitocervical synostosis, those with a single normal intervertebral disk between two long fused segments, and those with a long fused segment caudal to an abnormal (but mobile) occipitocervical junction. The timing and nature of operative treatment can be variable.

In cases of occipitocervical synostosis, there is an association with atlantoaxial instability in over half of cases. If instability is showed, occiput to C2 fusion with or without laminectomy may be indicated.

Complications and Outcomes

Complications of pain and neurologic compromise, including complete tetra- and paraplegia, rarely occur in the neonatal period.

Congenital spinal anomalies carry widely variable long-term prognoses. Whereas certain types of congenital scoliosis may require only observation and entail no functional deficits in the developing child, spinal dysraphism can present an enormously complex challenge, necessitating an aggressive team approach toward management in the hope of providing the patient with the maximum possible function.

Thoracic insufficiency syndrome (TIS) (the inability of the thorax to support normal lung growth and function) is common in complex congenital spinal deformities in which a large section of spine or major anomalies are present. Although the infant may have normal respiratory function, the absence of adequate thoracic volume though growth may lead to eventual respiratory insufficiency. Major chest wall anomalies, rib fusions, congenitally short spines, and early fusion may be associated with TIS.

Congenital Upper Extremity Problems

EMBRYOLOGY

Limb buds begin to form between 4 and 6 weeks of gestation as ventrally migrating dermatomyoblasts induce a thickening in the ectoderm, known as the apical ectodermal ridge (AER). Induced by the AER, the primitive upper limb bud bulges from the lateral body wall at approximately 4 weeks' gestation, arising from the eighth through tenth somites. This takes place 1 week before formation of the primitive lower limb bud. This AER then promotes appositional growth in the underlying mesoderm, as well as differentiation into cartilage (which, in turn, provides a basis for endochondral ossification and appendicular skeletal formation), skeletal muscle, and connective tissue elements.

Proximodistal patterning from the shoulder to the hand is mediated by the fibroblast growth factor (FGF) family of proteins in the AER. Dorsoventral patterning is determined by the ectoderm covering the limb and is mediated by Wnt-7a protein. Anterio-posterior patterning (radial to ulnar) is mediated by the zone of polarizing activity (ZPA) at the posterior margin of the limb. Sonic hedgehog (shh) is the primary regulatory signaling molecule in this process, which works in conjunction with other gene products such as the *Hox* genes.

At week 5 of gestation, hand paddles form, and by week 8, there is segmentation of hand and footplates into the typical five-ray pattern, which involves a process of physiologic necrosis and programmed cell death through both the overlying AER and underlying mesoderm. By week 9, actual finger motion begins and skin creases begin to develop. The majority of limb development and differentiation occurs between 4 and 8 weeks after fertilization, and by the twelfth week primary ossification centers have appeared in nearly all bones of the limbs.

Consideration of this timeline is important in light of the fact that musculoskeletal deformities, whether of the upper or lower extremities, are often immediately obvious. Prompt investigation into the possibility of concomitant, and much more serious abnormalities in the cardiac and renal systems should be initiated, as these systems develop simultaneously with the developing limbs in utero.

Incidence and Etiology

GENERAL CONSIDERATIONS

Congenital anomalies affect 1 to 2% of newborns, and approximately 10% of these will have upper limb abnormalities, and the estimated incidence of upper limb anomalies is 0.16%. Only 10% of these will require surgical treatment.

CONGENITAL AMPUTATIONS

Considered to be transverse deficiencies, the level of involvement may be anywhere from the finger to the complete arm, with the proximal third of the forearm being most common. This has been called the "short below-the-elbow" defect. Incidence is 1 in 20,000 live births for proximal forearm and 1 in 270,000 for complete arm amputation. Autosomal recessive transmission has been reported, but more often than not, cases are sporadic, with unknown etiology. Associated abnormalities are rare.

Disruption of the AER during limb development and/or a vascular insult likely leads to limb truncation. Early chorionic villous sampling and failed attempts at pregnancy termination by dilation and curettage have been associated with transverse limb deficiencies, lending support to vascular disruption as a potential cause.

CONSTRICTION BANDS

Amniotic disruption sequence or constriction band syndrome may result in congenital amputations, and most commonly affects the digits (hands or toes). This anomaly occurs in 1 in 15,000 births and mandates urgent orthopedic consultation. The central digits are most commonly affected, and the location of the constriction bands is most commonly distal. Presentation with other hand anomalies is not infrequent. Additionally, an estimated 40% of neonates with manifestations of constriction band syndrome of the upper extremities will have congenital malformations affecting other body parts, such as clubfoot or craniofacial defects.

The etiology is postulated to be a combination of intrinsic and extrinsic causes. The intrinsic concept believes that the amniotic bands represent a localized lack of mesodermal development. The extrinsic theory postulates that an amniotic band or membrane traps or encircles an affected part leading to a variable amount of injury. Severe damage can lead to complete vascular ischemia and truncation of the affected part.

PHOCOMELIA

This disorder comprises 1% of all upper extremity congenital deformities. A variable segment is absent between the shoulder and hand. Contemporary cases are usually sporadic, but previously many cases were associated with the use of thalidomide during pregnancy.

RADIAL CLUBHAND

The incidence of this anomaly is approximately between 1:55,000 and 1 in 100,000 births, with a 50% incidence of bilaterality. The majority of cases are sporadic without any definable cause. However, exposure to teratogens such as radiation or thalidomide can yield radial deficiencies. Familial incidence includes 5 to 10% of cases. There is a high incidence of associated conditions such as thrombocytopenia absent radius (TAR), Fanconi's anemia, Holt-Oram syndrome, or VACTERL syndromes. The degree of deformity is related to the degree of AER malfunction.

CENTRAL RAY (METACARPAL) DEFICIENCY

Cleft hand is a longitudinal deficiency of the central rays of the hand (index, long, and ring), which differentiate at a separate time from the radial and ulnar rays. This anomaly comprises 4% of all upper extremity congenital deformities. Many cases are sporadic but autosomal dominant transmission has been observed in some and, when present, typically produces bilateral deformity (typical cleft hand). Familial cases frequently are also associated with cleft lip or cleft palate. On the contrary, in an atypical cleft hand, cases are sporadic, unilateral, and associated with Poland's syndrome (ipsilateral anomaly of the chest wall, commonly absence of a portion of the pectoralis major muscle). The deficiency may be a result of fusion of digital rays or by necrosis of mesenchymal tissue with attempts at regeneration.

SYNDACTYLY

This is the most common congenital hand deformity, occurring in 1 in 2,000 to 2,500 live births. Fifty percent of cases are bilateral, and the most frequently reported site is between the long and ring fingers. This autosomal dominant trait has variable expression or reduced penetrance. The etiology includes failure of interdigital necrosis and cell apoptosis, regulated largely by factors secreted by the AER. It may be associated with Poland's syndrome, as well as syndactyly of the toes, polydactyly of the toes, and cleft feet.

THUMB HYPOPLASIA

Major developmental defects of the thumb constituted 10 to 16% of upper limb congenital abnormalities. The incidence of thumb hypoplasia is approximately 4% of all congenital hand anomalies. This deformity can be syndromic in nature or occur sporadically. An ataxic insult to the ZPA from chemical or viremia or abnormalities in the AER may affect thumb development.

Thumb hypoplasia is often can be associated with radial club hand. Therefore, this diagnosis should prompt consideration of the presence of additional congenital abnormalities, in particular those of the cardiovascular, spinal, and/or gastrointestinal systems.

THUMB DUPLICATION

This anomaly occurs with an approximate frequency of 1 in 100,000 births, is typically unilateral, and is more common in males and in white and Asian individuals. The cause of thumb polydactyly is unknown, and most cases are sporadic in origin.

POSTAXIAL POLYDACTYLY

Duplication of the small finger occurs in 1 in 300 blacks and 1 in 3,000 whites. This is one of the most frequently encountered upper extremity anomalies. Duplication of the small finger is genetically determined, and when it occurs in isolation, it is usually inherited in the dominant mode with variable penetrance. When there is an associated syndrome, it is often inherited in the recessive mode.

CENTRAL POLYDACTYLY

This anomaly presents with a frequency of 1% of all hand deformities. The ring finger is most frequently affected followed by the long and index fingers. It is often bilateral although contralateral hand deformities of different types can also be found. It is often associated with some degree of syndactyly between the digits, as well as other musculoskeletal deformities. The neural axis, genitourinary, or cardiovascular systems are involved rarely.

OVERGROWTH/MACRODACTYLY

This anomaly may involve isolated enlargement of various parts or may present as diffuse hypertrophy of the entire limb. Macrodacytly most commonly affects the index finger, and this anomaly presents with a frequency of 1% of all hand deformities. It is typically unilateral. Potential causes of overgrowth involve vascular abnormalities or malformations. Overgrowth may also be a constituent of a variety of syndromes such as neurofibromatosis or Klippel–Trenaunay–Weber syndrome. The true etiology of macrodactyly remains unknown. It may be static or progressive.

Prenatal Diagnosis and Treament

With improved sensitivity and familiarity with prenatal ultrasound, many congenital abnormalities of the hand can be diagnosed prenatally. Anomalies of the hand may present along a wide spectrum of defects, and should prompt evaluation for other systemic abnormalities on ultrasound. Defects including shortening very early in pregnancy often are lethal, and may be seen in achondrogenesis, osteogenesis imperfecta, and thanatophoric dwarfism. Avoidance of toxins during the critical period of limb development may reduce the number of limb anomalies; however; this critical period often passes before a woman discovers she is pregnant.

Postnatal Diagnosis

GENERAL CONSIDERATIONS

Plain radiographs may be necessary to confirm or further classify certain upper extremity congenital deformities, such as radial clubhand, central ray deficiency, or thumb duplication. These studies need not be obtained on an emergent basis.

One should always keep in mind the possible presence of additional congenital malformations or syndromes when a baby presents with a congenital upper extremity deformity. Common associations include the VACTERL (vertebral, anal, cardiac, tracheal, esophageal, renal, and limb) association and thrombocytopenia or Fanconi's anemia with radial clubhand.

CONGENITAL AMPUTATIONS

These cases present with either rudimentary or completely absent limb formation beyond the point of amputation. When at the level of the proximal third of the forearm, it is referred to as short below-the-elbow defect. Often rudimentary digits or dimpling can be located at the end of the amputation stump and represent an attempt at limb recovery.

CONSTRICTION BANDS

The affected neonate will present with what appears to be a deep skin crease surrounding the digit at a given level in a circumferential manner. Varying degrees of vascular compromise of the part of the digit distal to the band may be present. A pseudosyndactyly is often present and is attributed to healing between affected digits after an injury. Patients commonly have clubfeet.

PHOCOMELIA

This condition of longitudinal deficiency falls into one of three types: complete, proximal, and distal. All forms are characterized by an intersegmental deficiency. In complete phocomelia, the infant's hand attaches directly to the trunk with an absent arm segment. Proximal phocomelia involves an absent brachium with direct forearm–body attachment. Distal phocomelia involves absence of the antebrachium with direct hand-arm-body attachment. Cleft lip and palate are associated anomalies.

RADIAL CLUBHAND

The fundamental abnormality in this condition is partial or complete absence of the radius, resulting in a short forearm with marked radial deviation of the hand. Severity is graded I through IV based on radiographic interpretation. Considerable thumb hypoplasia may be present, and abnormalities in the cardiac, vertebral, gastrointestinal, or renal systems may be present such as in Holt-Oram syndrome, TAR, VACTERL, or Fanconi's anemia. The ulna, although present, is often deformed with thickening and bowing toward the absent radius. Radial sided musculature as well as vascular and neurologic structures are variably disturbed.

CENTRAL RAY DEFICIENCY

Cleft hand was formerly known as "lobster-claw hand" and involves a V shaped defect with absence of the central rays of the hand (metacarpals), resulting in a hand with the appearance of a lobster claw. Often called symbrachydactyly, there may be a component of syndactyly as well. Patients should be evaluated for the presence/absence of cleft lip or palate as well as the pectoralis major muscle.

SYNDACTYLY

This common anomaly presents as a failure of one or more digits to separate. The digits can be joined together by soft tissue and/or bone, depending on the degree of failure of programmed cell death that occurs during embryonic development and hand paddle differentiation. A simple classification scheme exists, describing either "complete" or "incomplete" defects, depending on whether a bridge extends all the way to the fingertip, and "simple" or "complex" defects, depending on whether a bridge consists only of soft tissue or has a bony element as well. It will most often be detected between the ring and long fingers, followed by the ring and small fingers. The least common location is between the thumb and index finger. Patients should be examined for the presence of Poland's syndrome.

THUMB HYPOPLASIA

This is partial or complete absence of the thumb. There are variable amounts of bony, muscular, and ligamentous deficiencies. The hypoplastic thumb may adopt a fixed adducted or abducted position or may involve absence of the metacarpal and remain attached to the hand by a soft tissue stalk, "pouce flottant." The presence or absence of a stable carpometacarpal joint is an important part of the assessment as well as the degree of extrinsic and intrinsic muscular deficiencies. The infant should also be evaluated for radial deficiency as well as for associated syndromes and systemic abnormalities (cardiac, renal, spinal, gastrointestinal, and hematologic).

THUMB DUPLICATION

Duplication of the thumb along with varying degrees of hypoplasia affecting both digits. The duplication can be partial or complete and has been classified into types based on the degree of skeletal duplication. The radial-based digit is typically more hypoplastic than the ulnar-based one. There are commonly eccentrically placed or split tendons as well as shared neurovascular structures, nailbeds, ligaments, and joints. Complete duplication of the proximal and distal phalanx is the most common presentation.

POSTAXIAL POLYDACTYLY

Presentation involves obvious duplication of the small digit, ranging from an apparent vestigial appendage to a relatively wellformed finger.

CENTRAL POLYDACTYLY

Presentation involves obvious duplication of any of the digits, ranging from an apparent vestigial appendage to a relatively well-formed finger. An extreme example is that of a "mirror hand" in which the hand possesses eight digits and no thumbs.

OVERGROWTH/MACRODACTYLY

In overgrowth, the presentation may include diffuse hypertrophy of the entire limb or isolated enlargement of isolated parts. Assessment for vascular malformations is critical. In macrodactyly, the affected digit is larger than its accompanying digits and can be stiff and angulated. The deformity typically progresses in one of two manners: either it grows at a rate commensurate with that of the rest of the hand or it grows disproportionately and continues to enlarge relative to the remaining digits.

Management

GENERAL CONSIDERATIONS

Orthopedic consultation should be obtained for all of the conditions described. Constriction band syndrome, which can be progressively limb threatening, is the only condition that requires urgent orthopedic attention.

CONGENITAL AMPUTATIONS

Treatment includes passive stretching exercises and fitting with a prosthetic device at age 6 to 9 months when independent sitting is achieved. Early fitting before 2 years of age increases the acceptance rate of upper limb prostheses. Surgery is usually not indicated, and only necessary if a small bone spicule or rudimentary nubbin irritates the residual stump. For those who do not have access to prostheses, or who have bilateral amputations, a surgical procedure can turn the arm into a pincer by separating the radius and ulna and allowing them to function independently.

CONSTRICTION BANDS

Depending on the degree of constriction, the band may need to be surgically released to prevent vascular compromise of the digit distal to the constriction on an emergent basis. More subtle presentations can have elective band excision. Multiple digit amputations require reconstruction or augmentation by a variety of techniques.

PHOCOMELIA

Treatment typically involves a specially designed prosthesis and limb training, although some centers have used limb-lengthening procedures combined with tendon transfer to improve function.

RADIAL CLUBHAND

Depending on the specifics and severity of the deformity, the patient may need anything from serial casting and stretching exercises to surgical soft tissue release, tendon transfer, and centralization of the carpus over the ulna. These procedures are typically performed, if necessary, between 6 months and 1 year of age. Treatment of other systemic conditions may be necessary.

CENTRAL RAY DEFICIENCY

Most patients function at a satisfactory level with this deformity and do not need surgery. Occasionally surgery will be used to close the defect to enhance grasp and improve appearance. Closure is usually not entertained until the age of 2 or 3.

SYNDACTYLY

Surgical separation of the involved digits is recommended and, depending on the severity of the deformity, should occur between ages 6 and 18 months. Border digits and digits of unequal length should be separated early (3 to 6 months) to prevent a tethering effect. Both sides of a digit should not be separated at the same time to prevent vascular compromise.

THUMB HYPOPLASIA

Depending on its severity and positioning, it may or may not need surgical correction. Pure reduction in size with maintenance of muscular function and joint stability can be treated with out an operation. Reconstruction can be performed with tendon transfers for intermediate cases. In cases where little functional anatomy remains, ablation with pollicization (rotation of the index finger to function as a thumb) should be pursued in the first 2 years of life.

THUMB DUPLICATION

Surgical correction of the deformity is recommended between 6 and 9 months of age. Generally the more hypoplastic thumb is ablated, with reconstruction of the remaining thumb with the remaining important parts.

POSTAXIAL POLYDACTYLY

In cases where there is a rudimentary nubbin, suture ligation at the base of the pedicle can be performed while the newborn is in the nursery. In more complex cases, surgical ablation is necessary.

CENTRAL POLYDACTYLY

Surgical ablation is recommended, with ablation of the duplicate digit with augmentation of the remaining digits. Surgical intervention may be necessary early (6 to 12 months of age) because of the tethering nature of many of the deformities.

MACRODACTYLY

This condition can require debulking procedures, which should take place around 3 months of age to avoid compromise of vascular structures. Arrest of the growth plates may be necessary. Enlargement that is progressive and uncontrollable may require amputation.

Complications and Outcomes

Although digits may remain stiff or dysfunctional after treatment, the long-term outcome of the vast majority of these cases is excellent as patients show a remarkable propensity for functional adaptation. Early acceptance and support of the family is crucial for those requiring prosthetic wear and who have residual differences after treatment.

Congenital Lower Extremity Problems

EMBRYOLOGY

The embryology of the limb bud has been described previously under congenital upper extremity problems. The embryology of the limb buds in the upper extremity are similar to those of the lower extremity.

Joints begin to develop during the sixth week, and by the end of the eighth week they resemble adult joints. Interzonal mesenchyme between developing bones differentiates into capsular and other ligaments peripherally. Centrally it disappears and the resulting space becomes the joint or synovial cavity. The mesenchymal cells disappear from the surfaces of the articular cartilages, likely as a result of fetal movements. Normal femoral acetabular movement and position in utero provides the physiologic stresses necessary to develop a normal acetabulum.

Incidence and Etiology

DEVELOPMENTAL DYSPLASIA OF THE HIP

Developmental dysplasia of the hip (DDH) occurs in approximately 10 in 1,000 live births and a dislocated hip occurs in approximately one in 1,000. Note that the term "DDH" is preferred over "congenital dysplasia or dislocation of the hip" because DDH encompasses a wide range of deformity from mild dysplasia to fixed dislocation and because DDH can occur prenatally, perinatally, or postnatally.

Genetic, hormonal, and mechanical factors have all been implicated in the etiology of DDH. Significant risk factors include female sex (female to male ratio of 5:1), family history, first born, breech positioning, white or European heritage, and increased birth weight. The left hip is affected three times as often as the right, and 50% of cases are bilateral. Firstborn females presenting in a breech position have the highest risk of DDH at 8%. The risk for DDH in subsequent pregnancies is 6% when neither parent has the condition, 12% when one parent has hip dysplasia, and 36% with both parents have the condition. As this condition is thought to be a mechanical phenomenon caused by intrauterine positioning, commonly associated conditions include torticollis, metatarsus adductus, and calcaneovalgus deformity of the foot.

Mechanistically, it is postulated that excessive laxity allows abnormal femoral head mobility. When the femoral head spends insufficient time within the acetabulum, the acetabulum may develop abnormally and show features of dysplasia. DDH is infrequently seen in premature infants. Delivery before the final weeks of pregnancy spares the fetus exposure to high levels of circulating hormones that give rise to the increased ligamentous laxity that in a cramped intrauterine environment is thought to attribute to DDH.

PROXIMAL FEMORAL FOCAL DEFICIENCY (CONGENITAL SHORT FEMUR)

This relatively uncommon deformity is the third most common type of longitudinal deficiency of the lower limb. It may include a spectrum of abnormalities ranging from hypoplasia of the femur to complete absence of the femur. Two-thirds of cases are associated with fibular hemimelia. These patients also often have knee ligamentous laxity or contractures.

POSTEROMEDIAL BOWING OF THE TIBIA

This relatively uncommon deformity occurs with no predilection for male or female, right or left. It is typically unilateral and associated with calcaneal valgus foot position. Correction tends to occur spontaneously, but osteotomy and leg equalization are often needed. Etiologies include abnormal intrauterine packing pressures and prenatal tibial physeal injury.

ANTEROLATERAL BOWING OF THE TIBIA (CONGENITAL PSEUDARTHROSIS)

Present in 1 in 140,000 live births and more common than posteromedial bowing, this condition is often associated with other pathologic processes, in particular, neurofibromatosis. The true etiology is not known, and the condition is not well defined pathologically. Between 40 and 80% of children with anterolateral bowing of the tibia eventual carry the diagnosis of neurofibromatosis, and most progress to a spontaneous pseudoarthrosis.

FIBULAR HEMIMELIA/DEFICIENCY

This is the most common congenital long bone deficiency and is often associated with the absence of lateral rays of the ipsilateral foot. Unlike tibial hypoplasia, which has a genetic inheritance pattern, fibular deficiencies generally are not inherited. It is likely because of abnormalities in the limb bud development, and is considered to be a postaxial hypoplasia. Other musculoskeletal anomalies may be present, such as shortening of the femur and tibia, femoral retroversion, valgus distal femur secondary to hypoplasia of the lateral femoral condyle, hypoplastic tibial spines, cruciate ligament deficiency, angular deformity of the tibia, tarsal coalition, and clubfoot deformity. However, it is commonly an isolated phenomenon rather than part of a syndrome or other generalized condition.

TIBIAL HEMIMELIA/HYPOPLASIA

Occurring with a frequency of 1 in 1,000,000 live births, this extremely rare anomaly is commonly bilateral and may be associated with additional limb deformities, such as central ray deficiency in the hand and developmental dysplasia of the hip. In addition, there is an association with hypospadias and imperforate anus. It is considered to be a longitudinal deficiency, and is likely a result of abnormal limb bud development. There is often an autosomal dominant pattern of transmission; however, spontaneous mutations do occur. Absence of the tibia may be partial or complete.

CONGENITAL KNEE DISLOCATION

This rare congenital condition (40 to 60 times less frequent than developmental dysplasia of the hip) presents more frequently in females and is commonly bilateral. Most often a subluxation is present, but a complete dislocation is also possible. Other musculoskeletal abnormalities occur in 40 to 100% of cases and may include hip pathology or clubfoot. Fetal molding because of oligohydraminos, or an extended breech position has been postulated as possible etiologies. Other theories include an abnormality in the ACL as well as a quadriceps contracture. Associated conditions include arthrogryposis and neuromuscular pathologies such as myelomeningocele and Down, Larsen's, and Turner's syndromes.

TALIPES EQUINOVARUS

Otherwise known as "clubfoot," this anomaly presents with a frequency of 1:250 to 1 in 1,000 live births. The male to female ratio is 2:1; the right side is affected more commonly than the left, and up to 50% of cases are bilateral. It is associated with other "packing" disorders such as DDH and torticollis.

The etiology of clubfoot is largely unknown, but is thought to be associated with multifactorial genetic inheritance and influenced by environmental factors. There is a seasonal variation, with a summer season peak incidence, suggesting a polio-like intrauterine enterovirus infection as an etiology.

CONGENITAL VERTICAL TALUS

Vertical Talus, also known as "rocker-bottom foot," occurs with a frequency of 1 in 10,000 births and has no male/female predilection. It is found in patients with severe chromosomal abnormalities such as Trisomy 13, 15, or 18. Associated conditions include neurofibromatosis, myelomeningocele, and arthrogryposis.

PES CALCANEOVALGUS

With an incidence of between 30 and 50% of live births, this represents the most common foot deformity observed in the neonate. The incidence is somewhat higher in firstborns; however, the incidence is unknown because of the variability in presentation of this disorder. The postulated etiology includes a mechanism of intrauterine packing pressure dorsally compressing the fetal feet.

Prenatal Diagnosis and Treatment

The relationship between the acetabulum and femoral head can be seen in the third trimester of pregnancy. Severe asymmetrical appearance of the limb and unilateral shortening of bones can be detected at the end of the first and in the early part of the second trimester. The diagnosis of proximal femoral deficiency can be possible as early as the fourteenth week of pregnancy. Both tibial and fibular hemimelia can be determined prenatally. Routine prenatal ultrasound has been shown to be highly effective in detecting clubfoot prenatally, with essentially no false negative predictions and a true positive predictive rate of around 80%. There may be a significant false positive rate (up to 30%), which is important to remember when counseling parents. Congenital vertical talus can be diagnosed prenatally with the presence of a prominent heel and dorsiflexion of the foot. The most obvious finding on prenatal exam may be an abnormality in the lower extremity, and may lead to the detection of associated anomalies frequently encountered in patients with lower extremity malformations.

Postnatal Diagnosis

DEVELOPMENTAL DYSPLASIA OF THE HIP

The baby is usually asymptomatic with minimal outward presentation until tested with clinical maneuvers. All newborns require clinical screening. Physical examination remains the mainstay of diagnosis, relying on three provocative maneuvers: the Ortolani test, the Barlow test, and hip abduction (Figure 1). The presence of a high-pitched "hip click" at or after birth does not indicate DDH. The Ortolani (low-pitched clunk, thud, or sensation as the hip reduces with abduction and elevation of the trochanter) and the Barlow (low-pitched clunk, thud, or sensation as the hip dislocates with adduction and gentle posterior pressure) tests are most reliable up to age 2 months. The Ortolani test can be

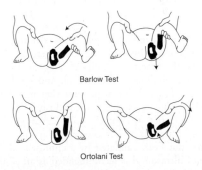

Barlow Test

Ortolani Test

Figure 1 Barlow and Ortolani tests.

performed, on one hip at a time, by placing the thumb over the proximal, medial aspect of the femur and the index and long fingers over the greater trochanter and gently abducting the hip, attempting to feel a palpable "thunk" as a subluxed or dislocated hip is reduced back into the acetabulum. The Barlow test can be performed with the opposite maneuver by adducting and applying gentle pressure along the longitudinal axis of the femur, attempting to subluxate or dislocate a reduced hip. The neonate must be relaxed for a reliable examination to take place. Minimal force is required. Eventually, the dislocated side will develop tightness of the adductors and show asymmetric abduction. When a unilateral dislocation is present, the Galleazzi test (one knee appears lower than the other with the hip flexed to 90 degrees) may be positive, or skin folds may be asymmetric.

At all ages, DDH is easily missed by physical examination, and in the older infant, fixed dislocation is easily missed as both the Ortolani and Barlow tests will be negative. Beyond age 2 months, limitation in hip abduction becomes the most sensitive finding. Repeated observation for DDH needs to continue through walking age as previously located hips may progress to subluxation or dislocation in the postnatal period, especially in patients with neuromuscular disorders.

Plain radiographs are not useful before 3 months of age. Dynamic ultrasonography is the preferred diagnostic imaging tool until about 6 months of age, when radiographs are necessary. Screening ultrasound should be used in patients at 4 to 6 weeks of age in patients with established risk factors. However, there is significant debate on the appropriate use of screening ultrasound for DDH. There are no clear guidelines defining the use of screening ultrasonography in the newborn period. The Pediatric Society of North America (POSNA) suggests that screening ultrasound for all infants is impractical, and results of studies attempting to define subsets of patients that may benefit from screening ultrasound have been inconclusive. The American Academy of Pediatrics in their clinical practice guideline states that screening all infants at 4 to 6 weeks of age is expensive and its benefit has not been validated by a clinical trial. It suggests that the use of ultrasound is recommended as an adjunct to the clinical evaluation, and should be used for assessing an infant at increased risk, to support a clinical finding, or to monitor DDH as it is being treated.

PROXIMAL FEMORAL FOCAL DEFICIENCY (CONGENITAL SHORT FEMUR)

The baby presents with a variable amount of shortening of the leg. The femur may be mildly hypoplastic or completely absent. The thigh will appear short, and the leg is often held in flexion, abduction, and external rotation. The position and stability of the knee and foot are variable. The major clinical problems include leg length discrepancy, malrotation of the extremity, and instability of the hip and/or knee. Assessment of the degree of shortening and the stability of the hip are important in guiding treatment options.

POSTEROMEDIAL BOWING OF THE TIBIA

The baby presents with a variable degree of bowing affecting the junction between the middle and distal third of the affected tibia. Angulation can vary from as little as 25 degrees to as much as 65 degrees and can be quite striking on presentation. The apex of the bow is located posteromedially. The affected tibia is shortened, and the ipsilateral foot, although structurally normal, is commonly smaller than the contralateral foot and is positioned in a hyperdorsiflexed and calcaneovalgus posture, appearing to fit within the affected tibia's anterior concavity. Diagnosis can be made by clinical examination and anteroposterior and lateral plain radiographs of the affected extremity.

ANTEROLATERAL BOWING OF THE TIBIA (CONGENITAL PSEUDARTHROSIS)

The affected tibia is bowed at the junction of the middle and distal thirds with the apex anterolateral. Café au lait spots may be present. Anteroposterior and lateral plain radiographs of the affected extremity should be obtained. The tibia will show bowing as observed clinically, and a sclerotic, narrow medullary canal may be present near the apex of the bow. The patient should be observed over time for development of other manifestations of neurofibromatosis.

FIBULAR HEMIMELIA

Severity ranges from partial to complete absence of the fibula. The ipsilateral tibia is commonly shorter than the contralateral tibia, and anterior bowing is not unusual. A dimple may be seen over the tibia. The ipsilateral foot may or may not be normal in appearance, and often a variable number of lateral rays may be missing. The ankle joint is typically unstable and the foot will be in equinus and valgus owing to the absence of lateral stabilizing structures. Degree of limb shortening and the stability of the ankle and foot joint are important in determining potential treatment options. In addition to a clinical examination, the diagnosis can be confirmed and further elucidated with plain radiographs.

TIBIAL HEMIMELIA

Marked limb shortening exists below the knee, and the knee joint itself is typically unstable with hypoplasia of the quadriceps muscle. The ankle may be in significant varus, and occasionally medial rays of the foot may be missing. Radiographs can be used to classify the degree of involvement. Examination for other musculoskeletal abnormalities is critical.

CONGENITAL KNEE DISLOCATION

The patient presents with varying degrees of hyperextension of the knee, ranging from mild subluxation to complete dislocation with an irreducible, markedly hyperextended position of the tibia on the femur. There may be evidence of DDH, and severe pes calcaneovalgus may be present. Although the physical examination is suggestive, anteroposterior and lateral radiographs may be necessary to differentiate between subluxation and complete dislocation, an important differentiation as treatment differs substantially between the two.

TALIPES EQUINOVARUS

The diagnosis is largely clinical, requiring no radiographic evaluation. The affected foot is smaller than the contralateral foot, with an adducted and supinated forefoot, inverted heel, and varus ankle.

The calf muscles may be weak, particularly the peroneal innervated muscles. The deformity is variable from a rigid deformity to one that is more passively correctable.

The diagnosis may be obvious based on physical examination, but plain radiographs consisting of anteroposterior, lateral, and oblique views of the affected foot can be helpful. The anteroposterior radiograph will show parallel alignment of the calcaneus and talus in the clubfoot, with lines drawn through the long axis of each being parallel. The navicular bone will be subluxed medially on the talus. On an anteroposterior radiograph of a normal foot, lines drawn through the long axes of the talus and calcaneus will cross at an angle of between 20 and 40 degrees, the "talocalcaneal angle." The talocalcaneal angle on the lateral radiograph of a clubfoot is also abnormal, measuring less than 20 degrees (normal again 20 to 40 degrees). The talus will be in an equinus position.

CONGENITAL VERTICAL TALUS

The infant presents with one or both affected hind feet fixed in equinus (plantarflexed), forefeet dorsiflexed, and pronated with deep skin creases along the dorsolateral aspect of the foot. There is a convex appearance to the plantar surface of the foot secondary to prominence of the malpositioned talar head.

The key to differentiating this deformity from those with similar appearance (eg, congenital calcaneovalgus) is that it is rigid. One cannot passively correct the deformity. Plain radiographs of the foot are essential and should include forced plantarflexion and dorsiflexion views. They will show a vertically oriented talus with the calcaneus in equinus position. However, it is not necessary to obtain these in the newborn nursery or ICU setting.

PES CALCANEOVALGUS

The affected foot is in a markedly dorsiflexed and everted position. At times, the dorsal aspect of the foot almost touches the anterior aspect of the leg. This is a flexible deformity, unlike congenital vertical talus, which can serve as an important clue when attempting to differentiate between the two. Plain radiographs can also be useful.

Management

DEVELOPMENTAL DYSPLASIA OF THE HIP

Treatment depends on two factors: the age at which the diagnosis is made and whether the hip is "dislocated" (Ortolani positive) or "dislocatable" (Barlow positive) and whether the hip can be easily passively reduced. The majority of dislocatable hips will spontaneously stabilize during the first 2 to 3 weeks after birth. Those that fail to resolve spontaneously can be treated initially with a Pavlik harness (Figure 2), a soft strap that maintains the hips in a flexed and abducted position. Initial treatment for a dislocated hip is also use of a Pavlik harness. Some hips fail to reduce with Pavlik harness treatment and require traction, casting, or even surgical reduction. Early diagnosis facilitates successful DDH treatment. The later and more established a dislocation, the more extensive surgical treatment becomes and the more likely a poor result with common complications of avascular necrosis, growth disturbance, stiffness, and premature arthritis.

PROXIMAL FEMORAL FOCAL DEFICIENCY

The absence of a hip joint results in limited reconstruction options. Fusion has not been shown to give advantage over leaving a flail articulation. Lengthening procedures may be effective in patients

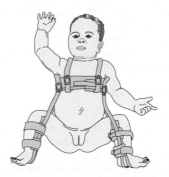

Figure 2   Pavlik harness.

with a stable hip joint. However, limb length correction is hampered by the deficiency of the hip and knee joints, leading to subluxation if not considered during lengthening procedures.

POSTEROMEDIAL BOWING OF THE TIBIA

Early passive stretching exercises may be instituted at a very early age to correct anterior compartment tightness. Although in most cases, the tibial deformity and foot position improve with growth and development, serial casting may be used in some cases. Depending on the degree to which angular deformity corrects spontaneously (average residual, 6 degrees) and the severity of leg length discrepancy (average 4.1 cm) at skeletal maturity, tibial osteotomy, and/or leg-lengthening, procedures may need to be employed.

ANTEROLATERAL BOWING OF THE TIBIA (CONGENITAL PSEUDARTHROSIS)

The natural history of this condition is fracture through the apex of the bow, followed by nonunion. Congenital pseudarthrosis of the tibia represents a difficult management problem. Eventually, patients should be fitted with a total contact orthosis to protect the intact tibia. Following fracture, which typically occurs later in life, multiple surgical options exist for treatment including intramedullary fixation, bone grafting, and vascularized graft, none of which are ideal.

FIBULAR HEMIMELIA

Treatment is determined based on the amount of predicted limb length inequality, the status of the ankle joint, and associated anomalies. Two primary modalities exist for treatment of this condition: tibial lengthening and early distal amputation with prosthetic fitting. If the ankle joint can be maintained and foot development is adequate for weight bearing, lengthening procedures should be considered. A recent study compared the two modalities and found that early amputation (before age of ambulation) yielded improved activity, pain, overall satisfaction, and fewer complications and procedures. Nevertheless, committing one's child to early amputation, albeit distal, is a difficult decision for parents to make. Education about treatment possibilities and outcomes must begin in the neonatal period.

TIBIAL HEMIMELIA

Management depends on the degree of tibial deficiency, stability of the knee, and severity of associated foot deformities. Complete absence of the tibia may be best treated with early knee disarticulation and prosthesis fitting. Marked shortening with an unstable knee or lack of an extensor mechanism may require early amputation with prosthesis fitting. The presence of an adequate tibia with a functional knee can be managed with tibiofibular synostosis and centralization.

CONGENITAL KNEE DISLOCATION

For simple hyperextension or subluxation, stretching with or without the use of serial casting or a Pavlik harness should begin in the neonatal period. Complete dislocation usually requires open surgical reduction with quadriceps or patellar tendon lengthening.

TALIPES EQUINOVARUS

The mainstay of treatment is manipulation and serial casting (the Ponseti method), typically begun while the patient is in the newborn nursery. Casts are changed on a weekly basis, and in 75 to 80% of cases, correction can be accomplished by 2 to 3 months of age. Percutaneous heel cord lengthening is frequently needed during infancy. Treatment after casting includes a prolonged period of bracing. Although some infants will fail this treatment ultimately, overall results of the Ponseti method appear superior to early surgical release.

CONGENITAL VERTICAL TALUS

This condition nearly always requires extensive surgical reduction of the talonavicular joint and other contracted tendons at approximately 1 year of age. Gentle manipulation begun in the neonatal period and serial casting can increase the compliancy of soft tissues and facilitate later surgery.

PES CALCANEOVALGUS

Passive stretching exercises begun in the neonatal period should suffice to correct this deformity. Recalcitrant cases can be treated with serial casting.

Complications and Outcomes

DEVELOPMENTAL DYSPLASIA OF THE HIP

Success rates with Pavlik harness use when begun in a timely fashion are 85 to 95% in patients with dysplasia or a reducible dislocation. The incidence of osteonecrosis with this treatment is low (< 5%). Excessive flexion and tight diapering must be avoided as this can cause femoral nerve palsy.

Failure of Pavlik harness treatment can lead to closed reduction with spica cast application up to 18 months of age. Closed reduction before 6 months of age leads to fewer reconstructive procedures at a later date. Closed reduction may be unsuccessful if there are anatomic obstacles to reduction. Excessive abduction may cause osteonecrosis. Children who fail treatment with the Pavlik harness or closed reduction and casting may require open reduction and casting, with or without pelvic and or femoral osteotomies. The rate of osteonecorsis following closed or open reduction ranges from 10 to 40%.

In general, successful outcome for treatment of the congenitally dislocated hip correlates with the preoperative grade of dislocation, the development of osteonecrosis, and the adequacy of reduction. Although most children with DDH are fully functional in childhood, those with residual deformity from incomplete acetabular or femoral development or the sequelae of avascular necrosis will develop early degenerative arthritis and typically require hip arthroplasty later in life.

PROXIMAL FEMORAL FOCAL DEFICIENCY

Although various methods of femoral pelvic arthrodesis and rotation of the distal limb to use the knee or ankle joint for motion have been described, fusion has not provided an advantage over a leaving a flail articulation. Lengthening is limited by instability in the remaining joints. Eventual function is correlated with the amount of deficiency present.

POSTEROMEDIAL BOWING OF THE TIBIA

This is a relatively benign condition and is not typically associated with more severe congenital abnormalities and tends to improve with skeletal growth. Most children ambulate at the appropriate age. The affected leg typically is several centimeters short, and compensating osteotomy and lengthening and/or contralateral growth plate arrest is frequently needed, but the functional outcome is excellent.

ANTEROLATERAL BOWING OF THE TIBIA (CONGENITAL PSEUDARTHROSIS)

Correction of this problem is quite challenging. Osteotomies before fracture commonly result in nonunion. The risk of fracture is much less after skeletal maturity. Some patients achieve enough healing to become brace free, with reasonable strength and motion. Many are plagued by recurrent fracture. Reconstructive procedures, regardless of technique, have relatively low success rates.

FIBULAR HEMIMELIA

Multiple studies have shown both tibial lengthening and early amputation with prosthesis fitting to be relatively effective treatments leading to functional, ambulating children but with residual deformity and weakness.

TIBIAL HEMIMELIA

The outcome is highly dependent on the severity of the deformity. In patients who have reconstruction, ligamentous instability, limited active motion, and contractures are common.

CONGENITAL KNEE DISLOCATION

The outcome is often complicated by associated conditions. There is no significant difference in outcomes comparing subluxated and dislocated knees when other associated musculoskeletal abnormalities are absent. Persistent instability or valgus alignment may cause persistent problems.

TALIPES EQUINOVARUS

With timely diagnosis and institution of treatment, current nonoperative measures are highly effective. Following a period of successful serial casting, parental participation will be required in the form of daily stretching exercises and maintenance of brace wear. Relapses are almost uniformly a result of noncompliance with brace wear. In one study, the relapse rate for patients who were compliant was 6%, whereas it was 60% for noncompliant patients. Within the subset of patients failing serial casting and progressing to surgical correction, between 15 and 50% will also fail surgical correction and require a salvage procedure. Long-term outcome includes diminished motion and strength.

CONGENITAL VERTICAL TALUS

Nonoperative treatment is rarely successful in treating these patients. Various surgical procedures exist for reduction of the talonavicular joint and correction of this deformity. With an early, appropriate procedure, a good outcome can be expected but with less than normal motion and strength.

PES CALCANEOVALGUS

Outcome is generally excellent when the appropriate stretching exercises are instituted in a timely fashion.

Recommended Readings

GENERAL REFERENCES

Abel MF. Orthopaedic knowledge update: pediatrics 3. Rosemont, IL: American Academy of Orthopaedic Surgeons; 2006.

Alexander M, Kuo KN. Musculoskeletal assessment of the newborn. Orthop Nurs 1997;16:21–31.

Drews U. Color atlas of embryology. New York, NY: Thieme Medical Publishers; 1993.

Fordham LA. Congenital abnormalities of the musculoskeletal system: perinatal evaluation and long-term outcome. Semin Roentgenol 2004;39:304–22.

Keller MS. Musculoskeletal sonogaphy in the neonate and infant.
    Pediatr Radiol 2005;35:1167–73.

Keret D, Bronshtein M, Wientraub S. Prenatal diagnosis of
    musculoskeletal anomalies. Clin Orthop Relat Res 2005;
    434:8–15

Miller MD. Review of orthopaedics. 3rd ed. Philadelphia, PA:
    WB Saunders; 2000.

Moore KL, Persaud TVN. The developing human: clinically ori-
    ented anatomy. Philadelphia, PA: WB Saunders; 1998.

Morrissy RT. Bone and joint infection in the neonate. Pediatr Ann
    1989;18:33–4,36–8,40–4.

Spivak JM, DiCesare PE, Feldman DS, et al. Orthopaedics, a
    study guide. New York, NY: McGraw-Hill; 1999.

Sweeney JK, Gutierrez T. Musculoskeletal implications of preterm
    infant positioning in the NICU. J Perinat Neonatal Nurs
    2002;16:58–70.

SKELETAL BIRTH TRAUMA

Beaty JH, Kasser JR. Rockwood and Wilkin's fractures in children.
    6th ed. Philadelphia PA: Lippincott Williams and Wilkins;
    2006.

Perlow JH, Wigton T, Hart J, et al. Birth trauma. A five-year
    review of incidence and associated perinatal factors. J Reprod
    Med 1996;41:754–60.

Sorantin E, Brader P, Thimary F. Neonatal trauma. Eur J Radiol
    2006;60:199–207.

BRACHIAL PLEXUS INJURY

Dodds SD, Wolfe SW. Perinatal brachial plexus palsy. Curr Opin
    Pediatr 2000;12:40–7.

Waters PM. Obstetric brachial plexus injuries: evaluation and
    management. J Am Acad Orthop Surg 1997;5:205–14.

MUSCULOSKELETAL INFECTION

Aroojis AJ, Johari AN. Epiphyseal separations after neonatal
    osteomyelitis and septic arthritis. J Pediatr Orthop 2000;
    20:544–9.

Baevsky RH. Neonatal group B beta-hemolytic streptococcus osteomyelitis. Am J Emerg Med 1999;17:619–22.

Barton LL. Neonatal group B streptococcal vertebral osteomyelitis. Pediatrics 1996;98:459–61.

Canale ST. Neonatal osteomyelitis of the os calcis: a complication of repeated heel punctures. Clin Orthop 1981;156:178–82.

Chattoraj MR, Barson W, McClead Jr RE. Radiological case of the month. Neonatal osteomyelitis. Arch Pediatr Adolesc Med 1994;148:1305–6.

Dan M. Neonatal septic arthritis. Isr J Med Sci 1983;19:967–71.

Dan M. Septic arthritis in young infants: clinical and microbiologic correlations and therapeutic implications. Rev Infect Dis 1984;6:147–55.

Dormans JP, Drummond DS. Pediatric hematogenous osteomyelitis: new trends in presentation, diagnosis, and treatment. J Am Acad Orthop Surg 1994;2:333–41.

Ho NK. Septic arthritis in the newborn—a 17 years' clinical experience. Singapore Med J 1989;30:356–8.

Kothari NA, Pelchovitz DJ, Meyer JS. Imaging of musculoskeletal infections. Radiol Clin North Am 2001;39:653–71.

Offiah AC. Acute osteomyelitis, septic arthritis and discitis: differences between neonates and older children. Eur J Radiol 2006;60:221–32.

Sucato DJ, Schwend RM, Gillespie R. Septic arthritis of the hip in children. J Am Acad Orthop Surg 1997;5:249–60.

CONGENITAL MUSCULAR TORTICOLLIS

Do TT. Congenital muscular torticollis: current concepts and review of treatment. Curr Opin Pediatr 2006;18:26–9.

CONGENTIAL SPINAL CONDITIONS

Copely LA, Dormans JP. Cervical spine disorders in infants and children. J Am Acad Orthop Surg 1998;6:204–14.

Farmer DL, von Koch CS, Peacock WJ, et al. In utero repair of myelomeningocele: Experimental pathophysicology, initial clinical experience, and outcomes. Arch Surg 2003;138:872–8.

Hedequist D, Emans J. Congenital scoliosis. J Am Acad Orthop Surg 2004;12:266–75.

CONGENITAL UPPER EXTREMITY CONDITIONS

Beredjiklian PK, Bozentka DJ. Review of hand surgery. Philadelphia, PA: Saunders; 2004.

Dao KD, Shin AY, Billings A, et al. Surgical treatment of congenital syndactyly of the hand. J Am Orthop Surg 2004;12:39–48.

Gallant GG, Bora W. Congenital deformities of the upper extremity. J Am Acad Orthop Surg 1996;4:162–71.

Graham TJ, Ress AM. Finger polydactyly. Hand Clin 1998; 14:49–64.

Marks TW, Bayne LG. Polydactyly of the thumb: abnormal anatomy and treatment. J Hand Surg 1978;3:107–16.

Shian-Chao T, Moran SL, Cooney WP, et al. The hypoplastic thumb. J Am Acad Orthop Surg 2006;14:354–66.

Watson T, Hennrikus WL. Postaxial type-B polydactyly. J Bone Joint Surg 1997;79:65–68.

CONGENITAL LOWER EXTREMITY CONDITIONS

Anonymous. American Academy of Pediatrics. Clinical practice guideline: early detection of developmental dysplasia of the hip. Pediatrics 2000;105:896–905.

Guille JT, Pizzutillo PD, MacEwen GD. Developmental dysplasia of the hip from birth to six months. J Am Acad Orthop Surg 1999;8:232–42.

Ko JY, Shih CH, Wenger D. Congenital dislocation of the knee. J Pediatr Orthop 1999;19:252–59.

Roye DP, Roye BD. Idiopathic congenital talipes equinovarus. J Am Acad Orthop Surg 2002;10:239–48.

Schoenecker PL, Capelli AM, Millar EA, et al. Congenital longitudinal deficiency of the tibia. J Bone Joint Surg 1989; 71:278–87.

THIRTEEN

Genetic Considerations

Charles F. Simmons Jr, MD

Up to 3% of newborns have one or more congenital malformations at birth; ultimately, up to 10% of newborns will exhibit at least one minor anomaly by 10 years of age. Of these newborns with major and minor anomalies, some will require surgical intervention. Surgery may occur in the immediate neonatal period for life-threatening abnormalities or may be deferred until later in life, with an emphasis on improved functional and cosmetic outcome. In this post-Human Genome Project era, an increasing number of surgical disorders are now known to result from specific genetic mutations. Knowledge of these mutations will impact the accuracy of genetic counseling and future prenatal diagnosis in affected families. In addition, careful attention to the genetic aspects of surgical disease, facilitated by the collaborative efforts of pediatric surgeons, neonatologists, and geneticists, will ensure that we continually improve our understanding of how genetic predisposition contributes to congenital abnormalities. Monogenetic, chromosomal, and multifactorial patterns of inheritance contribute to the molecular mechanisms of surgical disease in the newborn. In addition, it is becoming evident that nonmendelian inheritance, including mitochondrial inheritance, mosaicism, uniparental disomy, and genetic imprinting, may play a significant role in the development of some surgical conditions in the newborn.

Genetic Assessment

Although, ideally, assessment begins with the prenatal obstetric care of a prospective mother, sometimes evaluation begins only after the birth of a child with an unexpected congenital anomaly that requires surgical intervention. Despite the belief that genetic assessment of a family leaves much uncertainty regarding the role of genetics in the causation of a congenital anomaly, it is only through the systematic genetic assessment of affected newborns and their families that we will improve our understanding of molecular mechanisms of surgical disorders in the newborn. In the future, the development of additional population-based and individual biochemical and genetic screening tests may help prospectively refine the risks of genetic abnormalities. The genetic assessment of newborns with surgically amenable congenital anomalies and their families requires the coordinated efforts of pediatric surgeons, neonatologists, and genetics professionals, including geneticists and genetic counselors.

HISTORY

Accurate assessment of the newborn with a surgical abnormality first requires a detailed family history, pedigree, and medical history. The construction of a pedigree will serve as a corner stone and may suggest mendelian or nonmendelian modes of inheritance. Any teratogenic exposures or potentially teratogenic maternal illnesses such as diabetes mellitus or infectious agents should be identified. Any triple screen data should be interpreted. Neonatal deaths, spontaneous abortions, infertility, or family history of other newborns with congenital anomalies should be elicited in a sensitive conversation with the parents and, potentially, after parental and familial consent, other family members. A comprehensive evaluation may warrant examination of the parents.

PHYSICAL EXAMINATION

Careful attention to all organ systems should be undertaken, including ophthalmologic examination as warranted. The presence of multiple major anomalies increases the likelihood of an underlying chromosomal disorder. Of note, the concept of physical examination must be extended to include any available obstetric ultrasonography or magnetic resonance imaging.

LABORATORY STUDIES

- Cytogenetic analysis should be performed in all instances of major anomalies or multiple minor anomalies.

- Fluorescence in situ hybridization analysis can provide diagnostic information for specific deletion disorders, such as the chromosome 22q11 microdeletion syndrome, leading to velocardiofacial syndrome with its associated cardiovascular abnormalities and DiGeorge syndrome with micrognathia, hypoparathyroidism, immunodeficiency, and posterior cleft palate.
- Molecular genetic analysis can be performed for specific disorders, allowing detection of mutations, insertions, deletions, imprinting, and triplet repeat abnormalities. Comparative array genomic hybridization is a new method that facilitates detection of subtle chromosomal abnormalities. Specific biochemical analysis may be warranted depending on the suspected abnormality.
- In the event of a neonatal death, arrangements should be made for potential skin, liver, and muscle biopsy for cryopreservation as well as tissue culture in selected instances. Deoxyribonucleic acid, protein, and histologic studies can be performed on frozen tissue, whereas fresh tissue or tissue culture is required for functional studies or cytogenetic analysis. Premortem genetics consultation can establish the optimal means of collection and storage of appropriate samples for later analysis.

IMAGING STUDIES

Radiographic studies of the axial skeleton and long bones should be performed as warranted. In addition, ultrasonography, echocardiography, computed tomography, and magnetic resonance imaging studies may be required to further define the internal anatomy of a newborn with congenital anomalies.

Diagnosis

Clinical genetic diagnosis has increasingly become a combination of the acumen of the individual clinician, coupled with an efficient process for timely electronic database search algorithms and updates from the burgeoning repositories of genetic knowledge represented in both classic and electronic media formats.

INFORMATIONAL RESOURCES

The fund of genetic knowledge is rapidly expanding. Consequently, clinicians must continuously supplement differential diagnosis through the consultation of appropriate databases.

Gene Tests and Gene Clinics

This combined Web site was originally developed by Dr Roberta Pagon, University of Washington, with resources from the department of energy, the Health Resources and Services Administration, and the National Institutes of Health. This comprehensive, merged Web site offers the clinician a summary of the genetic condition, clinical description, differential diagnosis, suggested management, genetic counseling issues, molecular genetics summary, testing locations, and links to other resources and references pertinent to the disorder. Currently, over 400 conditions are summarized (for instance, congenital diagphragmatic hernia, Hirschsprung disease, and Beckwith-Wiedemann syndrome and associated omphalocele) with plans for progressive expansion of content (www.genetests.org).

Genetic and Rare Conditions

This University of Kansas Web site provides genetic disease information and links to support groups nationwide (such as Hirschsprung disease) (www.kumc.edu/gec/support).

PubMed—Online Mendelian Inheritance in Man

This site, supported by the National Library of Medicine, provides the clinician with the ability to rapidly search the literature for new data regarding a particular diagnosis. In addition, clinicians can access Online Mendelian Inheritance in Man, the catalog of human genes and genetic disorders developed by Dr Victor McCusick and colleagues at Johns Hopkins University (www.ncbi.nlm.nih.gov/omim). The database is searchable using the National Center for Biotechnology Information Entrez interface and facilitates access to both text information and references.

RESEARCH

To improve future health care, we need to identify, and rectify, gaps in our understanding of the etiologies of surgical disease in the newborn. It is incumbent on all health care professionals to become aware of local, regional, and national studies that seek to further understand the genetic basis of surgical disease in the newborn. Although critical to the advancement of medical and surgical diagnostic and treatment modalities, genetic research must not be coercive and must meet all ethical standards for the participation of the proband and family members as research subjects.

Treatment

In addition to treatment of the surgical disorder by the pediatric surgeon (detailed in each appropriate section of this book), concomitant medical disorders may require a multidisciplinary approach to patient care. The neonatal intensive care unit is an environment conducive to successful, collaborative multidisciplinary efforts.

Genetic Counseling

COLLABORATIVE APPROACH

To provide the best possible care for families, the integrated efforts of a team of individuals, including the obstetrician, perinatologist, neonatologist, pediatric surgeon, and genetics professionals, are required. The initial medical genetics referrals for such evaluations may come from obstetricians, neonatologists, or pediatric surgeons. Although risk assessment is based on mendelian principles in many conditions, conversely, many disorders have empiric risk calculations that are based on population-based incidence of disease.

FOLLOW-UP

Depending on the time at which genetic counseling is undertaken, the nondirective recommendations of genetics professionals may be pertinent during a current pregnancy or may be of future use to the reproductive planning of a family at risk.

Specific Disorders

Although up to 10 to 15% of all newborns eventually have a minor malformation detected in the first 10 years of life, approximately 3 to 5% of newborns have abnormalities detected within the newborn period. These abnormalities may be the result of environmental exposures, genetic abnormalities, or combinations of genetic and environmental etiologies. The following section summarizes genetic considerations for these common surgical disorders of the newborn.

CENTRAL NERVOUS SYSTEM

Neural Tube Defects, Including Anencephaly, Encephalocele, Myelomeningocele

Periconceptional folate has significantly decreased the incidence of neural tube defects. In addition, improved preconceptional control of diabetes mellitus has decreased the risk of spina bifida in this maternal condition. Single gene disorders include Meckel syndrome caused by mutation in a gene encoding a component of the flagellar apparatus basal body proteome. Walker-Warburg syndrome is caused by mutation in the genes encoding protein O-mannosyltransferase-1 and 2. Robert syndrome is caused by mutation in the ESCO2 gene whose protein product facilitates establishment of sister chromatid cohesion during S phase.

Hydrocephalus

The majority of cases result from neural tube defects; an X-linked form has been identified owing to mutations in the L1CAM gene on chromosome Xq28, although not all families with X-linked aqueductal stenosis map to this locus.

CRANIOFACIAL

Cleft Lip, Cleft Palate

This disorder is associated with major trisomies and over 50 mendelian disorders, some of which have had the causal gene identified. Maternal diabetes mellitus is associated with this disorder, as well as maternal ethanol ingestion.

Craniosynostosis

Mutations of the MSX2 gene, the FGFR2 gene (with syndactyly, Apert syndrome), Crouzon disease and FGFR2 mutations, and Pfeiffer syndrome with mutations in FGFR1 and FGFR2, all result in craniosynostosis.

PULMONARY

Congenital Diaphragmatic Hernia

Congenital diaphragmatic hernia can occur as an isolated, nonsyndromic anomaly, or as part of a syndrome. A chromosomal abnormality may be detected. Autosomal dominant, recessive, and X-linked patterns of inheritance have been reported in various pedigrees. The recurrence risk ranges from 1 to 2% for sporadic occurrence to 25 to 50% for autosomal recessive or dominant inheritance, respectively. Genes have not yet been identified for Fryns syndrome (autosomal recessive), Simpson-Golabi-Behmel syndrome, and Brachmann-de Lange syndrome, all of which can result in diaphragmatic hernia. Tetrasomy 12p can also result in diaphragmatic hernia.

CONGENITAL HEART DISEASE

Congenital heart disease often develops in combination with other serious congenital anomalies.

22q11 Microdeletion Syndrome

Commonly associated with DiGeorge syndrome or velocardiofacial syndrome, these infants can display hypocalcemia owing to hypoparathyroidism, immunodeficiency owing to deficient T-cell development in the thymus, posterior cleft palate, micrognathia, and pharyngeal muscle coordination difficulties.

Connexin 43 Mutations

These mutations can be associated with cardiac anomalies and heterotaxy but are still being evaluated for causal role in the molecular mechanism of the cardiac anomalies.

Heterotaxy: X-linked and Sporadic

Visceral heterotaxy includes a variable group of congenital anomalies that include complex cardiac anomalies and situs inversus or situs ambiguous. Zic3 transcription factor gene deletion or mutation has been found in some patients with sporadic heterotaxy.

CFC1 Mutations and Transposition of the Great Arteries or Double Outlet Right Ventricle With or Without Heterotaxy

Loss of function of CFC1 mutations have been defined in patients with heterotaxy syndromes, as well as transposition of the great arteries and double outlet right ventricle. EGF-CFC proteins act as cofactors in the nodal signaling pathway that controls left-right axis development in vertebrates including humans.

Tbx5 Mutations

Loss of function of Tbx5 mutations leads to a dominant haploinsufficiency state. Holt-Oram syndrome results from certain Tbx5 mutations and consists of upper limb malformations, atrial septal defects, and other cardiac anomalies.

NKX 2.5 (CSX) Mutations

Mutations in the CSX homeobox gene can result in tetralogy of fallot.

JAG1 Mutations

JAG1 mutations can result in right sided obstructive lesions, including tetralogy of fallot and isolated pulmonic stenosis, in addition to haploinsufficiency states that include Alagille syndrome.

DSCAM

DSCAM is a gene in the Down syndrome critical region and encodes a neural cell adhesion like molecule. DSCAM is a candidate gain of function gene for trisomy 21–related congenital heart disease and duodenal atresia.

Noonan Syndrome

Mutations in PTPN11, encoding the protein tyrosine phosphatase SHP-2, cause up to 50% of cases of autosomal dominant, gain of function Noonan syndrome (pulmonic stenosis).

GASTROINTESTINAL TRACT

Hirschsprung Disease

Monogenic, Syndromic Hirschprung Disease Syndromic Hirschprung disease presents with GI tract involvement associated with other anomalies. Of note,

- RET mutations are the most common mutations associated with Hirschsprung disease, thus far. RET is located on chromosome 10q11.
- EDNRB mutations are the second most common cause of Hirschsprung disease. They are usually associated with a short-segment disease phenotype and are autosomal dominant.
- SOX10 mutations result in Hirschsprung disease and Waardenburg syndrome.
- Bardet-Biedl syndrome: associated with Hirschsprung disease and the unknown gene
- Cartilage hair hypoplasia: associated with Hirschsprung disease and RMRP
- Congenital central hypoventilation syndrome is associated with Hirschsprung disease and PHOX2B, RET, GDNF, EDN3, and BDNF.
- Familial dysautonomia: associated with Hirschsprung disease and IKBKAP
- Fryns is associated with Hirschsprung disease and unknown gene.

- Goldberg-Shprintzen syndrome: associated with Hirschsprung disease and KIAA1279
- L1 syndrome: associated with Hirschsprung disease and L1CAM
- MEN2A: associated with Hirschsprung disease and RET
- MEN2B: associated with Hirschsprung disease and RET
- Mowat-Wilson syndrome: associated with Hirschsprung disease and RET
- Neurofibromatosis 1: associated with Hirschsprung disease and NF1, GDNF
- Smith-Lemli-Opitz syndrome: associated with Hirschsprung disease and DHCR7
- Waardenburg syndrome type 4: associated with Hirschsprung disease and EDNRB, EDN3, SOX10

Nonsyndromic Hirschsprung Disease

Isolated Hirschsprung disease is due to mutations in the RET ligand-receptor signaling pathway and EDNRB and related genes:

- RET: tyrosine protein kinase receptor
- GDNF: glial cell-derived neurotrophic factor
- NRTN: Neurturin
- EDNRB: Endothelin B receptor
- EDN3: Endothelin 3
- ECE1: Endothelin converting enzyme
- EDNRB mutations are the second most common cause of Hirschsprung disease. They are usually associated with a short-segment disease phenotype and are autosomal dominant.

Imperforate Anus

Cat eye syndrome (coloboma and inverted duplication of chromosome 22q11), VACTERL (vertebral, anal, cardiac, tracheal, esophageal, renal, and limb) association, trisomy 18, Pallister-Hall syndrome (GLI3 mutations), and Townes-Brocks syndrome (SALL1 transcription factor gene mutations) can all result in imperforate anus.

Duodenal Atresia

This is associated with trisomy 21, as well as with autosomal recessive inheritance. No genes have been identified. DSCAM is a candidate gene in the Trisomy 21 critical region.

Esophageal Atresia/VACTERL Association

There are sporadic cases owing to mitochondrial mutations and suspected GLI mutations.

Pyloric Stenosis

The recurrence risk is 10% in male sibs of an affected infant, but no pattern of inheritance, genetic loci, or susceptibility loci have been established.

VENTRAL WALL DEFECTS

Gastroschisis

This anomaly is usually isolated and rarely associated with aneuploid states. Autosomal recessive inheritance is suspected in some families.

Omphalocele

An association with Beckwith-Wiedemann syndrome and duplications or imprinting of region 11p15.5. Up to 50% of infants with omphalocele have associated anomalies.

Bladder Exstrophy

This is rarely associated with Opitz syndrome and mutations of MID1.

Cloacal Exstrophy

This genitourinary anomaly is occasionally seen as the OIES complex with omphalocele, imperforate anus, cloacal exstrophy, and spinal defects.

GENITOURINARY/RENAL

Vesicoureteral Reflux

This is likely autosomal dominant with linkage to chromosome 1p13. Mutations in the ROBO2 gene cause another variant of vesicoureteral reflux, VUR2.

HEMATOLOGIC

Thrombophilic states can contribute to surgical morbidity owing to complications in the perioperative period or secondary to catheter thrombosis. Mutations in the following genes promote a thrombophilic state:

Factor V Leiden

Approximately 2 to 5% of the population carries the Factor V Leiden mutation.

Protein C

Autosomal dominant; heterozygotes constitute 0.2 to 0.5% of the population.

Protein S

Autosomal dominan; numerous protein S mutations have been described.

Antithrombin III

There are many mutations, and the prevalence is 0.3% of the population.

Prothrombin 20210 mutation

The prevalence is 2 to 3% of the population.

MTHFR C677T mutation

Predisposes to hyperhomocysteinemia and thrombophilia.

Death of an Infant or Fetus with Anomalies

As noted above, the death of an infant with congenital anomalies is a tragic event but also represents a critical decision point regarding the extent of molecular and genetic analysis. Sensitive discussion with families at an appropriate time will lead to consideration of additional testing that may contribute to better understanding certain anomalies and their likelihood of recurrence.

DNA Banking

Storage of DNA for possible future use should be considered for families with children affected by various unexplained congenital anomalies, particularly if the anomaly may be lethal. Many laboratories offer this service (see www.GeneTests.org).

Fibroblast Culture

A skin biopsy, umbilical cord sample, or placental sample can provide sufficient cells for culture and later analysis.

Autopsy

Postmortem analysis of any infant with congenital anomalies should be considered with the family.

Imaging

Postmortem imaging has been suggested to provide additional information, particularly if autopsy permission is not granted.

Genetics Consultation

Medical genetic consultation can be invaluable to facilitate proper diagnosis, additional studies if warranted, and feedback regarding recurrence risks of various surgical anomalies.

Recommended Readings

Bianchi DW, Crombleholme T, D'Alton M. Fetology: diagnosis and management of the fetal patient. McGraw Hill; 2000.

Jones KL, Fletcher J. Smith's recognizable patterns of human mal-
    formation. 6th ed. WB Saunders; 2006.

Rimoin DL, Conner JM, Pyeritz R, Korf B, (eds). Emery and
    Rimoin's principles and practice of medical genetics. 5th ed.
    Churchill Livingstone; 2006.

FOURTEEN

Anesthesiology

Part 1: Anesthesia for Neonatal Surgical Emergencies

Roland Brusseau, MD, and Babu Koka, MD

Introduction

Newborns undergoing emergency operations present several difficult challenges for the anesthesiologist. Many surgical emergencies in the neonate are life-threatening and are frequently accompanied by multiple organ system failure. In the neonatal period, the stress from this degree of illness, in addition to the simultaneous adjustments to extrauterine life, can cause severe disturbances in an already precarious physiology. For the caregivers, there is often minimal time for adequate evaluation and proper preparation of the infant for surgery. Communication and cooperation between the entire health care team, including surgeons, anesthesiologists, and neonatologists, are of the utmost importance to ensure the best possible care of the neonate.

General Preoperative Evaluation

PRENATAL HISTORY

Obtaining an adequate prenatal history is an important first step in the preoperative assessment of the neonate. Significant information includes the following parameters:

Gestational Age

This is the single most important factor in determining survival. In general, the more premature the neonate, the higher the incidence of complications of prematurity (intraventricular hemorrhage, respiratory distress syndrome, apnea and bradycardia of prematurity, electrolyte and glucose imbalance, hyperbilirubinemia, and sepsis).

Presence of Polyhydramnios or Oligohydramnios

Polyhydramnios may indicate bowel obstruction from duodenal atresia or stenosis, annular pancreas, congenital diaphragmatic hernia (CDH), airway obstruction from cervical teratoma/cystic hygroma, tracheoesophageal fistula, anencephaly, cystic adenomatoid malformation of the lung, pulmonary sequestration, or immune or nonimmune hydrops.

Oligohydramnios is associated with renal agenesis or dysgenesis and symptoms may include marked deformation of the fetus due to intrauterine constraint (Potter syndrome) and may also adversely affect fetal lung development, resulting in pulmonary hypoplasia and severe respiratory insufficiency.

Mode of Delivery

Vaginal versus cesarean section, emergency cesarean section, variable or late decelerations during labor, presence of nuchal cord, forceps or vacuum delivery, and presence of meconium are important variables in the preoperative assessment and may provide insight into level of hemodynamic and physiologic stability of the infant.

Apgar Scores

A score of 0 to 10 is based on the newborn's heart rate, respiratory effort, muscle tone, reflex irritability, and color. Lower numbers suggest increased degree of perinatal depression.

Extent of Newborn Resuscitation

Meconium aspiration, ventilatory assistance/intubation, use of surfactant, ventilator settings, and hemodynamic stability.

PHYSICAL EXAMINATION

General Appearance

Gross anomalies (eg, omphalocele, gastroschisis), activity level (excessive or lethargic), state of nutrition, evidence of dehydration, cry (high-pitched, hoarse), presence or absence of cyanosis, jaundice, or edema.

Respiratory

Tachypnea, flaring of alae nasi, expiratory grunt, intercostal retractions, and rales.

Cardiac

Presence of heart murmur, rate and rhythm, palpation of femoral and radial pulses, or low blood pressure.

Signs of Impending Cardiovascular Collapse

Signs of cardiovascular collapse can vary significantly and often are insidious in onset. The earliest indicators include pallor, tachycardia (as neonatal cardiac output is rate-determined), collapsed veins, and listlessness. Initially, vital signs can remain stable followed by a sudden drop as compensatory mechanisms fail. Hypotension is a late and ominous sign.

EVALUATION OF ONGOING TREATMENT

Intake and Output of Fluids

The amount and type of replacement fluids given should be noted. Urine output is often calculated by weighing diapers as most infants will not have urinary catheters in place during the preoperative period.

Signs of Fluid Overload

Signs of fluid overload are often subtle and may include decreased oxygen saturation, decreased lung compliance, rales, increased cardiac size on chest radiography, and increased central venous pressure.

Electrolytes

Abnormalities depend on existing pathophysiology. Given their immature renal function, neonates are prone to hyponatremia, hypocalcemia, and hypokalemia.

Hematologic Evaluation

Minimal hematologic evaluation should include a complete blood count. For major surgical procedures, coagulation profile, recent transfusions, and the availability of blood products should be noted.

Medications

All current medications must be carefully noted, including the dosage and the rate of administration of all drugs, vasopressors, and inotropic agents.

Respiratory Assistance

Oxygen requirement, arterial blood gases, ventilator settings, type of ventilator used, and use of special techniques (high-frequency ventilation, nitric oxide).

Response to Treatment

Favorable changes in blood pressure, heart rate, and oxygen saturation measurements in response to treatment indicate a good general condition of the infant prior to surgery.

EVALUATION OF MONITORING AND INTRAVENOUS ACCESS

Mandatory Monitors

- Pulse oximetry (preductal and postductal)
- Blood pressure
- Heart rate
- Temperature

Invasive Monitors

- Indwelling arterial catheter: Continuous pressure display and timely measurements of arterial blood gases, electrolytes, and hematocrit are imperative for the care of critically ill neonates. Placement often is difficult and may require a surgical cutdown.
- Central venous catheter: Central venous catheter provides large-bore venous access for resuscitation, provision of

vasoactive and/or inotropic medications and access for anticipated long-term intravenous (IV) requirements. Central venous pressure monitoring may be helpful in evaluating fluid status.

IV Access

- Venous access is frequently difficult to obtain in the newborn period, especially in the setting of dehydration.
- Commonly, 24 gauge and 22 gauge are the largest IV catheters that can be inserted peripherally.
- Consider a central venous or a femoral vein catheter as an alternative.

CARDIOVASCULAR SYSTEM

Changing Cardiovascular Physiology

Perinatal cardiovascular physiology is an evolving process. Respiration initiates circulatory changes, which unfold over the first few hours to days of extrauterine life.

- Fetal circulation: In utero circulation is primarily a parallel circuit. Fluid-filled lungs are bypassed via the foramen ovale and ductus arteriosus.
- At birth: The pulmonary vascular resistance (PVR) drops allowing blood to flow through pulmonary vasculature. The ductus arteriosus and foramen ovale generally close physiologically.
- Extrauterine life: After birth, circulation changes to a series type of circuit. This transition can be disrupted by hypoxia, hypercarbia, acidosis, hypothermia, stress, and prematurity. These occurrences are frequently unavoidable during transport and surgery and consequently produce deleterious effects on the transitional physiology of circulation, leading to persistent fetal circulation.

Congestive Heart Failure

- The newborn is susceptible to congestive heart failure.
  1. The myocardium has limited compliance at birth.
  2. Histologic features include 50% reduction and chaotic arrangement of myofibrils, absent transverse tubular system, and immature sarcoplasmic reticulum.

3. The heart grows primarily by myocyte cell number expansion (hyperplasia) prior to birth; postnatally, heart growth is predominantly by myocyte cell enlargement (hypertrophy).
4. Left ventricular mechanics including wall motion and shortening fraction are impaired in the preterm infant.
5. Cardiac output is rate dependent, therefore any bradycardia should be aggressively treated to prevent a fall in cardiac output.

- Signs of congestive failure are usually nonspecific and include pallor, tachycardia, tachypnea, poor peripheral circulation, rising core temperature relative to peripheral temperature, acidosis, hypothermia, and oliguria.
- Management consists of diagnosing the underlying physiology, fluid restriction, diuretics, and inotropic agents.

Congenital Cardiac Defects

There is an increased incidence of congenital cardiac defects in neonates with other congenital anomalies.

- Signs: Cyanosis, cardiac failure, presence of murmur, dyspnea, decreased oxygen saturation, and hypotension with decrease femoral pulses
- Relatively common lesions: Patent ductus arteriosus, ventricular and atrial septal defects, tetralogy of Fallot, coarctation of the aorta, transposition of the great arteries, and pulmonic stenosis
- Diagnostic studies: Electrocardiography, chest radiography, and echocardiography are the most common and accessible preoperative cardiac examinations. Other studies, including Doppler ultrasonography, computed tomography, magnetic resonance imaging (MRI), cardiac catheterization, and selective angiocardiography, require further planning and personnel and may not be available in the immediate preoperative period.

NEONATAL AUTONOMIC NERVOUS SYSTEM

Sympathetic System

The sympathetic system is immature at birth in preterm and term infants; however, there is progressive maturation after birth. Newborns may need vasopressors/fluid to maintain hemodynamic stability.

Parasympathetic System

The parasympathetic system is predominant in preterm and term infants. Consequently, any stimulation or stress (including hypoxemia) may lead to bradycardia. Atropine (20 to 30 µg/kg IV/IM/PO/PR) may be needed prior to stressful interventions, such as laryngoscopy.

Neonatal Somatosensory System

- This system is functional extremely early in fetal life.
- By 16 weeks' of gestation, the fetus is capable of a reflex response to stress.
- Somatosensory pathways continue to develop after birth.
- A considerable body of evidence now indicates that preterm and term infants require anesthesia and analgesic medications to adequately suppress the stress response to surgical intervention and improve surgical outcomes.

Respiratory System

Physiology

- Type II pneumocytes that are responsible for surfactant production differentiate at 24 weeks of gestation, but surfactant synthesis is not adequate until 34 to 36 weeks of gestation. Maternal preterm betamethasone therapy (for up to 48 hours prior to delivery) has been shown to improve lung maturation in preterm neonates.
- Oxygen consumption of neonate is twice that of an adult on a per weight basis; hence, alveolar ventilation in neonates needs to be twice that of adults.
- Infants have relatively lower functional residual capacity than adults.
- Even modest decreases in ventilation or fraction of inspired oxygen (FiO_2) will predispose newborns to rapidly desaturate.
- Airway obstruction cannot be overcome by neonates because of a compliant chest wall and weak muscles of respiration.

This obstruction can occur when infants are sedated or during mask ventilation.

- Any impediment to diaphragmatic movement (eg, owing to abdominal distention or secondary to gastric insufflation) can cause significant respiratory compromise.
- Central control of ventilation is not fully developed, and responses to hypoxia are immature in the neonate. Peripheral feedback mechanisms likewise are not sufficiently matured.
- The respiratory control mechanisms are unstable, and oxygenation can oscillate between hyperoxia and hypoxemia.
- Apnea often results from airway obstruction, hypoxemia, or hypothermia.
- Methylxanthines (caffeine) have been used to treat apnea of prematurity and to reduce the rate of bronchopulmonary dysplasia for the past 30 years. Recent work has demonstrated improved survival rate without neurodevelopmental disability from this treatment method.

Respiratory Failure

Premature infants are especially prone to respiratory failure owing to the fragile physiology described above.

- Causes include pleural effusions, hemothorax, meconium aspiration syndrome, pneumonia, atelectasis, pulmonary edema, and abdominal compression of the diaphragm.
- Signs include tachypnea, tachycardia, chest retractions, cyanosis, nasal flaring, and decreased oxygen saturation.
- Evaluation may include chest radiography and arterial blood gases.
- If intubation and controlled ventilation are required, oxygen requirements, respiratory rate, tidal volume, positive end-expiratory pressure, and the type of ventilator and the settings used should be noted. In case of severe prematurity or critical respiratory failure, it is highly advantageous to use an identical ventilator with comparable settings during the operation.

Endotracheal Tube Size

- The cricoid cartilage is the narrowest portion of the larynx in a pediatric patient.

- Despite the size of the endotracheal tube, an audible air leak should exist when positive pressure is applied at 20 to 40 cm H_2O.
- Uncuffed tubes remain preferable, unless prolonged ventilation, poor pulmonary compliance, or increased postoperative intraabdominal pressure (ie, closure of gastroschisis) are expected.

Weight	Internal Diameter (mm)
1 kg	2.5 uncuffed
1.5 kg	3 uncuffed
2 kg	3 uncuffed
3 kg (preterm)	3 uncuffed
3 kg (term)	3 to 3.5 uncuffed

Intubation Techniques

The following differences exist in the neonatal airway compared with the adult's:

- Large head and tongue
- Mobile, "U"-shaped epiglottis
- Anterior position of the larynx
- Cricoid cartilage narrowest point in the airway

For these reasons, intubation of the trachea is easier with the head in a slightly flexed or neutral position than with the head hyperextended. Laryngoscopy is performed with straight blades that aid in maneuvering under the epiglottis so that the vocal cords can be visualized. Commonly used blades include Miller 0, Miller 1, and Wis-Hipple blades. The availability of more than one type of blade is recommended in the event that intubation is more difficult than expected. Laryngeal mask airways can also be used in neonates (usually size 1 or 1 1/2) but offer limited protection for the lungs from the risk of aspiration.

Renal Physiology

Sodium Regulation

- Preterm and term infants cannot concentrate urine; they are obligate sodium losers.
- By contrast, the urine-diluting capacity is well developed.

- When the infant is fluid deprived, urine osmolality reaches only 680 osm/L (the adultís can rise to 1,400 osm/L).
- Adequate exogenous sodium and water must be provided during the perioperative period.

Glomerular Filtration Rate

- This rate is greatly decreased in preterm and term infants.
- It increases fourfold by 3 to 5 weeks of age.
- Excretion of drugs dependent on glomerular filtration rate may be delayed.

HEMATOLOGIC CONSIDERATIONS

- Coagulation tests, except bleeding time, are abnormal in the neonate.
- Prothombin time and partial thromboplastin time are prolonged.
  1. Concentration of vitamin K-dependent factors (II, VII, IX, X) is decreased.
  2. In case of vitamin K deficiency, 1 mg of vitamin K should be given intravenously, with clinical effects usually seen 4 hours after administration.
- Fibrinogen and Factor V concentrations are similar to those of adults.
- Term neonates often coagulate at an increased rate owing to decreased amounts of naturally occurring anticoagulants.
- Acutely ill neonates may develop bleeding disorders. Signs include generalized petechiae, large soft tissue and subcutaneous hemorrhages, and oozing from the puncture site.
- Preterm infants (< 35 weeks) are at risk for intraventricular hemorrhage.

THERMOREGULATION

Causes of Hypothermia

Infants, especially preterms, are extremely susceptible to hypothermia for several reasons:

- Large body surface area relative to body weight

- Thin layer of insulating subcutaneous fat
- Decreased ability to produce heat. The primary mechanism is nonshivering thermogenesis mediated by brown fat.

Prevention of Hypothermia

The utmost care is taken to prevent heat loss during the transport and the intraoperative period.

- Provide a neutral thermal environment (warm operating room).
- Transport the neonate in a heated module.
- Humidify and warm inspired gases.
- Warm solutions to clean skin and for intraoperative irrigation.
- Warm blood and IV solutions.
- Heated mattress
- Radiant warmer
- "Bair Hugger" warmers. Heated hot air circulation under the drapes.

Need for Anesthesia

In the past, anesthesia and analgesia for operations and painful procedures on premature and term infants were often withheld because of the false perception that the neonate cannot sense pain. A growing body of evidence demonstrates that the developing fetus can mount a stress response to noxious stimuli as determined by measured serum catecholamines as early as 16 weeks of gestation. Studies in neuroanatomy and physiology indicate that nociception is functional in preterm neonates. Recent studies also suggest that PVR increases in response to stress, placing the neonate at increased risk of shunting of blood at the level of the foramen ovale and/or ductus arteriosus with resultant hypoxemia. Preterm neonates "anesthetized" with only nitrous oxide and curare mount a significant hormonal stress response when compared with premature neonates receiving fentanyl as the primary anesthetic. For these reasons, anesthesia and analgesia should be and can be safely administered to neonates, even those who are critically ill, provided that the following are considered:

Effects of Anesthetic Agents

- Volatile anesthetic agents produce a dose-dependent depression in cardiac output and function to a greater degree in neonates than in adults.
- Neonates require lower concentrations of volatile anesthetics than do infants 1 to 6 months of age. This may be attributable to elevated levels of progesterone and β-endorphins.
- Preterm infants need even lower anesthetic concentrations than required by the term infants.
- Preterm and term infants are more likely than older children to develop hypotension during administration of an anesthetic agent.
- Volatile anesthetic agents may place the infant at risk for bradycardia and diminished cardiac output secondary to nodal and conduction depression.
- Opioids produce minimal hemodynamic changes in the preterm and term infant. However, these cause substantial respiratory depression, making postoperative ventilatory support necessary.

Anesthetic Management of Specific Neonatal Conditions

CDH

Pathology

- The incidence is 1 in 5,000 live births.
- Defective formation of the diaphragm results in failure of the gut to return to the abdominal cavity.
- The diaphragmatic defect varies in size and location. The foramen of Bochdalek (left posterolateral hernia) comprises 80% of cases.
- Compression by abdominal contents results in unilateral or bilateral lung hypoplasia and possible mediastinal shift.
- The presence of liver in the chest is associated with very high mortality.
- The amount of lung surface available for gas exchange will ultimately determine neonatal outcome (eg, less than

15% predicted lung volume (determined by MRI) suggests poor prognosis).

Clinical Presentation

- CDH is often diagnosed in utero by ultrasonography.
- Classic features include respiratory distress, scaphoid abdomen, increased anteroposterior diameter of the chest, detection of bowel sounds during auscultation of the chest, and profound arterial hypoxemia.
- Chest radiograph: Loops of bowel in thorax, mediastinal shift, and compression of lungs
- Differential diagnosis includes lung cysts, hemopneumothorax, and pneumonia.

Associated Congenital Defects

- Cardiac defects: Present in 25 to 30% of patients
- Gastrointestinal (GI): Malrotation of intestines, intestinal obstruction
- Skeletal abnormalities

Ventilation

- If there is obvious respiratory failure, ventilate with 100% Fio_2. In the presence of pulmonary hypoplasia, ventilation with small tidal volume and faster respiratory rates will lower mean airway pressure and avoid pulmonary barotrauma.
- As mask ventilation will introduce air into the GI tract, as well as the lungs, early intubation should be considered.
- Nasogastric decompression aids in decreasing the gas content of the bowel and further diminution of lung volume and should be performed early.
- Inflating pressures should be less than 30 cm H_2O with continuous monitoring of airway pressure.
- Pulmonary barotrauma can lead to devastating complications, such as pneumothorax, pneumomediastinum, soft tissue emphysema, and air embolism.
- Equipment to place a chest tube should be immediately available at all times, including during the transport of the infant.

- Turning the infant on the side of the hernia may help ventilation and oxygenation.
- Intraoperative use of muscle relaxants will facilitate intubation, positive pressure ventilation, and avoidance of coughing or straining on the endotracheal tube. This will also prevent swallowing of air that might further distend the stomach and intestines in the chest.
- With all of the above measures, there may be an initial improvement; however, this is often followed by deterioration of respiratory status.

Pulmonary Hypertension

Some degree of pulmonary hypertension is usually present in these infants, and, in the past, every possible step was taken to prevent further rises in PVR. Since hypercarbia and hypoxemia increase PVR, infants were hyperventilated to decrease arterial partial pressure of carbon dioxide ($PaCO_2$), and the FiO_2 was increased to maintain arterial partial pressure of oxygen (PaO_2) above 100 torr.

This technique has been associated with increased pulmonary barotrauma and a higher morbidity in these infants. The preferred approach at present is a "kinder and gentler" ventilation with permissive hypercarbia and lower PaO_2 levels. This helps minimize iatrogenic lung injury in those infants who cannot afford any further compromise in lung parenchyma.

OPERATIVE CONSIDERATIONS

Surgery Versus Extracorporeal Membrane Oxygenation

There remains considerable debate about the timing of surgery. Currently, more than 30% of CDH neonates are being managed with extracorporeal membrane oxygenation (ECMO) before undergoing surgical repair. Patients with liver herniation or significantly reduced predicted pulmonary volumes are often given a trial of ventilation followed by ECMO for respiratory failure, whereas patients with particularly severe diminutions of pulmonary volume are now frequently placed directly onto ECMO with an ex utero intrapartum treatment (EXIT) to ECMO procedure (see below) prior to surgical correction. Although outcomes for patients with without liver herniation and associated anomalies are impressive (with survival rates greater than 90%), the survival rates for infants with significant disease who do not respond to aggressive therapy remain quite low.

EXIT

EXIT procedures have become a treatment option for certain fetuses with CDH diagnosed in utero at several pediatric institutions. EXIT procedures for CDH entail delivering the fetal head through a controlled hysterotomy either to intubate the fetus and assess oxygenation or place the fetus onto ECMO prior to umbilical cord clamping. In this way, the fetus receives an uninterrupted supply of oxygen from the mother via the umbilical cord until another form of adequate oxygenation can be established for extrauterine life. In some circumstances, fetal gas exchange can be supported by ex utero placental circulation for over 60 minutes, affording ample time to make appropriate management decisions for the infant. Such EXIT to ECMO procedures are performed on those infants with no hope of survival if delivered by traditional means.

Low Oxygen Saturation

Hypoxia and acidosis might be aggravated owing to surgical manipulations in the chest, cardiac failure, fluid overload, or hypothermia. Pulmonary barotrauma should be avoided by careful monitoring of the airway pressures. Lung compliance might deteriorate during intraoperative fluid resuscitation owing to increased lung water.

Increased Intra-abdominal Pressure

During the operation, the defect in the diaphragm is repaired, and the abdominal viscera are returned to their original location. Intra-abdominal pressure may increase excessively at the time of abdominal closure. Patients will require higher ventilating pressures.

Ventilation

Infants with CDH have limitations in lung function and compliance, as discussed previously. For these reasons, several important points need to be considered when providing controlled ventilation for these patients.

- Respiratory failure and acidosis may be aggravated owing to surgical manipulations in the thorax.
- Pulmonary barotrauma should be avoided by careful monitoring of airway pressure (< 30 cm H_2O maximum pressure).
- Infants with CDH will require higher ventilating pressures owing to increased intra-abdominal pressure when the abdominal viscera are returned to their original location.
- Lung compliance may deteriorate during intraoperative fluid resuscitation due to increased lung water.

Monitors

- Central venous pressure catheter is useful for venous access and for ensuring adequate right ventricular preload.
- An arterial line is necessary for continuous pressure monitoring during surgical manipulations, to observe the effects of pressors when needed, and for blood gas measurements.

Drugs

Inotropic agents (dopamine, dobutamine) may be necessary to improve myocardial performance and right ventricular output.

Venous Access

It is of the utmost importance to obtain adequate venous access prior to undergoing surgical repair. Access for drug resuscitation and blood transfusion may be needed emergently. Central venous access may be considered if peripheral access is limited.

Anesthesia and Ablation of Stress Response

- Narcotics: A growing body of evidence indicates that opioids (fentanyl) can profoundly suppress fetal and newborn catecholamine levels in response to painful stimuli. In addition, large doses of narcotics probably minimize the pulmonary vasoconstrictor responses to stress and painful stimuli.
- Thoracic epidural: An epidural catheter is usually placed via the caudal approach and threaded to the midthoracic region.

Preemptive analgesia with local anesthetics (bupivacaine) has been shown to substantially suppress catecholamine and cortisol levels in response to surgical stimuli. In addition, the presence of a thoracic epidural can be of invaluable assistance in the postoperative period to minimize the requirements for sedation and muscle relaxants in the intensive care setting.

ESOPHAGEAL MALFORMATIONS

Esophageal malformations can occur in several forms: tracheoesophageal fistula, isolated esophageal atresia with or without tracheal communication, or double fistulae. The incidence is estimated at one in 4,000 live births. In the vast majority of cases (87%), there is a blind upper pouch with fistulous communication to the trachea or the bronchus.

Prenatal diagnosis can be made with ultrasonography. Signs noted soon after birth include drooling, aspiration, choking spells, and abdominal distention. A gastric tube cannot be passed beyond the atretic esophagus. Contrast radiographic studies are often conclusive. The clinical course can be complicated by the consequences of prematurity, pulmonary aspiration, and abdominal distention.

Preoperative Considerations

Apart from the anatomic considerations, there are other factors that influence surgical therapy.

- Aspiration and presence of pneumonia
- Air leak through the fistula, abdominal distention, and loss of tidal volume
- Degree of prematurity: Almost half of affected infants are premature.
- Associated anomalies of other organs found in more than 50% of cases. Often there is a combination of vertebral, anal, cardiac, tracheal, esophageal, renal, and limb anomalies. Cardiac anomalies are found in 15 to 40% of cases.

Intraoperative Considerations

- Primary closure of the fistula and anastomosis: This is the primary goal of therapy in all infants because this prevents further aspiration and abdominal distention. Often the general condition and the presence of other anomalies determine the timing and the extent of the surgical intervention.

- Type of operation: Depending on the general condition of the patient, surgical options include primary closure of the fistula, gastrostomy before or after the ligation of the fistula, or a delayed primary closure.

- Timing of gastrostomy: The decision to perform a gastrostomy depends on the condition of the infant. In most situations, primary repair is preferable without a preliminary gastrostomy. Children repaired with this technique generally do better because gastrostomy by itself carries a degree of morbidity.

- Abdominal distention: If there is significant gastric distention causing respiratory compromise, it is advisable to perform a gastrostomy under local anesthesia to vent the stomach prior to induction.

- Preliminary tracheobronchoscopy is very useful in locating the opening of the fistula. In approximately 5% of cases there may in fact be a second fistula present. Some authors propose that TEF occlusion by placement of a Fogarty arterial embolectomy catheter should be used before beginning the surgical procedure, minimizing the time during which there is a conduit between the GI and respiratory tracts.

- Induction and intubation: During induction of anesthesia, extreme care should be taken to prevent abdominal distention and pulmonary aspiration. In ill premature infants, an awake intubation is preferred. Alternatively, intubation following a deep inhalational induction may be considered. To minimize the air escape through the fistulous connection, some reports suggest the feasibility of placing the tip of the endotracheal tube beyond the fistula so that the opening can be sealed off. However, the length of the newborn trachea is so small that it is not practical to place the endotracheal tube in the exact position. In addition, even a small movement of the head can dislodge the tip of a well-placed tube. In many cases, the fistulous opening is at the carina, in which case it is not possible to try to obstruct the opening.

- Maintaining O_2 saturation: Retraction of the lung is necessary for adequate exposure during the intraoperative period. Maintaining adequate O_2 saturation is the main problem during this period. Difficulties with oxygenation are not surprising in an open chest procedure with collapsed lung, especially in a premature infant. Close communication with the surgeon is essential. There are reports of successful single lung ventilation following deliberate left mainstem intubation, particularly when thoracoscopic surgical techniques are used.

- Blockage of the endotracheal tube: Bleeding into the trachea during surgical manipulations can cause blockage of the endotracheal tube. This also can lead to dramatic episodes of desaturation. Often it is difficult to distinguish between tube obstruction and lung retraction as the cause of desaturation. The retracted lung should be reinflated and the endotracheal tube suctioned. The endotracheal tube should be replaced if the blockage cannot be cleared.

- Prevention of excess airway pressures: Airway pressures should be carefully monitored and kept to a minimum during the entire procedure. This precaution is essential prior to the ligation of the fistula to prevent gastric distention. This is also important in the intraoperative and postoperative period as excessive airway pressures may disrupt the repair.

- Prevention of fluid overload: During the repair of the fistula, there should be only minimal loss of blood or fluids. Hence, IV fluids should be used with caution. Even modest excess of lung water may cause severe respiratory failure in the presence of prematurity, aspiration, or congestive failure.

OMPHALOCELE AND GASTROSCHISIS

Omphalocele Pathology

The major abdominal wall defects that present at delivery are omphalocele and gastroschisis. Both lesions are caused by failed closure of the anterior wall, thus allowing herniation of abdominal viscera. The incidence of omphalocele is one in 3,000 to 10,000 live births. Classically, an omphalocele is a periumbilical defect of the abdominal wall. Herniation of viscera covered with a translucent layer of peritoneum and amniotic membrane is the hallmark of the lesion although this membrane can rupture during a traumatic delivery.

Omphalocele Preoperative Considerations

Coexisting anomalies associated with omphalocele include malrotation of the intestine, congenital heart defects (tetralogy of Fallot, atrial septal defect), chromosomal abnormalities, diaphragmatic hernia, trisomies, meningocele, microcephaly, and Beckwith-Wiedemann syndrome.

Gastroschisis Pathology

The defect in gastroschisis is caused by the absence of a portion of the right abdominal wall. Although the etiology of this lesion is not clear, most attribute this lesion to the disappearance of the right umbilical vein in utero. Lack of regional blood flow leads to an atretic right abdominal wall. Associated GI malformations, such as intestinal atresia and infarcts, occur with this lesion. However, defects in other organs are rare.

Intraoperative Considerations

Although the etiology of the two lesions is different, intraoperative considerations are similar for both.

- Prevention of infection: The defect is wrapped in sterile wet dressing to prevent infection. If the defect is large, it is usually covered with a bulky dressing. If proper attention is not paid, intestine at the base of the defect might get twisted and compromise blood supply. This is especially true during transportation or during the preparatory period in the operating room.
- Hypothermia: Heat loss can be a problem because a large surface of the intestine is exposed. Measures to prevent heat loss and to keep the baby warm must be initiated vigorously.
- Fluid loss: This extensive exposed surface of the intestines also leads to large insensible fluid losses. Aggressive fluid replacement is essential in these cases.
- Increased intra-abdominal pressure: If the edges of the abdominal defect are closed too tightly, intra-abdominal pressure will increase. This can lead to respiratory compromise and diminished blood flow to abdominal organs and to the lower extremity, as well as decreased central venous return and diminished cardiac output. Close communication between the surgeon and the anesthesiologist during the closure will avoid this problem.

EXSTROPHY OF THE BLADDER

Exstrophy of the bladder or of the cloaca is a rare disorder affecting one in 30,000 to 40,000 live births. Males are affected three to four times more than females. These defects are best closed during the neonatal period to minimize fluid loss and to prevent infections. Surgery can be lengthy and complicated because of the revision of the bladder, small bowel, colon, and sometimes the bony pelvis. Blood loss and hypothermia are the major anesthetic problems associated with the surgical repair of this lesion.

INTESTINAL OBSTRUCTION

Obstructive lesions of the GI tract create surgical emergencies in the neonate. The site of obstruction can occur anywhere from the esophagus to the anus. Causes of neonatal intestinal obstruction are (1) congenital, including atresias, stenosis, or webs of the esophagus, pylorus, duodenum, jejunum, ileum, or colon; (2) mechanical, including malrotation, intussusceptions, incarcerations, perforations, or volvulus of the bowel; and (3) functional, including meconium ileus or Hirschsprung's disease.

Preoperative Considerations

The signs and symptoms of intestinal obstructions consist of vomiting, abdominal distention, and failure to pass stools. Hypovolemia, dehydration, and electrolyte imbalances can be attributed to loss of gastric, biliary, and pancreatic secretions.

Intraoperative Considerations

There is a significant risk of pulmonary aspiration during induction of anesthesia in patients with these lesions. Rapid sequence induction with cricoid pressure is preferred for most patients. In severely debilitated neonates, awake intubation should be considered. Abdominal distention can precipitate respiratory or cardiovascular collapse. Therefore, preoperative gastric decompression with a nasogastric tube is essential; the nasogastric tube should remain on suction during induction of anesthesia and intubation to minimize the amount of gastric contents in the oropharynx. The degree of dehydration should be carefully assessed and corrected.

NECROTIZING ENTEROCOLITIS

Necrotizing enterocolitis (NEC) is the most common surgical emergency in newborns. It is the leading cause of death among neonates who undergo surgical procedures. Mortality is 50% in the presence of sepsis. Given the improving survival rate of very-low-birth-weight neonates owing to aggressive respiratory support, NEC has become a leading determinant of neonatal morbidity.

Preoperative Considerations

The causes of NEC are still not clear and are likely multifactorial. Risk factors for NEC are prematurity, enteral feedings, hypoxemia, patent ductus arteriosus, and cyanotic heart disease. Ischemic damage of intestine, bacterial colonization, and release of toxic substrate have all been implicated in the pathogenesis of this disease.

A total of 3 to 8% of low-birth-weight neonates (< 1,500 g) develop NEC. These patients usually have immature respiratory function and require intubation and mechanical ventilation. Full-term neonates with concurrent disease, such as congenital heart disease and polycythemia are at risk for NEC. NEC is heralded by mild intestinal distress, followed by ileus, hematochezia, and sometimes fulminant sepsis and shock. The characteristic abdominal radiographic findings are of pneumatosis coli and free peritoneal air.

Medical Treatment

- Discontinue oral feedings.
- Decompress the stomach with a nasogastric tube.
- Administer broad spectrum antibiotics.
- Replace intravascular volume with normal saline. Use component blood therapy, such as packed red blood cells (15 mL/kg) and fresh frozen plasma (10 mL/kg) if needed.
- May need to support circulation with vasopressors, such as dopamine or epinephrine if necessary.

Surgical Treatment

Surgical intervention becomes necessary in some cases.

- The absolute indication for surgery is pneumoperitoneum.

- Relative indications include positive paracentesis, erythema of the abdomen, fixed abdominal mass, persistent dilated loop of bowel, or persistent metabolic acidosis.
- The lesion is usually localized to one segment of bowel; however, any part can be involved. Therefore, it is important to assess the entire length of the intestine.

Intraoperative Considerations

Anesthetic management is quite exacting given the fragile state of the neonate with NEC. By the time surgery is warranted, these newborns are often on the verge of hemodynamic collapse and require aggressive fluid resuscitation and mechanical ventilation. Before the start of surgery, an arterial catheter is very helpful to monitor blood pressure, blood gases, and hematocrit. Adequate venous access is mandatory. Anesthesia can be maintained with narcotics and low-dose isoflurane. A disproportionate amount of blood can be rapidly lost. Insensible fluid loss can be extreme because of bowel manipulation. These deficits should be aggressively replaced with blood products and 5% albumin.

MENINGOMYELOCELES AND MENINGOCELES

Failure of the closure of the caudal end of the neural tube is characterized by a sac that contains neural contents. A growing body of evidence supports a dual causation for the loss of spinal cord function, consisting of the initial embryonic defect and a secondary injury of the neural tissue exposed to amniotic fluid throughout gestation. The contribution of the secondary injury relative to the initial embryonic defect remains unknown and is difficult to establish in human studies. Care should be taken to prevent contamination, drying, or injury of exposed structures during induction of anesthesia. Hydrocephalus and increased intracranial pressure are usually present and are indications for surgical insertion of a ventriculoperitoneal shunt.

NEONATAL TUMORS

- Typical abdominal tumors include neuroblastomas, ovarian cysts, and mesenteric cysts. Frequently, surgical emergencies develop because the tumors cause bleeding, torsion of the

mesentery, airway compression or significant pressure on the vital structures.
- Sacrococcygeal teratoma is the most common neoplasm of the newborn. These tumors are highly vascularized and can hold a large volume of blood and fluid. The high incidence of mortality with this lesion has been associated with spontaneous hemorrhage, obstruction of umbilical vessels in utero, and high-output cardiac failure.

Intraoperative Considerations

Excision of a large tumor is associated with enormous amounts of blood and heat loss. Given the high cardiac output state associated with lesions, large fluid shifts during the surgical resection of this tumor can provoke fulminant congestive heart failure.

Conclusion

The responsibility of treating such severity of illness in such small patients is challenging. Numerous permutations and combinations can occur with congenital defects leading to variations in the presentation and severity of neonatal surgical illness. However, even the smallest and sickest infants can be successfully anesthetized with adequate knowledge of newborn physiology, careful planning, and attention to minute detail.

Recommended Readings

Anand KJ, Hall RW. Pharmacological therapy for analgesia and sedation in the newborn. Arch Dis Child Fetal Neonatal Ed 2006;91:F448–53.

Atzori P, Iacobelli BD, Bottero S, et al. Preoperative tracheobronchoscopy in newborns with esophageal atresia: does it matter? J Pediatr Surg 2006;41:1054–7.

Cote CJ, et al. A practice of anesthesia for infants and children. 4th ed. Elsevier; 2008.

Fine GF, Borland LM. The future of the cuffed endotracheal tube. Paediatr Anaesth 2004;14:38–42.

Kunasaki SM, Barnewolt CE, Estroff JA, et al. Ex utero intrapartum treatment with extracorporeal membrane oxygenation for severe congenital diaphragmatic hernia. J Pediatr Surg 2007;42:98–106.

Spitzer AR, ed. Intensive care of the fetus & neonate. 2nd ed. Mosby; 2005.

TABLE 1 Pharmacologic Agents

		Single Dose‡	Infusion§
Local Anesthetics			
Lidocaine 0.5%*		Maximum dose: 5 mg/kg SQ	(1 mL/kg of 0.5% solution) (0.5 mL/kg of 1% solution)
EMLA 5% cream†		33 to 37 wk PMA and > 1.8 kg	Maximum dose: 0.5 g for 1 to 2 h (then remove excess)
		> 37 wk PMA and > 2.5 kg	Maximum dose: 1 g for 1 to 2 h (then remove excess)
Analgesics			
Morphine	Intubated	0.05 to 0.15 mg/kg IV or SQ	0.01 to 0.03 mg/kg/h
	Nonintubated	0.025 to 0.05 mg/kg IV or SQ	not recommended
Fentanyl¶	Intubated	2 to 5 mg/kg (over 5 min) IV	0.2 to 0.5 mg/kg/h
	Nonintubated	0.25 to 0.5 mg/kg (over 5 min) IV	not recommended
Acetaminophen		10 to 15 mg/kg PO/PG/PR every 6 hours prn Maximum dose 40 mg/kg/24 h	

Local Anesthetics

Sedatives

Short-term
Midazolam# 0.05 to 0.1 mg/kg IV or intranasal

Long-term
Phenobarbital Loading dose: 5 to 10 mg/kg
PO, PG, or IV

Maintenance dose: 3 to 4 mg/kg
PO, PG, or IV

PMA = postmenstrual age; SQ = subcutaneous; IV = intravenous; PO = by mouth; PG = per gastrum; PR = per rectum; prn = as needed.

*Lidocaine toxicity may cause cardiac arrhythmia or seizure. 0.5% solution can be made by 1:1 dilution of 1% lidocaine with normal saline.

†EMLA should be limited to a single dose per day and must be removed within 2 hours. It takes 40 to 60 minutes following application to achieve the maximum effect of EMLA. Prilocaine (in EMLA) may cause methemoglobinemia. Swelling associated with the use of EMLA might distort anatomic structures.

‡May repeat dosing at 10- to 15-minute intervals until initial therapeutic effect is achieved.

§May titrate above this dosing range to achieve a therapeutic effect.

Morphine may cause hypotension.

¶Rapid infusion of fentanyl may cause chest wall rigidity.

#Midazolam is recommended for use only in full-term infants. Abnormal myoclonic movements have been described in premature infants treated with midazolam.

TABLE 2 Postoperative Analgesia

	Intubated and Ventilated Infants	Nonintubated Infants
Herniorraphy	Acetaminophen 10 to 15 mg/kg PO/PG/PR q4 to 6h Morphine 0.05 to 0.1 mg/kg q2 to 4h prn IV q4h prn or fentanyl* 1 to 3 *g/kg q2 to 4h prn	Acetaminophen† 10 to 15 mg/kg PO/PG/PR q6h or morphine 0.025 to 0.05 mg/kg IV q4h prn or fentanyl*0.25 to 0.5 µg/kg IV q4h prn
Laparotomy	1st 24 h: Morphine 0.1 mg/kg q2 to 4h or fentanyl* 1 to 3 mg/kg q2 to 4h Then: Morphine 0.05 to 0.1 mg/kg q2 to 4h prn or fentanyl* 1 to 3 mg/kg q2 to 4h prn	Morphine 0.025 to 0.05 mg/kg IV q4h prn or fentanyl* 0.25 to 0.5 mg/kg IV q4h prn
Thoracotomy	1st 24 h: Morphine 0.05 to 0.1 mg/kg or fentanyl* 1 to 3 mg/kg q2 to 4h Then: Morphine 0.05 to 0.1 mg/kg q2 to 4h or fentanyl* 1 to 3 mg/kg q2 to 4h	Acetaminophen† 10 to 15 mg/kg PO/PG/PR q6h prn or morphine 0.025 to 0.05 mg/kg IV q4h prn or fentanyl* 0.25 to 0.5 mg/kg IV q4h prn
Laser surgery	Acetaminophen† 15 mg/kg 2 h before and acetaminophen† 10 mg/kg q6h after the procedure (24 h), then q6h prn	Acetaminophen† 10 mg/kg PO/PG/PR q6h after the procedure (1st 24h), then q6h prn
Neurosurgery	Fentanyl* 1 to 3 mg/kg q2 to 4h prn or morphine 0.05–0.1 mg/kg q² to 4h prn	Acetaminophen† 10 to 15 mg/kg PO/PG/PR q6h prn or fentanyl* 0.25 to 0.5 mg/kg IV q4h prn or morphine 0.025 to 0.05 mg/kg IV or SQ q4h prn

IV = intravenous; PO = by mouth; PG = by gastrum; PR = per rectum; prn = as needed; SQ = subcutaneous.
*Fentanyl should be infused at ≤1 mg/kg/min (eg, 3 mg/kg) infused over >3 minutes).

Part 2: Pain Assessment and Management

Linda J. Van Marter, MD, MPH, and
Corinne Pryor, BA, RNC

Background

Both scientific evidence and humanitarian considerations favor management strategies to prevent pain and stress whenever possible and, when discomfort is unavoidable, to provide prompt and appropriate treatment. These principles are as relevant to the treatment of newborn infants as they are in managing pain in older children and adults.

FETAL AND NEONATAL PHYSIOLOGIC RESPONSES TO PAIN

Because sensory nerve terminals exist on all body surfaces by 22 to 29 weeks of gestation, the fetus is capable of perceiving painful stimuli. Early in development, overlapping nerve terminals create local hyperexcitable networks, enabling even low-threshold stimuli to produce an exaggerated pain response.

Physiological responses to painful or stressful stimuli include increase in circulating catecholamines, increased heart rate and blood pressure, and elevated intracranial pressure. Although the fetus is capable of mounting a stress response beginning at approximately 23 weeks of gestation, the autonomic and other markers of the stress response of the immature fetus or preterm infant are less competent than that of the more mature infant or child. Therefore, among immature infants, the common vital sign changes associated with pain or stress (eg, tachycardia, hypertension, agitation) are not reliable indicators of painful stimuli. Even when the infant's stress response is intact, persistence of painful stimuli for hours or days fatigues or deactivates the sympathetic nervous system response, obscuring signs of pain or discomfort. Repeated noxious stimuli alter sensitivity to painful stimuli and appear to lower the pain threshold, slow recovery, and adversely effect long-term outcomes.

MEDICAL AND DEVELOPMENTAL OUTCOMES

Neonatal Medical and Surgical Outcomes

Neonatal responses to pain contribute to compromised physiologic states such as hypoxia, hypercarbia, acidosis, hyperglycemia, respiratory dyssynchrony, and pneumothorax. Early studies of surgical responses to pain suggest an infant's intraoperative course is more stable and postoperative recovery is improved when the infant receives adequate surgical analgesia and anesthesia. Pain causes both increased intrathoracic pressure due to diaphragmatic splinting and vagal responses that can affect oxygenation and cerebral blood flow.

Neurodevelopmental Outcomes

Behavioral and neurological studies suggest that preterm infants who experience numerous painful procedures and noxious stimuli are less responsive to painful stimuli at 18 months corrected age. However, at 8 to 10 years of age, unlike their normal birthweight peers, infants born at or below 1,000 g birth weight rated medical pain intensity greater than measures of psychosocial pain. These data provide evidence that neonatal pain and stress influence neurodevelopment and affect later perceptions of painful stimuli and behavioral responses and that prevention and control of pain are likely to benefit infants. There are few large randomized clinical trials of pain management. One such trial (ie, NEOPAIN trial) evaluated preemptive analgesia with morphine infusion up to 14 days among ventilated preterm infants and showed no difference overall in the primary composite outcome (ie, neonatal death, severe intraventricular hemorrhage [IVH], or periventricular leukomalacia) between placebo and preemptive morphine treated groups. Concerns were raised, however, when post hoc analyses revealed an increased risk of severe IVH among morphine infusion treated babies in the subgroup born at 27 to 29 weeks of gestation. Subsequent analyses suggested the adverse outcomes were limited to infants who were hypotensive before morphine therapy was initiated. These data suggest that treatment with prophylactic morphine infusion should be limited to infants who are normotensive.

Principles of Prevention and Management of Neonatal Pain and Stress

PRINCIPLES OF PAIN MANAGEMENT

The initial management guideline of the Committee on the Fetus and Newborn of the American Academy of Pediatrics offered number of principles relevant to newborn pain and stress.

- Neuroanatomical components and neuroendocrine systems of the neonate are sufficiently developed to allow transmission of painful stimuli.
- Exposure to prolonged or severe pain may increase neonatal morbidity.
- Infants who have experienced pain during the neonatal period respond differently to subsequent painful events.
- Severity of pain and effects of analgesia can be assessed in the neonate using validated instruments.
- Newborn infants usually are not easily comforted when analgesia is needed.
- A lack of behavioral responses (including crying and movement) does not necessarily indicate the absence of pain.

CURRENT AAP RECOMMENDATIONS

In 2006, the Committee on the Fetus and Newborn of the American Academy of Pediatrics provided expanded guidelines for assessment and management of pain and stress in the newborn.

Assessment of Pain and Stress in the Newborn

a. Caregivers should be trained to assess neonates for pain using multidimensional tools.
b. Neonates should be assessed for pain routinely and before and after procedures.
c. The chosen pain scales should help guide caregivers in the provision of effective pain relief.

Reducing Pain From Bedside Care Procedures

a. Care protocols for neonates should incorporate a principle of minimizing the number of painful disruptions in care as much as possible.

b. Use of a combination of oral sucrose/glucose and other non-pharmacologic pain-reduction methods (nonnutritive sucking, kangaroo care, facilitated tuck, swaddling, developmental care) should be used for minor routine procedures.

c. Topical anesthetics can be used to reduce pain associated with venipuncture, lumbar puncture, and intravenous catheter insertion when time permits but are ineffective for heel-stick blood draws, and repeated use of topical anesthetics should be limited.

d. The routine use of continuous infusion of morphine, fentanyl, or midazolam in chronically ventilated preterm neonates is not recommended because of concern about short-term adverse effects and lack of long-term outcome data.

Reducing Pain from Surgery

a. Any health care facility providing surgery for neonates should have an established protocol for pain management. Such a protocol requires a coordinated, multidimensional strategy and should be a priority in perioperative management.

b. Sufficient anesthesia should be provided to prevent intraoperative pain and stress responses to decrease postoperative analgesic requirements.

c. Pain should be routinely assessed using a scale designed for postoperative or prolonged pain in neonates.

d. Opioids should be the basis for postoperative analgesia after major surgery in the absence of regional anesthesia.

e. Postoperative analgesia should be used as long as pain-assessment scales document that it is required.

f. Acetaminophen can be used after surgery as an adjunct to regional anesthetics or opioids, but there are inadequate data on pharmacokinetics at gestational ages less than 28 weeks to permit calculation of appropriate dosages.

Reducing Pain From Other Major Procedures

1. Analgesia for chest-drain insertion comprised all of the following:

   a. general nonpharmacologic measures,

   b. slow infiltration of the skin site with a local anesthetic before incision unless there is a life-threatening instability, and

   c. systemic analgesia with a rapidly acting opiate such as fentanyl

2. Analgesia for chest drain removal comprises the following:
   a. general nonpharmacologic measures and
   b. short-acting, rapid onset systemic analgesia
3. Although there are insufficient data to make a specific recommendation, retinal examinations are painful and pain-relief measures should be used. A reasonable approach would be to administer local anesthetic eye drops and oral sucrose.
4. Retinal surgery should be considered major surgery, and effective opiate-based pain relief should be provided.

Evaluating Neonatal Pain and Stress

There are a number of validated and reliable scales of pain assessment. Behavioral indicators (eg, facial expression, crying, body/extremity movement) and physiological indicators (eg, tachycardia or bradycardia, hypertension, tachypnea or apnea, oxygen desaturation, palmar sweating, changes in vagal tone, plasma cortisol or catecholamine levels) often are useful in assessing the infant's level of comfort or discomfort.

Physiological responses to painful stimuli include release of circulating catecholamines, heart rate acceleration, blood pressure increase, and a rise in intracranial pressure. Because the stress response of the immature fetus or preterm infant is less competent than that of the more mature infant or child, gestational age must be considered in evaluating the pain response. Among preterm infants experiencing pain, the vital signs associated with the stress response (eg, tachycardia, hypertension) and agitation are not consistently evident. Even among infants with an intact response to pain, a painful stimulus that persists exhausts sympathetic nervous system output and obscures the clinician's ability to objectively assess the infant's level of discomfort.

RECOMMENDED ASSESSMENT TOOLS

Selecting the most appropriate tool for assessment of neonatal pain must take into consideration the infant's gestational age and other clinical factors, such as severity of illness. A number of useful tools exist; we recommend three; the Premature Infant Pain

Profile (PIPP), the Behavioral Pain Score (BPS), and the Neonatal
Infant Pain Scale (NIPS).

Intensive Care Infants: PIPP

Pain assessment must consider the influence of gestational age on
the pain response. The Premature Infant Pain Profile (PIPP), a
method that includes assessment of facial expression as well as
physiological measures in the context of gestational age and neonatal state, is the only method that has been validated for assessment
of pain among preterm infants. Although PIPP mainly has been
used for preterm infants, because it adjusts for gestational age, it
also can be used to assess pain and discomfort in term infants.

Intermediate Care or Well Nursery
Infants: BPS or NIPS

For full-term or growing former preterm infants, there are a number
of pain assessment scales. We recommend the Behavioral Pain Score,
a method that assesses motor activity, cry, consolability, and sleep. An
alternative is the Neonatal Infant Pain Scale, a research tool that has
been used to assess pain preinterventions and postinterventions.

Management: Pain Prevention and
Treatment

ENVIRONMENTAL AND BEHAVIORAL
APPROACHES

Painful or stressful procedures should be minimized and coordinated with other aspects of the newborn's care.

1. During the procedure, the following environmental and devel-
   opmentally-supportive measures might prove useful to reduce
   infant pain and stress:

   - Clustering painful interventions prior to a comforting event
     (eg, feeding)
   - Swaddling during the procedure
   - Nonnutritive sucking; pacifier
   - Use of mechanical lancets for heel-stick blood draws

2. Following the procedure, other measures are helpful:

- Reducing noise and light
- Touch or massage
- Parent-infant skin-to-skin contact or Kangaroo Care
- Holding the baby following the procedure
- Positional nesting or containment using blanket rolls

PHYSIOLOGICAL INTERVENTIONS

There are 2 primary approaches to physiological pain management. These are sucrose analgesia and competitive stimulation.

1. Sucrose analgesia (0.12 to 0.36 g) (0.5 to 1.5 mL of 24% sucrose solution) given orally approximately 2 minutes prior to the painful procedure and
2. Competitive stimulation (eg, gently rubbing, tapping, or vibrating one extremity before and/or during painful stimulus to another)

Pharmacological Management

A number of considerations are relevant to the pharmacological management of neonatal pain.

1. Complementary therapies: Environmental and behavioral interventions should be applied to all infants experiencing painful stimuli. These measures and sucrose analgesia often are useful in conjunction with pharmacological treatments.
2. Prophylaxis versus pain treatment: Narcotic analgesia given prophylactically on a scheduled basis results in a lower total dose and improved pain control compared with "as needed" dosing. In acute illness in which pain is ongoing and repeated narcotic dosing is needed, a continuous narcotic infusion might achieve effective pain control at a lower cumulative dose than accomplished by intermittent dosing.
3. Gestational maturity: A prophylactic approach is appropriate in the immature acutely ill infant who must be assumed to be incapable of mounting a detectable stress response to signal his/her discomfort. The inability of the infant to mount an appropriate response is especially relevant when the infant is extremely immature or the painful stimulus is severe and/or prolonged.

4. No long-term adverse effects of the use of opioid analgesia among ventilated infants have been reported. These include long-term studies assessing intelligence, motor function, and behavior.

Pharmacological Treatment of Procedure-Related Pain

ANALGESIA FOR MINIMALLY-INVASIVE PROCEDURES

When the infant is full-term, sucrose analgesia is recommended for once or twice-daily blood draws, at a dose of sucrose 0.12 to 0.36 g total dose (24% sucrose solution 0.5 to 1.5 mL) approximately 2 minutes prior to the procedure. Studies of sucrose analgesia are largely limited to full-term infant populations. Evidence is scanty in support of the use of sucrose analgesia among premature infants, and one investigator raised caution concerning the use of sucrose analgesia among infants below 31 weeks of gestation. However, some centers use smaller doses of sucrose solution to treat moderately preterm infants (30 to 36 weeks gestational age) who were undergoing minimally invasive procedures. Among preterm infants, we recommend lower doses: sucrose 24% solution, 0.1 to 0.5 mL (0.024 to 0.12 g), with the option to repeat this dose 2 minutes before and after the procedure.

ANALGESIA FOR INVASIVE PROCEDURES

Narcotics (eg, morphine or fentanyl) and sedatives (eg, midazolam or phenobarbital) are useful in treating critically ill newborns undergoing invasive or very painful procedures. Alleviating pain is the most important goal. Therefore, treatment with analgesics is recommended in preference to sedation without analgesia. The addition of a short-acting muscle relaxant might decrease the time and number of attempts needed for intubation and reduce the rate of severe oxygen desaturation.

1. For most invasive procedures, pharmacological premedication is recommended. Except in instances of emergency intubation, newborns should be premedicated for invasive procedures. Examples of procedures for which premedication is indicated include elective intubation, mechanical ventilation, chest tube

insertion or removal, arterial catheter placement, laser surgery, and circumcision.

2. For intubation and the first few days of mechanical ventilation, we recommend around-the-clock medication with fentanyl 1 to 3 µg/kg IV or Morphine 0.05 to 0.15 mg/kg IV every 4 hours. Thereafter, we recommend dosing these medications on an as needed basis. Among infants who are not intubated, we recommend fentanyl 0.25 to 1 µg/kg IV of fentanyl with repeated dosing as needed. Fentanyl must be infused slowly (no faster than 1µg/kg/min) to avoid the complications of chest wall rigidity and impaired ventilation. Among infants at or near term gestation undergoing an isolated procedure, such as intubation, midazolam 0.1mg/kg IV may be used in addition to narcotic analgesia. Before adding a short-acting muscle relaxant for intubation, airway control and the ability to perform effective bag-mask ventilation must be ensured.

3. For circumcision, we recommend treatment with oral 24% sucrose analgesia and 15 mg/kg of acetaminophen preoperatively and, for the procedure, ring or dorsal penile block with a maximum dose of 0.5% 0.5 mL/kg of lidocaine. Following the procedure, the infant might benefit from 10 mg/kg of acetaminophen every 6 hours for 24 hours (total dose not to exceed 40 mg/kg).

4. Sedatives and narcotics cause respiratory depression and should be used in newborns only in settings in which respiratory depression can be promptly treated by medical staff who have expertise in airway management.

PERIOPERATIVE ANALGESIA

We recommend premedicating intubated infants undergoing surgery with 1 to 3 µg/kg of fentanyl or 0.1 mg/kg of morphine 1 hour before transfer to the operating suite. Infants who are not intubated receive perioperative analgesia and sedation in the operating room just prior to intubation. Postoperative analgesia should be provided, and guidelines are provided in Table 3.

NALOXONE FOR REVERSAL OF OPIOID SIDE EFFECTS

Naloxone (Narcan) is not routinely used to treat infants receiving narcotic analgesia. Instead it is used only to treat the side effects of excessive opioid dosing, most commonly respiratory depression.

In neonatal resuscitation, a relatively large dose (0.1 mg/kg or more) is used. This is appropriate in the infant with profound respiratory depression. However, in an infant receiving narcotic analgesia, the optimal goal is to block the adverse effects without exacerbating pain. If the baby's clinical status permits, an alternative approach can be used, titrating administration, to administer naloxone in increments of 0.05 mg/kg until the side effects are reversed.

Suggested Readings

American Academy of Pediatrics Committee on Fetus and Newborn and Section on Surgery and Canadian Paediatric Society Fetus and Newborn Committee. Prevention and management of pain in the neonate: an update. Pediatrics 2006;118:2231–41.

Anand KJ, Aranda JV, Berde CB, et al. Summary proceedings from the neonatal pain-control group. Pediatrics 2006;117:S9–22.

Anand KJS, Stevens BJ, McGrath PJ. Pain in neonates and infants. Edinburgh: Elsevier; 2007.

Belleini C, Bagnoli F, Perrone S, et al. Effect of multisensory stimulation on analgesia in term neonates: a randomized clinical trial. Pediatr Res 2002;51:460–3.

Bhutta A, Anand KJS. Vulnerability of the developing brain: neuronal mechanisms. Clin Perinatol 2002;29:357–72.

Buskilla D, Neumann L, Zemora E, et al. Pain sensitivity in prematurely born adolescents. Arch Pediatr Adolesc Med 2003;157:1079–82.

Hall RW, Kronsberg SS, Barton BA, et al; NEOPAIN Trial Investigators Group. Morphine, hypotension, and adverse outcomes among preterm neonates: who's to blame? Secondary results from the NEOPAIN trial. Pediatrics 2005;115:1351–9.

Johnston CC, Filion F, Snider L, et al. Routine sucrose analgesia during the first week of life on neonates younger than 31 weeks' postconceptional age. Pediatrics 2002;110:523–8.

Lemyre B, Hogan D, Gaboury I, et al. How effective is tetracaine 4% gel before a venipuncture in reducing procedural pain in infants: a randomized double-blind placebo controlled trial. BMC Pediatrics 2007;7:7.

Puchalski M, Hummel P. The reality of neonatal pain. Adv Neonatal Care 2002;2:233–47.

Roberts KD, Leone TA, Edwards WH, et al. Premedication for nonemergent neonatal intubations: a randomized, controlled trial comparing atropine and fentanyl to atropine, fentanyl, and mivacurium. Pediatrics 2006;118:1583–91.

Stevens B, Yamada J, Ohlsson A. Sucrose for analgesia in newborn infants undergoing painful procedures. Cochrane Database Syst Rev 2004;CD 001069.

Winberg J. Do neonatal pain and stress program the brain's response to future stimuli? Acta Paediatr 1998;87:723–5.

TABLE 1   Analgesics, Sedatives and Local Anesthetic Medication

Local Anesthetics

Lidocaine 0.5%*	Maximum dose: 5 mg/kg SQ	(1 mL/kg of 0.5% solution) (0.5 mL/kg of 1% solution)
EMLA 5% Cream†	33 to 37 weeks PMA and > 1.8 kg	Maximum dose: 0.5 g for 1 to 2 h (then remove excess)
	>37 weeks PMA and >2.5 kg	Maximum dose: 1 g for 1 to 2 h (then remove excess)

Analgesics

		Single dose‡	Infusion§
Morphine##	Intubated	0.05 to 0.15 mg/kg IV or SQ	0.01 to 0.03 mg/kg/h
	Not Intubated	0.025 to 0.05 mg/kg IV or SQ	Not recommended
Fentanyl#	Intubated	1 to 3 µg/kg IV (over 5 minutes)	0.2 to 0.5 µg/kg/hour
	Not Intubated	0.25 to 1 µg/kg IV (over 5 minutes)	Not recommended**
Acetaminophen	10 to 15 mg/kg PO/PG/PR every 6 hours PRN maximum dose 40 mg/kg/24 h		

Continued

TABLE 1 *Continued*

Sedatives	
Short-Acting	
Midazolam[††]	0.05 to 0.1 mg/kg IV or intranasal
Chloral hydrate[‡‡]	20 to 30 mg/kg PO or PG
Long-Acting	
Phenobarbital	Loading dose: 5 to 15 mg/kg PO, PG, or IV
	Maintenance dose: 3 to 4 mg/kg/day PO, PG, or IV

EMLA = Eutectic Mixture of Local Anesthetic; IV = intravenous; PMA = postmenstrual age; PO = by mouth; PG = ; PR = per rectum; PRN = as needed; SQ = subcutaneous.

[|] Lidocaine toxicity may cause cardiac arrhythmia or seizure. 0.5% solution can be made by 1:1 dilution of 1% Lidocaine with normal saline.

[†] EMLA should be limited to a single dose per day and it must be removed within 2 hours. It takes 40 to 60 minutes following application to achieve the maximum effect of EMLA. Prilocaine (in EMLA) may cause methemoglobinemia. Swelling associated with the use of EMLA might distort anatomical structures.

[‡] May repeat dosing at 10 to 15 minute intervals until initial therapeutic effect is achieved.

[§] May titrate above this dosing range to achieve a therapeutic effect.

[##] Morphine may cause hypotension.

[#] Rapid infusion of fentanyl may cause chest-wall rigidity.

[||] Rapid fentanyl tolerance (tachyphylaxis) might require significantly higher infusion rates.

[††] Midazolam is recommended for use only in full-term infants. Abnormal movements have been described in premies treated with midazolam.

[‡‡] Chloral hydrate is metabolized to trichloroethanol, which competes for glucuronidation and may exacerbate hyperbilirubinemia.

TABLE 2   Analgesia for Invasive Procedures in Preterm and Term* Infants

Procedure	Intubated and Ventilated Infants	Nonintubated Infants
Procedure		
Intubation (emergency)	None	None
Intubation/reintubation (elective)	Fentanyl† 0.5 to 2 µg/kg IV (infused over 2 min) IV **or** Morphine 0.05 to 0.1 mg/kg IV or SQ	Fentanyl† 0.25 to 2 µg/kg IV (infused over 2 min) IV **or** Morphine 0.025 to 0.05 mg/kg IV or SQ
Mechanical Ventilation		
First 24 h	Fentanyl† 1 to 3 µg/kg Q 4 h and PRN **or** Morphine 0.05 to 0.15 mg/kg IV Q 4 h and PRN **or** Fentanyl infusion 0.2 to 2 µg/kg/h (start at low rate and increase PRN)	N/A
>24 h	Fentanyl† 1 to 3 µg/kg Q 4 h and PRN **or** Morphine 0.05 to 0.15 mg/kg Q 4 h and PRN **or** Fentanyl infusion 0.2 to 2 mg/kg/h	N/A

Continued

TABLE 2 Continued

Procedure	Intubated and Ventilated Infants	Nonintubated Infants
Chest Tube		
Insertion	Lidocaine 0.5% (max: 1 mL/kg) SQ and Fentanyl† 2 to 5 μg/kg IV 1 time **or** Morphine 0.1 to 0.2 μg/kg IV (titrate PRN)	Lidocaine 0.5% (max: 1 mL/kg) SQ and Fentanyl† 1 to 2 μg/kg IV **or** Morphine 0.05 to 0.1 μg/kg IV (titrate PRN)
In-place	Morphine 0.05 to 0.15 mg/kg Q 2 to 4 h PRN **or** Fentanyl† 1 to 3 μg/kg IV Q 2 to 4 h PRN	Morphine 0.025 to 0.05 mg/kg IV or SQ **or** Fentanyl† 0.25 to 1 μg/kg IV
Removal	Morphine 0.05 to 0.15 mg/kg **or** Fentanyl† 1 to 3 μg/kg IV 1 time	Morphine 0.025 to 0.05 mg/kg IV or SQ **or** Fentanyl† 0.5 to 2 μg/kg IV
Umbilical catheter placement	Morphine 0.05 to 0.1 mg/kg IV PRN Fentanyl† 1 to 3 μg/kg IV PRN	Morphine 0.025 to 0.05 mg/kg IV or SQ **or** Fentanyl† 0.25 to 1 μg/kg IV

Continued

TABLE 2 *Continued*

Procedure	Intubated and Ventilated Infants	Nonintubated Infants
Peripheral arterial catheter placement	Morphine 0.05 to 0.1 mg/kg Q 2 to 4 h **or** Fentanyl[†] 1 to 3 µg/kg IV Q 2 to 4 h **or** EMLA (if ≥ 34 weeks)	Morphine 0.025 to 0.05 mg/kg IV or SQ **or** Fentanyl[†] 0.25 to 1 µg/kg IV **or** EMLA (if ≥ 34 weeks)
Percutaneously inserted central catheter placement	Morphine 0.05 to 0.1 mg/kg Q 2 to 4 h **or** Fentanyl[†] 1 to 3 µg/kg IV Q 2 to 4 h **or** EMLA (if ≥ 34 weeks)	Morphine EMLA (if ≥ 34 weeks) **or** Fentanyl[†] 0.25 to 1 µg/kg IV **or** EMLA (if ≥ 34 weeks)

EMLA = Eutectic Mixture of Local Anesthetic; IV = intravenous; PO = by mouth; PG = ; PR = per rectum; PRN = as needed; SQ = subcutaneous.

* Full-term infants only also may receive 0.05 to 0.1 mg/kg of midazolam for anxiety.

† Fentanyl should be infused at ≤ 1 mg/kg/minute (e.g., 3 mg/kg infused over ≥ 3 minutes).

TABLE 3 Analgesia for Minimally Invasive Procedures

Procedure	Intubated and Ventilated Infants	Nonintubated Infants
Arterial puncture		24% Sucrose 0.5 to 1.5 mL PO; may repeat
Venipuncture		24% Sucrose 0.5 to 1.5 mL PO; may repeat
Heelstick blood draw		24% Sucrose 0.5 to 1.5 mL PO; may repeat
Intravenous placement		24% Sucrose 0.5 to 1.5 mL PO; may repeat
Lumbar puncture	Morphine 0.05 to 0.15 mg/kg IV or SQ **or** Fentanyl† 1 to 3 µg/kg IV and/or if ≥ 34 weeks: EMLA‡ **or** buffered lidocaine 0.5% (max: 0.5mL/kg) SQ	24% Sucrose 0.5 to 1.5 mL PO; may repeat and if ≥ 34 weeks: EMLA‡ **or** buffered lidocaine 0.5% (max: 0.5mL/kg) SQ
Dressing change	Morphine 0.05 to 0.1 mg/kg IV **or** Fentanyl† 1 to 3 µg/kg IV	24% Sucrose 0.5 to 1.5 mL PO; may repeat and/**or** Morphine 0.025 to 0.05 mg/kg IV **or** SQ **or** Fentanyl† 0.25 to 1 µg/kg IV

Continued

TABLE 3 *Continued*

Procedure	if ≥ 34 weeks:	if ≥ 34 weeks:
Endotracheal suctioning (mechanically ventilated)	Morphine 0.05 to 0.15 mg/kg **or** Fentanyl† 1 to 3 µg/kg IV	N/A
Immunization injection "(EMLA should be used only in infants ≥ 34 weeks' PMA)	N/A	24% Sucrose 0.5 to 1.5 mL PO; may repeat and/or EMLA‡ (if ≥ 34 weeks)

EMLA = Eutectic Mixture of Local Anesthetic; IV = intravenous; PMA = postmenstrual age; PO = by mouth; SQ = subcutaneous.

ᶦ Competitive stimulation may be used for any of these procedures, except suctioning.

† Fentanyl should be infused at ≤ 1 mg/kg/min (eg, 3 mg/kg infused over ≥ 3 min).

‡ Only one application per day of EMLA should be used. It takes 40 to 60 min to reach peak effect and should be removed within 2 h of application.

TABLE 4 Perioperative Analgesia

	Intubated and Ventilated Infants	Nonintubated Infants
Preoperative (ie, intubated infants under-going general anesthesia)	Fentanyl* 1 to 3 μg/kg IV 1 h before in preparation for transfer to the OR for the procedure	N/A
Laser Surgery	2 h before the procedure: Acetaminophen 15 mg/kg and during the procedure: Morphine 0.05 to 0.1 mg/kg IV Q 1 to 2 h PRN **or** Fentanyl* 1 to 3 μg/kg IV Q 1 to 2 h PRN and, if ≥ 34 weeks: midazolam 0.1 mg/kg IV Q 1 to 2 h PRN	N/A
Circumcision	N/A	24% sucrose 0.5 to 1.5 mL/kg PO and Acetaminophen 10 to 15 mg/kg 2 h PO/PG before and Q 6 h after the procedure (×24 h) and either ring block (lidocaine 0.5%) (max: 0.5 mL/kg) or dorsal penile block (lidocaine 0.5%) or if ≥ 34 weeks PMA and >1.8 kg: EMLA

Continued

TABLE 4 *Continued*

	Intubated and Ventilated Infants	Nonintubated Infants
Herniorrhaphy	Acetaminophen 10 to 15 mg/kg PO/PG/PR Q 4 to 6 h Fentanyl* 2 to 3 µg/kg Q 2 to 4 h PRN **or** Morphine 0.05 to 0.1 mg/kg Q 2 to 4 h PRN	Acetaminophen 10 to 15 mg/kg PO/PG/PR Q 6 h **or** Fentanyl* 0.25 to 0.5 µg/kg Q 4 h PRN **or** Morphine 0.025 to 0.05 mg/kg IV or SQ Q 4 h PRN
Laparotomy	First 24 h: Fentanyl* 1 to 3 µg/kg Q 4 to 6 h **or** Morphine 0.1 mg/kg Q 4 to 6 h; >24h post-operatively: Morphine 0.05 to 0.1 Q 2 to 4 h PRN **or** Fentanyl* 1 to 3 µg/kg Q 2 to 4 h PRN	Fentanyl* 0.25 to 0.5 µg/kg Q 4 h PRN **or** Morphine 0.025 to 0.05 mg/kg IV or SQ Q 4 h PRN
Thoracotomy	First 24 h: Fentanyl* 1 to 3 µg/kg Q 4 h **or** Morphine 0.05 to 0.1 mg/kg Q 4 h;	Acetaminophen 10 to 15 mg/kg Q 6 h Q 6 h PRN **or** Fentanyl* 0.25 to 0.5 µg/kg Q 4 h PRN **or** Morphine 0.025 to 0.05 mg/kg IV or SQ Q 4 h PRN

	Intubated and Ventilated Infants	Nonintubated Infants
Laser Surgery	≥24h post-operatively: Morphine 0.05 to 0.1 mg/kg Q 2 to 4 h PRN **or** Fentanyl* 1 to 3 µg/kg Q 2 to 4 h PRN	
	Acetaminophen 15 mg/kg PG/PR 2 h before and Acetaminophen 10 mg/kg Q 6 h after procedure (×24 hours); then Q 6 h PRN	Acetaminophen 10 mg/kg Q 6 h after the procedure (×24 hours); then Q 6 h PRN
Neurosurgical (Cranial)	Fentanyl* 1 to 3 µg/kg Q 2 to 4 h PRN **or** Morphine 0.05 to 0.1 mg/kg Q 2 to 4 h PRN	Acetaminophen 10 to 15 mg/kg Q 6 h PRN **or** Fentanyl* 0.25 to 0.5 µg/kg Q 4 h PRN **or** Morphine 0.025 to 0.05 mg/kg IV or SQ Q 4 h PRN
Neurosurgical (Lumbar)	Fentanyl* 1 to 3 µg/kg Q 2 to 4 h PRN **or** Morphine 0.05 to 0.1 mg/kg Q 2 to 4 h PRN	Acetaminophen 10 to 15 mg/kg Q 6 h Q 4 h PRN **or** Fentanyl* 0.25 to 0.5 µg/kg (over 2 min) **or** Morphine 0.025 to 0.05 mg/kg IV or SQ Q 4 h PRN

EMLA = Eutectic Mixture of Local Anesthetic; IV = intravenous; PMA = postmenstrual age; PO = by mouth; PG = ;
PR = per rectum; PRN = as needed; SQ = subcutaneous.
* Fentanyl should be infused at ≤ 1 mg/kg/min (eg, 3 mg/kg infused over ≥ 3 min).

FIFTEEN

Health Maintenance/Discharge Planning

Sarah Stewart de Ramirez, MD, MPH, MSc, and Anne R. Hansen, MD, MPH

Overview

Infants with corrected surgical conditions often need complex home care, including the administration of medications, management of medical devices such as gastrostomy tubes (GTs) or central venous lines (CVLs), the use of specialized equipment such as pumps and monitors, skilled nursing, home health aides, and coordination of multiple follow-up appointments. The optimal discharge process involves an interdisciplinary approach, often requiring extensive parent education and communication with many subspecialty services, the primary physician, home care, and insurance companies. Newborns with chronic conditions or multiple congenital abnormalities may be eligible for state or federal assistance. Social workers should be available to assist families in applying for specific support such as supplemental security income or Medicaid.

Educational material, either borrowed or developed internally, can be an efficient and an effective part of discharge teaching. Lists of support groups and specific references can also be helpful for some families. Where appropriate, we have included such material in this chapter.

Routine Newborn Screening

Services and regulations vary by region and change over time.

Newborn Screening

All states have a newborn screening program. Practitioners should familiarize themselves with conditions that are (and are not) screened for and should know the results of these tests for all patients discharged to home. If results are pending, this incomplete information must be communicated to the physician who will be assuming care of the infant after discharge. A list of conditions screened for in each state can be found at <www.aap.org/advocacy/archives/augscreenreport.htm>.

Hearing Screening

- Approximately 1 infant per 1,000 is deaf, and an additional 2 to 3 per 1,000 have partial hearing loss, 90% of whom have hearing parents. Only half of infants with a hearing deficit have identifiable risk factors at birth.
- Some states mandate universal hearing screens for all newborns. Whether required or optional, hearing can be screened when an infant is medically stable. If not universally required, risk categories that should prompt a hearing screen include the following:
  1. Family history of hearing disorders
  2. Prematurity
  3. Congenital viral infection
  4. Craniofacial anomalies
  5. Bacterial meningitis
  6. Receipt of more than 72 hours of an aminoglycoside and/or vancomycin
  7. Admission to a neonatal intensive care unit (NICU)
- Infants with a known risk factor for a hearing deficit should be screened with a diagnostic brainstem auditory evoked response (BAER) test.

- Infants without an identified risk of hearing deficit can be screened with either a screening BAER or an otoacoustic emission (OAE) test. If a baby does not pass this hearing screen, she/he should be referred for a diagnostic BAER evaluation. Both the BAER and the OAE tests are noninvasive and can generally be performed at the bedside under quiet conditions.
- Many hearing conditions can be improved or corrected. Early institution of appropriate speech and language intervention is well documented to minimize delays in speech, language, social, cognitive, and emotional development.
- For more information, contact the Marion Downs Center for Infant Hearing (<www.colorado.edu/slhs/mdnc>) or the National Center for Hearing Assessment and Management (<www. infanthearing.org>).

Immunizations

HEPATITIS B VACCINE

Correct treatment depends on accurate knowledge of maternal hepatitis B status.

- Infants born to hepatitis B surface antigen (HBsAg) negative mothers should receive the first dose of hepatitis B vaccine by 2 months of age. The second dose should be at least 1 month after the first dose. Premature infants should receive their first dose of hepatitis B vaccine when they achieve 2 kg, 2 months of age, or at time of discharge to home, whichever comes first.
- Infants born to HBsAg positive mothers should receive hepatitis B vaccine and 0.5 mL of hepatitis B immune globulin (HBIG) at separate sites within 12 hours of birth. The second dose of hepatitis B vaccine is recommended at 1 to 2 months of age. No further doses of HBIG are indicated.
- Infants born to mothers whose HBsAg status is unknown should receive hepatitis B vaccine within 12 hours of birth. Maternal blood should be drawn at the time of delivery to determine the mother's HBsAg status. If the HBsAg test is positive, the infant should receive HBIG as soon as possible (no later than 1 week of age). For infants less than 2 kg, if the

maternal HBsAg results are not known by 12 hours of age, HBIG should be administered.

TWO-MONTH IMMUNIZATIONS

- Currently, the 2-month immunization series consists of the second hepatitis B vaccine; diphtheria, tetanus toxoids, and acellular pertussis vaccine; *Haemophilus influenzae* type b; inactivated poliovirus vaccine; pneumococcal 7-valent conjugate vaccine (Prevnar); and oral rotavirus vaccine.

  Rotavirus vaccine is a live virus but has an accumulating safety record of administration in the inpatient setting and should be considered if the benefits outweigh the risks (eg, SBS in hospital through 12 weeks of age). The first dose should be given at 2 months of age and not later than 12 weeks of age. Because of the association between rotavirus vaccine and intussusception, if the first rotavirus vaccine cannot be given by 12 weeks of age, the baby becomes ineligible for this vaccine series.[1] Please refer to the CDC Web site for revisions: <www.cdc.gov/od/science/iso/concerns/rotavirus.htm>.

- The Pediarix vaccine combines DTaP, HepB, and IPV to facilitate the vaccination series at 2 months of age for babies who are either receiving their first HepB vaccine, or who received their first HepB vaccine at least 1 month prior.

  Premature infants should receive immunizations 2 months after birth (not 2 months after their due date).

- Please refer to the American Academy of Pediatrics' (AAP) guidelines (<www.AAP.org/healthtopics/immunizations.cfm>) for the most current immunization schedule and recommendations.

PALIVIZUMAB (SYNAGIS)

Indication

Palivizumab is a human monoclonal antibody that reduces the severity of symptoms of respiratory syncytial virus (RSV) infection in high-risk pediatric patients. Intramuscular palivizumab is preferred over intravenous RespiGam (respiratory syncytial virus immune globulin intravenous [human]) for most high-risk children because of its ease of administration, safety, and effectiveness.

Eligibility Criteria

The eligibility criteria are adapted from the AAP guidelines.[2]

- Palivizumab should be given to infants in the following circumstances:
  1. With residual chronic lung disease (CLD) of significant severity as evidenced by discharge from hospital on supplemental oxygen or diuretic therapy
  2. With severe chronic disorders compromising lung function (congenital diaphragmatic hernia [CDH], chest wall disorders, congenital lung malformation)
  3. Of gestational age 29 to 32 weeks and less than 6 months postnatal age at the onset of the RSV season, or gestational age ≤ 28 weeks and less than 1 year of age at the onset of the RSV season
- Palivizumab may be given to infants in the following circumstances:
  1. Born between 32 and 35 weeks' gestation without CLD who are less than 6 months of age at the start of the RSV season and who have at least two additional risk factors including school-age siblings, crowding in the home, day care attendance, exposure to tobacco smoke in the home, and multiple births
  2. Regardless of gestational age at birth, those who are predisposed to respiratory complications; those with significant respiratory disease, immunodeficiency, neurologic impairment, skeletal dysplasia, and metabolic disorders

Indications for Use During an Infant's Second RSV Season

These indications are based on limited data. Infants with CLD requiring medical therapy or supplemental oxygen within 6 months before the anticipated RSV season may benefit from treatment during their second RSV season. See the AAP guidelines for further details and updates.

Congenital Heart Disease

Currently, we give palivizumab to infants with congenital heart disease who meet the above-described pulmonary criteria or who have (1) serious recurrent lower respiratory tract disease or symptoms (ie, reactive airway disease, bronchiectasis), (2) left to right shunt (in which case, early repair is recommended if possible), (3) pulmonary hypertension, or (4) status-postheart transplant (adapted from Mary Mullen, MD, with permission).

Dosage

Give 15 mg/kg intramuscularly once each month during the RSV season (typically mid-November to April, although it can be defined functionally based on documented cases of RSV in the community).

Inpatient and Outpatient Screening

NEUROLOGY

The two most common neurologic conditions that require outpatient follow-up are intraventricular hemorrhage (IVH) and periventricular leukomalacia (PVL), conditions generally seen in infants born preterm. Infants with IVH or PVL should be followed as outpatients by a neurologist/neurodevelopmentalist.

Intraventricular Hemorrhage

See Chapter 9, "Neurological Disorders".

- Etiology: The hemorrhage originates most commonly in the germinal matrix, a vascular structure that involutes by approximately 36-weeks gestation.
- Incidence: IVH occurs in approximately 10% of prematurely born infants. Thus, it is a relatively frequent complication of prematurity, decreasing in incidence with improvement in NICU care. The incidence and severity of IVH are inversely related to gestational age and directly proportional to the severity of the illness.
- Population at risk: We generally screen all infants for IVH by head ultrasonography if born at gestational age less than 32 weeks gestation or with a birth weight less than 1500 g, or as clinically indicated.

- Sequelae are as follows:
    1. A severe IVH can obstruct cerebrospinal fluid flow and/or resorption, causing posthemorrhagic hydrocephalus (PHH) (see Chapter 9, "Neurological Disorders").
    2. Blood can extend into, or originate in, the parenchyma of the brain, causing neuronal injury.
- Outcome is as follows:
    1. Isolated germinal matrix hemorrhage (grade I) and lateral ventricular blood that does not distend the ventricle (grade II) generally do not increase the risk of neurologic sequelae above that predicted by degree of prematurity and severity of illness alone.
    2. Hemorrhage that distends the lateral ventricle (grade III) and parenchymal hemorrhage (grade IV) are associated with a worse neurologic outcome.
    3. Of note, a small proportion of infants with resolving PHH will develop late progressive PHH. Primary physicians should follow all infants with a history of IVH for excessive head growth or any signs or symptoms consistent with elevated intracranial pressure during the first year of life.

Periventricular Leukomalacia

- Etiology: Injury to the white matter surrounding the lateral ventricles may or may not be associated with IVH.
- Incidence: As with IVH, the incidence of PVL decreases as NICU care improves, with current rates of 3 to 8% for infants less than 32 weeks and/or less than 1500 g.
- Population at risk: As with IVH, generally, infants should be screened for PVL by head ultrasonography if born at gestational age less than 32 weeks or birth weight less than 1500 g, or as clinically indicated.
- These neuropathologic lesions may be seen on ultrasonography, first as areas of echodensity and then at about 1 month of age as echolucencies. Although not currently recommended for routine screening, magnetic resonance imaging is a more sensitive imaging technique for diagnosing PVL and can be useful in selected cases.

- PVL generally predicts a worse neurodevelopmental outcome than IVH, with predominantly motor deficits (eg, spastic diplegia), although cognitive function may also be affected.

OPHTHALMOLOGY

- Retinopathy of prematurity (ROP) is a potential complication of prematurity (see Chapter 10, "Retinopathy of Prematurity"). The AAP recommends infants of gestational age less than 30 weeks and/or birth weight less than 1,500 g, as well as selected infants between 1500 and 2000 g with an unstable clinical course should be screened for ROP prior to discharge.[3] Follow-up will usually be determined by the ophthalmologist based on the extent of ROP.

  1. An infant with active ROP at the time of discharge will require an outpatient visit in 1 to 3 weeks. The combination of dilating eye drops and the eye examination itself can prompt recurrence of respiratory symptoms in medically fragile infants with minimal respiratory reserve and a recent history of apnea/bradycardia of prematurity. Specifically, the α-adrenergic agent phenylephrine can cause decreased compliance, tidal volumes, and peak airflow in infants with bronchopulmonary dysplasia.[4] Therefore, if such an infant will require an outpatient eye examination within 1 to 2 weeks of discharge, consideration should be given to postponing discharge until after the examination or readmission after examination for observation and monitoring.

  2. Infants who meet screening criteria but who do not develop ROP should be seen by an ophthalmologist at approximately 8 months of age.

EARLY INTERVENTION PROGRAM

This community-based service is available to children up to 3 years of age who are at risk of developmental delay due to identified disabilities or other medical concerns. Referrals should be made early in the infant's hospital stay as centers may have waiting lists.

INFANT FOLLOW-UP PROGRAM

An infant follow-up program coordinates multidisciplinary services to assess and to manage sequelae associated with prematurity and provides referrals as appropriate. The team of care providers generally consists of a pediatrician, someone skilled in assessing cognitive and motor development, and a social worker. These clinics often work in collaboration with subspecialists such as neurologists and ophthalmologists.

Discharge Teaching

WELL BABY CARE

- In addition to learning specialized medical care, parents need to be comfortable with routine well baby care including feeding, bathing, changing diapers, cleaning of the umbilical cord, and circumcision care.
- Parents should be encouraged to participate in the care of their infant as soon as possible. A 24-hour per day visiting policy supports this process.

NUTRITION

- Ideally, preterm infants should gain 10 to 15 g/kg/d, and term infants should gain 20 to 30 g/d. Consistent weight gain should be established prior to discharge.
- Most infants will grow adequately on 100 to 120 kcal/kg/d. Exceptions to this are patients with high metabolic demands (CLD, cardiac disease, CDH), poor absorption (short gut), or the need for catch-up growth (infants born prematurely or growth restricted).

Breast-Feeding

- Refer to a lactation consultant if indicated.
- Infants may need breast milk to be fortified to increase caloric density and provision of specific nutrients. Additives such as formula powder, corn oil, medium-chain triglycerides (MCT), and polycose can be used to supplement calories and specific nutrients. A nutritionist should generally be involved if an infant is to be discharged home on high-caloric density milk. Prescriptions are needed to obtain some nutritional supplements (ie, polycose, MCT oil) on an outpatient basis.
- The following are recipes for supplementing breast milk (courtesy of Deanne Kelleher, RD):

1. 22 kcal/oz: add 1/8 tsp formula powder to 1 oz of breast milk
2. 24 kcal/oz: add 1/4 tsp formula powder to 1 oz of breast milk
3. 26 kcal/oz: add 1/2 tsp formula powder to 1 oz of breast milk
4. 28 kcal/oz: add 1/2 tsp formula powder and 1/4 tsp glucose polymers (polycose, moducal) powder to 1 oz of breast milk
5. 30 kcal/oz: add 1/2 tsp formula powder and 1/2 tsp polycose powder to 1 oz of breast milk

Formulas

Many formulas have been developed to accommodate the needs of infants with various surgical conditions. See Chapter 8, "Genitourinary Disorders," for specific nutritional advice for infants with this condition.

- Some formulas can be obtained (or covered by insurance) only with a prescription.
- The Special Supplemental Nutrition Program for Women, Infants, and Children is a federally funded program that provides supplemental formula to high-risk children up to 5 years of age.

Weight Checks

Infants at risk for poor growth must have their weight followed closely as an outpatient. A goal and plan should be designed prior to the patient's discharge. Typically, these infants are initially weighed weekly or biweekly in the primary physician's office or by a visiting nurse.

Visiting Nurse

A visiting nurse is usually needed if parents are taking home a baby with complex medical issues. Referral should be considered for infants with these special needs:

- First-time or adolescent parents
- Breast-feeding mother with limited experience
- Feeding difficulties
- Nutritional needs/risks, requirement for frequent weight checks
- Healing wound, dressing changes

- Home monitor for apnea/bradycardia and/or supplemental oxygen
- History of seizures, discharge on anticonvulsant
- Ostomy
- GT or jejunostomy tube (JT) feedings
- CVL
- Tracheostomy

COMMUNICATION

Parents should be provided with concrete written information about the circumstances for which they should contact their primary physician, surgeon, or other health care provider. They should be given emergency and nonemergency telephone numbers and other methods of communication (electronic mail, fax, etc). They should be told to clarify the infant's underlying surgical condition to any care provider unfamiliar with their infant's medical history. Depending on the underlying surgical condition and the parents' judgment, they should call the primary physician and/or the surgeon for the following conditions:

- Fever over 100°F
- signs and symptoms (s/s) of wound infection (redness or drainage from wound)
- s/s bowel obstruction (vomiting, abdominal distention, no stooling, lethargy)
- s/s esophageal stricture (difficulty feeding, vomiting, coughing, choking with feeds)
- s/s respiratory distress (increased work of breathing, increased respiratory rate, grunting, nasal flaring, retractions, color changes, difficulty in feeding)
- Feeding intolerance or gastrointestinal infection (vomiting, diarrhea)
- s/s dehydration (decreased activity level, decreased urine output, decreased stool output for breast-fed infants, depressed anterior fontanelle)
- Skin breakdown issues (peristomal or perianal) (see Addendum for "Diaper Dermatitis Algorithm," adapted with permission from Sandy Quigley, RN, CETN)

Home Safety

Before parents leave the hospital with a medically complex infant, the following general safety measures should be taken:

- Teach cardiopulmonary resuscitation (CPR) to parents and all other caregivers (It is helpful if this is offered by hospital staff). This is especially critical for any infant with potential airway compromise (ie, CDH, tracheoesophageal fistula, subglottic stenosis, cardiac disease, lymphatic malformations of the neck, tongue, and tracheostomy).
- Ensure that the car seat is appropriate and that parents know its proper placement and use. The AAP recommends the following for the transportation of an infant with risks of respiratory compromise:
  1. Any infant less than 37 weeks' gestation should have a period of observation in his/her car seat before hospital discharge. An appropriate hospital staff person should conduct the observation.
  2. Travel for infants at risk should be minimized.
  3. Infants who fail the car seat test should be transported in the supine or prone position in an alternate device such as a car bed.
  4. Infants who require home monitoring should be monitored during travel.
     <www.aap.org/healthtopics/carsafety.cfm>.
- Notify the local emergency medical service or fire department of an at-risk infant at home.
- Notify local utilities of the need for service (telephone and electrical) for an infant with special needs to ensure that necessary services are not discontinued.

Specific Medical Devices

GASTROSTOMY TUBES

See also Chapter 8, "Gastrointestinal Disorders."

- Gastrostomy tubes (GTs) (Mic-Key, skin-level tubes, malecots) are placed in neonates for feeding and/or gastric decompression.

These infants are discharged with the GT in place for use at home.

- The GT must be well secured for the first 6 weeks after placement. Initially, it will be sutured in place and should be secured with tape as well. If the tube is inadvertently dislodged in the first weeks, it must be replaced by a skilled health care provider.
- When no longer needed, the GT can be removed by a surgeon during an outpatient visit. Although most sites will then close spontaneously, some will need surgical closure.
- Parents' teaching needs to include the following:
  1. Providing daily skin care, observing for skin breakdown (versus granulation tissue)
  2. Securing the tube with tape for first 6 weeks
  3. Checking balloon volume weekly
  4. Planning for a replacement if the GT falls out at home (this plan should be made with the individual surgeon; if the tube is over 6 weeks old, parents may be instructed to replace the GT at home)
  5. Administering feedings via the GT (bolus by gravity versus continuous by pump)
  6. Administering medications through the GT
  7. Flushing the GT (after medications and feedings)
  8. Instruction to contact a health care provider for persistent vomiting, dislodgment of the tube in the first 6 weeks after placement, GT site skin breakdown, or excessive leakage
- Home equipment needs to include the following:
  1. A prescription for a replacement GT, including type, size, and length
  2. A syringe for checking the balloon weekly
  3. Other supplies including dressings, feeding bags, pumps
- Refer the patient to a home care agency that can supply the above-listed equipment.

JEJUNOSTOMY TUBES

- A combination GT/JT is sometimes required for infants with severe gastroesophageal reflux or gastric emptying problems.

The GT is used for gastric decompression and the JT for feedings.

- Generally, infants fed through a nasojejunal tube will remain hospitalized as these tubes are difficult to maintain at home owing to frequent problems with dislodgment or clogging.
- JTs are particularly prone to clogging. All medications should be given in liquid form, and the tube must be flushed after administration of any medication or feeding. If the JT does become clogged, sometimes instillation of warm water will restore patency.
- If a JT is dislodged or permanently clogged, it must be replaced by a skilled health care professional, often under fluoroscopic guidance.
- Parents' teaching needs are similar to those for GTs and are as follows:
  1. Skin care, balloon check, feedings, securing the JT with tape
  2. Instructions to contact a health care provider for persistent vomiting, clogged tube, dislodgment of the tube regardless of interval since placement, skin breakdown, and leakage of any volume
- Home equipment needs and referrals are similar to those for infants with GTs.

OSTOMIES

- Families should begin learning to care for an ostomy as soon as possible after surgery. Parents' teaching needs are as follows:
  1. Checking stoma and skin condition
  2. Emptying the pouch routinely
  3. Changing the pouch
  4. Assessing stool output and developing a sense of what is normal for their infant
  5. Instructions to call a health care provider if increased or no stool output, persistent emesis, discoloration (pale or dusky) or prolapse of stoma, and significant skin breakdown
- Home equipment needs are as follows:
  1. Ostomy pouch, with specific brand and size specified

2. Skin barriers and pastes
3. Topical antifungal therapy in anticipation of localized fungal infections
- The patient should be referred to a home care agency, preferably one with an enterostomal therapist on staff.

CENTRAL VENOUS LINES

- Infants who will need long-term central access (ie, total parenteral nutrition, chemotherapy, prolonged antibiotic course, frequent blood draws) may go home with a tunneled (Broviac) or percutaneous central line.
- Parents' teaching needs are as follows:
  1. Heparin flush
  2. Routine dressing
  3. Cap change
  4. Initial management of blockage/dislodgment/breakage of line/infiltration
  5. Recognition of signs and symptoms of infection
  6. Instruction to call a health care provider if there is fever, line breakage, inability to flush/infuse the line, erythema/tenderness at the insertion site, or neck or chest swelling
- Home equipment needs are as follows:
  1. Flushes
  2. Medication
  3. Infusion pump
  4. Emergency clamp
- The patient should be referred to a home care agency familiar with management of CVLs.

TRACHEOSTOMY

- Occasionally, an infant will require a tracheostomy to manage the airway. This is usually in place for several weeks to months prior to discharge home. It is essential that this time be used to provide parents (and any other anticipated care providers) with intensive training in both tracheostomy care and cardiopulmonary assessment and resuscitation prior to hospital discharge.
- Parents' teaching needs are as follows:

1. Anatomy and physiology
2. Signs and symptoms of respiratory distress (possibly caused by dislodgment or obstruction of the tube)
3. Use and interpretation of a home monitor
4. Use of oxygen and humidity
5. Suctioning the tracheostomy tube
6. Skin care
7. Changing the tracheostomy tube
8. Traveling with a tracheostomy tube, oxygen, and other equipment
9. CPR
10. Instructions to call a health care provider for respiratory distress, increased oxygen requirement, purulent drainage, erythema, or tenderness at the tracheostomy insertion site

- Home equipment needs are as follows:
  1. Monitor (cardiac/apnea, possibly oximeter)
  2. Spare tracheostomy tube
  3. Portable suction machine, gloves, catheters, saline bullets
  4. Humidity: artificial nose, compressed air or oxygen, tracheostomy collar
  5. Skin care equipment: sponges, tracheostomy ties, bandage scissors, antibiotic ointment
  6. Oxygen if needed
  7. Anesthesia (eg, Ambu) bag and mask
  8. Nebulizers
- Refer the patient to a home care agency familiar with the management of tracheostomies.

References

1. AAP Committee on Infections Diseases. Prevention of rotavirus disease: guidelines for use of rotavirus vaccine. Pediatrics 2007 Jan;119:171–82.
2. AAP Committee on Infectious Diseases and AAP Committee on Fetus and Newborn. Revised indications for the use of palvizumab and respiratory syncitial virus immune globulin intravenous for the prevention of respiratory scyncitial virus infections. Pediatrics 2003 Dec;112:1442–6.

3. AAP section on Ophthalmology. American Academy of Pediatrics: Screening examination of premature infants for retinopathy of prematurity. Pediatrics 2001 Sept;108:809–11.
4. Mirmanesh SJ, Abbasi S, Bhutani VK. α-adrenergic bronchoprovocation in neonates with bronchopulmonary dysplasia. J Pediatr 1992;121:622–5.

Index